THE BLACK DEATH IN THE MIDDLE EAST

THE BLACK DEATH IN THE MIDDLE EAST

MICHAEL W. DOLS

PRINCETON UNIVERSITY PRESS
PRINCETON, NEW JERSEY

Published by Princeton University Press, Princeton, New Jersey
In the United Kingdom: Princeton University Press, Guildford, Surrey

Library of Congress Cataloging in Publication Data
will be found on the last printed page of this book

This publication was supported in part by NIH Grant LM 02700
from the National Library of Medicine

Printed in the United States of America
by Princeton University Press, Princeton, New Jersey

Princeton Legacy Library edition 2019
Paperback ISBN: 978-0-691-65562-8
Hardcover ISBN: 978-0-691-65704-2

To my mother and father

PREFACE

When I began my work on the Black Death in the Middle East, Professor Richard Ettinghausen described my project with inimitable good humor as "a great undertaking!" The subject has indeed proved to be greater than I first imagined but not the morbid task that one might suppose. The result is this monograph, which sets out to recount and to explain an important phenomenon in medieval Islamic history: the drastic destruction of Middle Eastern population and the subsequent impoverishment of Muslim society by plague epidemics. The epidemics clearly began with the outbreak of the great pandemic or universal epidemic of plague in the mid-fourteenth century known as "the Black Death." It was undoubtedly the worst disaster that has ever befallen mankind. "Oh, happy posterity," wrote Petrarch of the Black Death in Florence, "who will not experience such abysmal woe and will look upon our testimony as a fable." The dimensions of the calamity challenge—almost defy—the imagination.

I know only too well that I have crossed the boundaries of many disciplines to tell the story of the Black Death in the Middle East. As the medical nature and the historical consequences of plague epidemics are complex, my indebtedness to others has been correspondingly great. It is a pleasure to express my gratitude to those who have given me their generous help during the lengthy preparation of this study. My thanks go first and foremost to Princeton University, its library, and the faculty of the Near Eastern Studies Department, especially Professors Philip K. Hitti, L. Carl Brown, Martin Dickson, Michel Mazzaoui, Roy Mottahedeh, and Andras Hamori. Among the community of scholars associated with Princeton, I am grateful for the assistance of Professors

Richard Ettinghausen, S. D. Goitein, and the late Bayard Dodge.

During my research in Egypt in 1969-1970, numerous men and institutions made my work there both profitable and enjoyable despite the political difficulties. I am particularly indebted to the following: Professors Sa'īd 'Āshour and Hassanien Rabie of Cairo University; Professor Ḥasan Ḥabishī of 'Ayn Shams University; the director and staff of the National Library; al-Azhar Mosque Library; Dr. 'Abd at-Tawwāb of the Egyptian Museum; the library and faculty of the American University in Cairo, especially Professor Adil Sulayman Gamal; the French Institute; and the German Institute, especially Professor Ulrich Haarmann. In addition, Dr. Harry Hoogstraal of the United States Naval Research Unit Number Three in Cairo and his staff, particularly Dr. Robert Maronpot, greatly aided me in understanding and interpreting the medical aspects of plague in the Middle East. Outside of Egypt, I wish to thank the 'Umayyad Mosque Library, Damascus, and the Süleymaniye Mosque Library, Istanbul, for permitting me to use their collections. With regard to the manuscripts in Istanbul, I am most appreciative of the help of Professor Joel Shinder, as well as his constant encouragement during the initial stages of my research.

My continued research on this topic was supported in 1973 and 1974 by faculty research grants from the California State University, Hayward. In 1974-1975 a fellowship from the American Research Center in Egypt gave me the opportunity to return to Cairo and to re-examine some of the manuscript material and make significant additions and corrections. Concurrently, a grant from the Joint Committee on the Near and Middle East of the American Council of Learned Societies and the Social Science Research Council enabled me to extend my work to other parts of the Middle East and Europe and to make a final revision of the monograph.

I am also pleased to acknowledge the generous assistance of various European libraries that allowed me access to their manuscript collections: the British Museum; Cambridge University Library; the Bodleian Library, Oxford; Staatsbibliothek, Berlin, West Germany; Universiteitsbibliotheek, Leiden; and the Library of San Lorenzo de El Escorial. I am particularly grateful to Dr. Jacqueline Sublet (Institut de Recherche et d'Histoire des Textes, Paris) for her help in dealing with the numerous difficulties of the oriental manuscript material. Yet any failure to locate relevant manuscripts is entirely my own. The interpretation of the Arabic sources is also clearly my own responsibility; because of the lack of previous study of a large part of this plague literature, I have been careful to document extensively my use of the sources.

Perhaps a few technical details should be mentioned here regarding the composition of the monograph. In the interests of brevity and economy, I have transliterated all Arabic citations. The system of Arabic transliteration follows that of the Library of Congress, with the single exception that the definite article preceding "sun letters" is transliterated as pronounced. Wherever an Arabic name or word has assumed a more familiar English form than in strict transliteration, such as Saladin for Ṣalāḥ ad-Dīn or Cairo for al-Qāhirah, I have adopted the former. Concerning dates of the Muslim calendar, I have designated their Christian equivalent in the text by placing the Muslim year first and then the Christian year, as in 852/1448-1449; otherwise a date refers to the Christian calendar. In the notes, Muslim dates are often cited as A.H., "anno hijrah." I should also explain that I have spelt *mamlūk* with a capital *M* when referring to the empire or period of hegemony in Egypt and Syria from 1250 to 1517; in all other instances, I have used a small *m*. Furthermore, parts of Chapters I and VIII of this book, in somewhat revised form, have appeared as articles in *The Journal of the American Oriental Society* and in *Viator: Medieval and Renaissance Studies* respectively.

Finally, I would like to express my profound thanks to those who have read all or part of the manuscript with great care, especially Professor Ira M. Lapidus, Professor Frank D. Gilliard, Dr. Richard S. Cooper, Mr. Steve Pellitiere, Mr. Nicholas L. Childs, Mrs. Mava Luther, and the late Muḥammad

Rashād ʻAbd al-Muṭṭalib. I also wish to thank Princeton University Press, particularly Mr. Lewis Bateman, for his constant guidance and support, and Mrs. Arthur Sherwood, for her meticulous editorial assistance. My deepest obligation is to Professor Abraham L. Udovitch of Princeton University, who first suggested this study to me. I am indebted to him as well for his extraordinary patience, courtesy, and encouragement through all the stages of its composition.

MICHAEL WALTERS DOLS

San Francisco, 1975.

CONTENTS

ABBREVIATIONS

AGM	*Archiv für Geschichte der Medizin*, ed. by Karl Sudhoff, Leipzig, 1908 ff.
Annales	*Annales: économies, sociétés, civilisations*, Paris, 1946 ff.
Badhl	Ibn Ḥajar al-ʻAsqalānī, *Badhl al-māʻūn fī faḍl aṭ-ṭāʻūn*, Dār al-Kutub al-Miṣrīyah MS no. 2353 *taṣawwuf*
al-Bidāyah	Ibn Kathīr, *al-Bidāyah wan-nihāyah fī t-taʼrīkh*, Cairo, n.d.
BIE	*Bulletin de l'Institut Égyptien*, Cairo, 1857 ff.
BIFAO	*Bulletin de l'Institut Français d'Archéologie Orientale*, Cairo, 1901 ff.
BSOAS	*Bulletin of the School of Oriental and African Studies*, London, 1917 ff.
Campbell	A. M. Campbell, *The Black Death and Men of Learning*, New York, 1931
Dafʻ an-niqmah	Ibn Abī Ḥajalah, *Dafʻ an-niqmah fī s-salāt ʻalā nabī ar-raḥmān*, Escorial MS no. 1772, fols. 1a-87b
Darrag	Aḥmad Darrag, *L'Égypte sous le règne de Barsbay 825-841/1422-1438*, Damascus, 1961
Durrat al-aslāk	Ibn Ḥabīb, *Durrat al-aslāk fī dawlat (mulk) al-atrāk*, Cairo University Library, photocopy no. 22961
EI[1]	*The Encyclopaedia of Islam*, 4 vols., Leiden-London, 1913-1934
EI[2]	*The Encyclopaedia of Islam*, new ed., Leiden-London, 1960-

"England to Egypt"	Robert Lopez, H. Miskimin and A. Udovitch, "England to Egypt, 1350-1500: Long-Term Trends and Long-Distance Trade," *Studies in the Economic History of the Middle East*, London, 1970, ed. by Michael A. Cook, pp. 93-128
Études et Travaux	*Études et Travaux de Centre d'Archéologie Méditerranéenne de l'Académie Polonaise des Sciences*, Warsaw, 1957 ff.
GAL	Carl Brockelmann, *Geschichte der Arabischen Litteratur*, 2 vols., 2nd ed. (Leiden, 1945-1949); *Supplement*, 3 vols. (Leiden, 1937-1942)
GAS	Fuat Sezgin, *Geschichte des Arabischen Schrifttums*, 3 vols. (Leiden, 1967-1971)
"La Grande Peste Noire"	Gaston Wiet, "La Grande Peste Noire en Syrie et en Égypte," *Études d'orientalisme dédiées à la mémoire de Lévi-Provençal*, vol. 1 (Paris, 1962), pp. 367-384
Hirst	L. Fabian Hirst, *The Conquest of Plague: A Study of the Evolution of Epidemiology*, Oxford, 1953
Ibn Iyās	Ibn Iyās, *Badā'i' az-zuhūr fī waqā'i' ad-duhūr*, 2 vols., Būlāq, A.H. 1311-1312
IJMES	*International Journal of Middle East Studies*, Cambridge, 1970 ff.
'Iqd al-jumān	al-'Aynī, *'Iqd al-jumān fī ta'rīkh ahl az-zamān*, Dār al-Kutub al-Miṣrīyah MS no. 1574 *ta'rīkh*
JA	*Journal Asiatique*, Paris, 1822 ff.
JAOS	*Journal of the American Oriental Society*, Baltimore, 1843 ff.
JESHO	*Journal of Economic and Social History of the Orient*, Paris, 1957 ff.
JRAS	*Journal of the Royal Asiatic Society*, London, 1834 ff.

al-Khiṭaṭ	al-Maqrīzī, *al-Mawā'iẓ wal-i'tibār bi-dhikr al-khiṭaṭ wal-athār*, 2 vols., Būlāq, 1854
Kitāb aṭ-ṭibb	Ibn Abī Ḥajalah, *Kitāb aṭ-ṭibb al-masnūn fī daf' aṭ-ṭā'ūn*, Dār al-Kutub al-Miṣrīyah MS no. 102 *majāmī' m*, fols. 141a-146a
Kunūz adh-dhahab	Sibṭ ibn al-'Ajamī, *Kunūz adh-dhahab fī ta'rīkh Ḥalab (Les Tresors d'Or)*, trans. by Jean Sauvaget, Beirut, 1950
Mā rawāhu l-wā'ūn	as-Suyūṭī, *Mā rawāhu l-wā'ūn fī akhbār aṭ-ṭā'ūn*, ed. by Alfred von Kremer, "Ueber die grossen Seuchen des Orients nach arabischen Quellen," *Sitzungsberichte der Kaiserlichen Akademie der Wissenschaften (Philosophisch-Historische Classe)*, vol. 96, book 1 (Vienna, 1880), pp. 144-156
Muqni'at	Ibn al-Khaṭīb, *Muqni'at as-sā'il 'an al-maraḍ al-hā'il*, Escorial MS no. 1785, fols. 39a-48b
Muslim Cities	Ira M. Lapidus, *Muslim Cities in the Later Middle Ages*, Cambridge, Mass., 1967
an-Nujūm	Ibn Taghrī Birdī, *an-Nujūm az-zāhirah fī mulūk Miṣr wal-Qāhirah*: (1) Cairo ed.: 16 vols., Cairo, 1929-1972 (2) Popper trans.: William Popper, *History of Egypt 1382-1469 A.D., University of California Publications in Semitic Philology*, vols. 5-7, 13-14, 17-19, 22-23, 24 (indices), Berkeley and Los Angeles, 1915-1963
"The Plague and Its Effects"	David Neustadt (Ayalon), "The Plague and Its Effects upon the Mamlūk Army," *Journal of the Royal Asiatic Society*, 1946, pp. 67-73
REI	*Revue des Études Islamiques*, Paris, 1906 ff.
Risālat an-naba'	Ibn al-Wardī, *Risālat an-naba' 'an al-waba'*, ed. by F. ash-Shidyāq, *Majmū'at al-jawā'ib*, Istanbul, A.H. 1300, pp. 184-188

Sublet	Jacqueline Sublet, "La Peste prise aux rêts de la jurisprudence: Le Traité d'Ibn Hağar al-'Asqalānī sur la peste," *Studia Islamica*, vol. 33 (Paris, 1971), pp. 141-149
as-Sulūk	al-Maqrīzī, *as-Sulūk li-ma'rifat duwal al-mulūk*, 4 parts in 12 vols., Cairo, 1936-1958, 1970-1973
Systematic Notes	William Popper, *Egypt and Syria Under the Circassian Sultans, 1382-1468* A.D.*; Systematic Notes to Ibn Taghrī Birdī's Chronicles of Egypt, University of California Publications in Semitic Philology*, vols. 15-16, Berkeley and Los Angeles, 1955, 1957
Taḥṣīl	Ibn Khātimah, *Taḥṣīl al-gharaḍ al-qāṣid fī tafṣīl al-maraḍ al-wāfid*, Escorial MS no. 1785, fols. 49a-105b
Ṭāshköprüzāde	Ṭāshköprüzāde, *Majmū'at ash-shifā' li-adwiyat al-wabā' ma' rasā'il lil-Bisṭāmī*, Berlin MS Landberg no. 999 (Ahlwardt no. 6378)
"Ueber die grossen Seuchen"	Alfred von Kremer, "Ueber die grossen Seuchen des Orients nach die arabischen Quellen," *Sitzungsberichte der Kaiserlichen Akademie der Wissenschaften (Philosophisch-Historische Classe)*, vol. 96, book 1 (Vienna, 1880), pp. 69-156
Ullmann	Manfred Ullmann, *Die Medizin im Islam*, Leiden, 1970
Ziegler	Philip Ziegler, *The Black Death*, London, 1969

LIST OF MAPS

THE BLACK DEATH IN THE MIDDLE EAST

A history more worthy of the name than the diffident speculations to which we are reduced by the paucity of our material would give space to the vicissitudes of the human organism. It is very naive to claim to understand men without knowing what sort of health they enjoyed.

Marc Bloch, *Feudal Society*
trans. by L. A. Manyon
(Chicago, 1964), vol. 1, p. 72

I

INTRODUCTION

In the middle of the fourteenth century a devastating pandemic of plague, familiarly known in European history as "the Black Death," swept westward over the Eurasian continent. While a controversy will always exist over the precise degree of depopulation caused by the disease, the mortality rate was indeed extraordinary. The historical importance of this sudden decline of population has been appreciated by European historians since the nineteenth century, and there can now be little doubt that it had a marked effect on late medieval European society.[1] The Black Death is, perhaps, our most forceful reminder that the history of epidemic disease must form an inseparable part of the history of mankind.

The European phase of the Black Death raises a number of pertinent questions about its comparable role in medieval Muslim society. Despite the existence of relevant historical material, there has been no general examination of the Black Death in the predominantly Muslim countries of the Middle East. This study, based on Arabic sources, therefore, attempts to establish the chronology and geographical distribution of the plague pandemic in this region in the mid-fourteenth century and to describe its impact upon Muslim society.[2]

[1] The extensive literature on the Black Death in Europe, with special attention usually being given to Great Britain, has been conveniently summarized by four recent surveys. *The Black Death* by Ziegler is a particularly good, concise account that includes a helpful bibliography. The three other studies are: George Deaux, *The Black Death 1347* (London, 1969); J.F.D. Shrewsbury, *A History of Bubonic Plague in the British Isles* (Cambridge, 1970); and Geoffrey Marks, *The Medieval Plague* (New York, 1971).

[2] The restriction of this study to primarily Arabic sources precluded intensive research in Turkish, Persian, and Chinese literature. These areas are touched upon with regard to the transmission of the Black

Moreover, the Black Death initiated a series of plague recurrences that substantially reduced Middle Eastern population. This prolonged reduction of population was the fundamental event in the social and economic history of Egypt and Syria during the later Middle Ages.

The present investigation has, then, somewhat betrayed its title not only by chronicling the occurrence of the Black Death but by considering the effects of the recurrent plague epidemics which began with the Black Death. Attention has been focused on the reappearances of plague during approximately the following one hundred and fifty years. Documentation of these epidemics shows that plague recurred in cycles, as in Europe. But unlike the European experience of plague, the recurrences in the Middle East had a far more damaging effect on population—a cumulative effect far greater than that of the Black Death itself.

Many of the more detailed treatises on plague and the informative historical reports of plague epidemics date from these recurrences after the Black Death.[3] None of the Arabic sources, however, refers to the first appearance of plague in the middle of the fourteenth century as "the Black Death," nor

Death through the Middle East. There is, however, considerable material for the study of later plague epidemics in the Ottoman Period. For the Turkish sources, one should begin with two papers presented at the Ninth International Congress of the History of Medicine (Bucharest, September, 1932), *Comptes-Rendus* edited by Victor Gomoin and Victorica Gomoin: Galip Ata, "Évolution de la médicine en turquie," pp. 95-131, and especially A. Süheyl Ünver, "Sur l'histoire de la peste en Turquie," pp. 479-483. (See Appendix 3 for plague treatises for the Ottoman Period.) For Persia, a point of departure is J.-D. Tholozan, *Histoire de la peste bubonique en Perse* (Paris, 1874). Another major area of source material that, unfortunately, had to be excluded is the Arabic Christian literature, particularly the Coptic sources from Egypt. Let us hope that further research will investigate this rich source, which might add important comparative data with regard to Muslim and Christian responses to plague as well as chronological and demographic information.

[3] See Appendix 3.

was this pseudonym used by medieval European chroniclers.[4] The genesis of the name is a minor mystery, but it may be due to the over-literal translation into European languages of the Latin *pestis atra* or *atra mors* in the sixteenth and seventeenth centuries.[5] The name has been retained here because it has

[4] To my knowledge, the only Oriental use of such an expression related to plague or to disease in general is the Persian term *ḳaraḳhalaḳ*: "According to the communication of N. I. Khodukin, haemorrhagic fever has also been known to the indigenous population of other districts of Uzbekhistan apparently over a fairly long period, since there exists a definite name for it: *ḳaraḳhaluḳ* (Black Death). This term, the author notes, is sometimes confused with the term for plague, but not with malaria which bears the name *ḳizdyrma*." (S. Ye. Shapiro and Z. S. Barkagan, "History of Haemorrhagic Fever in Central Asia," *Voprosy Virusologii* [in Russian], vol. 5, no. 2 [Moscow, 1960], p. 245.)

[5] The contemporary Latin chroniclers designated the pandemic as "the Great Mortality," "the Great Pestilence," "the Plague of Florence," and so forth (see Ziegler, pp. 17-18; F. A. Gasquet, *The Black Death of 1348 and 1349* [London, 1908], pp. 7-8; Hirst, p. 32; Shrewsbury, *A History of Bubonic Plague*, p. 37; and especially Stephen d'Irsay, "Notes to the Origin of the Expression 'arta mors,'" *Isis*, vol. 8 [1926], pp. 328-332). The Muslim witnesses referred to the pandemic as: (1) "the Universal Plague" (*aṭ-ṭāʿūn al-ʿām: Badhl*, fol. 123b; Ibn Hajar al-ʿAsqalānī, *ad-Durar al-ḳāminah* [Hyderabad, 1348-1350 A.H.], vol. 3, pp. 192, 382; *ʿIqd al-jumān*, chap. 24, part 1, fol. 85; *Durrat al-aslāḳ*, p. 358; *Mā rawāhu l-wāʿūn*, p. 155; adh-Dhahabī and al-Ḥusaynī, *Min dhuyūl al-ʿibar* [Kuwait, n.d.], p. 270); (2) "the Plague of the Kindred" (*ṭāʿūn al-ansāb: Durrat al-aslāḳ*, p. 358; *idem, Tadhḳirat an-nabīh fī ayyām al-Manṣūr wa banīh*, British Museum Or. Add. MS no. 7335, fol. 145b; *Risālat an-nabaʾ*, p. 186; *Kunūz adh-dhahab*, vol. 2, p. 10); (3) "the Great Destruction" (*al-fanāʾ al-ḳabīr: al-Khiṭaṭ*, vol. 1, p. 637; *ʿIqd al-jumān*, chap. 24, part 1, p. 85; also *fanāʾ ʿaẓīm biṭ-ṭāʿūn*: Sālih ibn Yahyā, *Taʾrīḳh Bayrūt*, 2nd ed. [Beirut, 1927], p. 140; *al-fanāʾ al-ʿaẓīm*: Ibn Ḥabīb, *Tadhḳirat an-nabīh*, fol. 144b; *an-Nujūm*, Cairo ed., vol. 10, p. 233); (4) "the Great Plague" (*at-tāʿūn al-ʿaẓīm*: al-Muʾminī, *Kitāb futūh an-naṣr min taʾrīḳh mulūḳ Miṣr*, Dār al-Kutub al-Miṣrīyah MS no. 2399 *taʾrīḳh*, vol. 2, fol. 295); (5) "the Great Pestilence" (*al-wabāʾ al-ʿaẓīm: an-Nujūm*, Cairo ed., vol. 10, p. 211); (6) "the Violent Plague" (*at-taʿūn al-jārif*: al-Qalqashandī, *Ṣubh al-aʿshā* [Cairo, 1914-1928], vol. 13, p. 79; Ibn Khaldūn, *at-Taʿrīf* [Cairo, 1951], p. 19); or (7) "the Year of the Annihilation" (*sanat al-fanāʾ: an-Nujūm*, Cairo ed., vol. 10, p. 211). These examples refer to the Black Death as a proper noun; for the common substantives for plague, see Appendix 2.

become the accepted historical term for the pandemic. It also serves to emphasize the universal nature of the disease.

Geographically, the study could not be neatly limited to the "Middle East"—also an awkward Western term. My investigation of all the possible Arabic sources dealing with plague has led me far afield to the three important plague tracts written in Andalusia during the time of the Black Death, which are particularly informative about contemporary medical practice in Muslim society. While concentrating on the pandemic in the Middle East, I have tried to survey the entire field in order to form a comprehensive framework for further research.

Despite the wide geographical and temporal ranges of this study, most of the pertinent historical material that has survived centers on the Mamlūk Sultanate of Egypt and Syria from the outbreak of the Black Death in 1347 to the middle of the fifteenth century. Although the source material for the Mamlūk Period (1250-1517) is relatively abundant and allows us to concentrate on this area, the general history of the period has been sorely neglected.[6] Recent scholarship has been devoted

[6] The following works in western languages are devoted in their entirety or in part to the general history of the Mamlūk Sultanate: Stanley Lane-Poole, *A History of Egypt in the Middle Ages* (London, 1968 reprint), pp. 242-357, the standard account of the period; John B. Glubb, *Soldiers of Fortune: the Story of the Mamlukes* (London, 1973), a poor popularization of the period with an emphasis on military history; Bernard Lewis, "Egypt and Syria" in *The Cambridge History of Islam*, ed. by P. M. Holt, A.K.S. Lambton, and B. Lewis (Cambridge, 1970), vol. 1, pp. 201-230; Wolfgang Niemeyer, *Ägypten zur Zeit der Mamluken* (Berlin, 1936), a geopolitical study based on secondary sources; Maurice Gaudefroy-Demombynes, *La Syrie au début de quinzième siècle* (Paris, 1923), prefaced by an excellent introductory survey; Sir William Muir, *The Mameluke or Slave Dynasty of Egypt, 1260-1517* (London, 1896), an outdated political history; Gaston Wiet, *L'Égypte Arabe de la conquête Arabe à la conquête Ottomane, 642-1517 de l'ère Chrétienne* in the collective work, *Histoire de la nation Égyptienne*, ed. by Gabriel Hanotaux, vol. 4 (Paris, 1937), pp. 387-636, comparable to Lane-Poole's account but lacking a bibliography; A. N. Poliak, *Feudalism in Egypt, Syria, Palestine, and the Lebanon, 1250-1900* (London, 1939); J. J. Saunders, *Aspects of the Crusades* (Christchurch, New Zealand, 1962), a good survey of the political circumstances of the Middle

largely to historiography, economic and urban history, and the mamlūk army. In such broad areas as literary, religious, social, agrarian, demographic, and art history, much work remains to be done.

Thus, it is not surprising that the Black Death in the Orient has attracted so little scholarly attention. Furthermore, the historical studies of plague in the Middle East by nineteenth-century scholars reveal that they were severely handicapped by their ignorance of the pathology of plague. This limited medical knowledge distorted their interpretations and partly accounts for their failure to distinguish among epidemic diseases.[7] The modern examination of the Black Death from the Arabic sources has been cursory: Gaston Wiet has trans-

East at the time of the mamlūk ascendancy in Egypt and Syria; Lapidus, *Muslim Cities*, a very valuable study of mamlūk urban history with an extensive bibliography; Popper, "Systematic Notes to Ibn Taghrī Birdī's Chronicles of Egypt," an excellent survey of the geography of the Mamlūk Empire and the government; Bertold Spuler, *The Muslim World; an Historical Survey*, vol. 2: *The Mongol Period*, trans. by F.R.C. Bagley (Leiden, 1960) places Mamlūk Egypt and Syria within the context of the general political history of the rest of the Middle East; Mustafa M. Ziada, "The Mamlūk Sultans to 1293" and "The Mamlūk Sultans, 1291-1517," *A History of the Crusades*, ed. by Kenneth Setton, vol. 2 (Madison, 1969), pp. 735-758 and vol. 3 (Madison, 1975), pp. 483-512; *EI*[1]: "mamlūks" (M. Soberheim); Ibn Khaldūn, *The Muqaddimah*, trans. by Franz Rosenthal, 3 vols. (Princeton, 1967), an invaluable source for the social and intellectual history of fourteenth-century Egypt; Hassanein M. Rabie, *The Financial System of Egypt* A.H. *564-741*/A.D. *1169-1341* (Oxford, 1972), a convenient summary of the financial administration; and the important articles of David Ayalon (Neustadt) primarily on the mamlūk army, see the Bibliography. For additional works on the Mamlūk Period, see Jean Sauvaget, *Introduction to the History of the Muslim East: A Bibliographical Guide*, ed. by Claude Cahen, trans. by von Grunebaum and Little (Berkeley and Los Angeles, 1965), pp. 176-183.

[7] See C. J. Lorinser, *Die Pest des Orient* (Berlin, 1837); "Ueber die grossen Seuchen," pp. 69-143 and the treatment of plague in von Kremer's *Culturgeschichte der Orients unter den Chalifen* (Vienna, 1877), vol. 2, pp. 489-493; G. Sticker, *Abhandlungen aus der Seuchengeschichte und Seuchenlehre*, vol. 1: *Die Pest* (Giessen, 1908), which relies heavily on von Kremer's work; and Enrico di Wolmar, *Abhandlungen über die Pest* (Berlin, 1827).

lated the most important (though not contemporary) historical text dealing with it in Egypt and Syria;[8] David Ayalon (Neustadt) has demonstrated the effects of recurrent plague epidemics on the mamlūk army;[9] and Abraham Udovitch has considered plague as a significant cause of the economic decline of Mamlūk Egypt.[10] Most recently, the Islamic legal principles regarding plague have been investigated, using the comprehensive Arabic plague treatise, *Badhl al-mā'ūn fī faḍl aṭ-ṭā'ūn*, by Ibn Ḥajar al-'Asqalānī (d. 852/1449).[11] Beyond this, nothing has been accomplished.[12]

Because the Muslims of the fourteenth and fifteenth centuries largely adopted the earlier religious and medical traditions concerning plague, I have begun by tracing briefly the previous history of plague in the Middle East from the Muslim conquests of the seventh century. Muslims of the later Middle Ages relied upon the previously established interpretations of the disease, Arabic terminology, plague symptomatology, and methods of prevention and treatment. The succession of plague epidemics in early Islamic history also poses the question of whether plague was endemic in the Middle East immediately before the Black Death.

As for the advent of the Black Death itself, most of the modern accounts of the pandemic in Europe begin by placing its origin rather indistinctly in the Orient and proceed quickly to its introduction into Sicily and Italy. Therefore, considerable attention has been paid to the transmission of plague from Central Asia through the Middle East, North Africa, and

[8] "La Grande Peste Noire en Syrie et en Égypte."

[9] "The Plague and Its Effects upon the Mamlūk Army."

[10] "England to Egypt," pp. 115-128.

[11] Sublet.

[12] Jean Marchika announced an exhaustive study of plague from the Black Death to modern times in his introduction to *La Peste en Afrique Septentrionale* (Algiers, 1927), p. 10. This thesis was to form only a part of the larger work; I have been unable to locate the author's proposed study.

Spain. A plague chronology and its geographical distribution have been determined, as well as the manner in which plague recurred in Muslim countries until the Ottoman conquest of Egypt in 1517.[13]

The nature and dissemination of the Black Death are no longer the gruesome mystery they were in the Middle Ages. Modern scientific research has disclosed the complex pathology of plague and set us comfortably apart from the past. It is essential, however, to summarize this knowledge in order to understand the medieval observations of the disease and to determine the existence of the various forms of plague. With an appropriate medical background, we can more fully appreciate the historical riddle of plague and the diverse medical explanations that persisted until the discovery of the plague bacillus, *Pasteurella pestis*, at the end of the nineteenth century and the subsequent establishment of plague pathology.

Without this knowledge, Muslims were no better equipped than others of their time to deal effectively with this disease; their desperately devised defenses form a major theme of the present inquiry. These defenses may be seen most vividly in the confusing medical explanations of the disease and in the futile attempts at prevention and treatment. More fundamental and perhaps more effective was the spiritual defense which the Muslims sought to formulate against this otherwise unaccountable scourge. The severe pandemic posed in acute form the basic theological problem of all Semitic religions: how to reconcile men's suffering with the justice and mercy of God. The abundant theological discussions in the plague treatises reflect the prevailing beliefs of contemporary Muslim scholars toward plague. In order to elucidate this literature and its religio-legal interpretations, I have chosen to analyze as representative the important plague treatise of Ibn Ḥajar al-'Asqalānī.

In one respect, Ibn Ḥajar's discussion of plague is atypical of the majority of Muslim treatises on plague. He argues against the predominant view that plague resulted from a

[13] See Appendix 1.

miasma or corruption of the air. Ibn Ḥajar believed that plague was inflicted on mankind by evil jinn or demons—a view not inconsistent with the Muslim belief that plague was sent directly by God. The plague-bearing jinn were simply agents of His design. This acceptable Muslim interpretation was the basis for a large number of superstitions and magical practices described in the plague treatises. Medically worthless, if not positively harmful, these measures of plague prevention and cure through exorcism are indicative of widespread popular belief in jinn and the efficacy of magic in the Middle Ages. As do the medical writings on the pestilence, the frequent advocacy of magic suggests that magical practices must have played an important part in the Muslim reaction to plague in the countryside and the major cities.

Regrettably, we have no Arabic equivalent of Boccaccio's *Decameron* that fully describes the responses of a Muslim community to the Black Death. Yet the actual reactions of specific communities, particularly Cairo and Damascus, have been fairly well documented by poets and historians, religious scholars and physicians. With the aid of supplementary information taken from later plague epidemics, we may arrive at a reasonably clear picture of the effects of the Black Death, especially in Egypt and Syria. In order for us to assess the consequences of the Black Death in these areas, I have attempted a very brief description of the political and social conditions of the Mamlūk Sultanate of Egypt and Syria before the Black Death. It would be an error to assume too great a familiarity by most readers with this period, although the specialist in medieval Islamic history may find this background unnecessary.

The immediate consequence of the pandemic was rural and urban depopulation, and this was recorded by Egyptian historians. While the medieval chronicles do not satisfy our curiosity about exact mortality figures, they indisputably document a significant decrease in general population. It is known that one class of urban society, the mamlūks, suffered severely from the Black Death. Since the mamlūks formed the military and governmental élite, they warrant our special attention. For this ruling class, as for Muslim society in general, the Black Death and the recurrences of plague had a damaging cumulative effect. To substantiate this claim, I have endeavored to draw together all the available demographic information relating to the Black Death and the recurrent plague epidemics. In this matter, I have been conscious of the recent skepticism about the demographic importance of plague recurrences in late medieval Europe. However, there is good reason to suggest an appreciable and sustained decline in Middle Eastern population from the mid-fourteenth century largely due to plague.

Faced with the tragic spectacle of the massive human destruction caused by the Black Death, Muslim society responded. We are particularly well informed about urban activity during the calamity because most of the chroniclers were residents in the plague-stricken cities. In the midst of frightening circumstances, the people were organized in communal supplications for alleviating the affliction, and large-scale funeral services as well as processions out to the cemeteries were arranged.

For the survivors, the Black Death influenced the conditions of daily life by changing the prices of commodities and the level of salaries. It is especially in the economic sphere, such as in land values and commerce, that we can discern the long-term as well as the immediate adjustments to demographic decline. The historical and literary sources are replete with information about the immediate and dramatic economic and social effects of the Black Death on Muslim communities. Indeed, this affliction of mankind has provided a powerful literary theme for writers as diverse as Boccaccio and Defoe, Hesse and Camus.[14]

These writers have employed the historical occurrences of

[14] Giovanni Boccaccio, *Decameron*, Florence, 1960; Daniel Defoe, *A Journal of the Plague Year*, London, 1928; Hermann Hesse, *Narcissus and Goldmund*, New York, 1968; and Albert Camus, *La Peste*, Paris, 1947. Other works could be added to this list, for example, Ingmar Bergman, *The Seventh Seal*, London, 1968.

plague for various reasons, but primarily to explore man's response to imminent death and to expose the frailty of human society. We can assume that the Black Death posed an intense personal dilemma for most Muslims. For medieval Muslim society as a whole, which is our main concern, the Black Death was a sharply focused and unavoidable stimulus that evoked defensive reactions in every sector of the community. These reactions provide us with material for the construction of a cross-section of communal relationships, economic interdependence, and cultural values and practices at one moment in time. This is not to imply that these aspects of Muslim life could not be studied individually or in a different manner. However, the plague pandemic offers a convenient, interesting, and effective method for studying some of the fundamental components of Muslim social organization and cohesiveness, as well as their adjustments to rapid change.[15]

In conclusion, I will attempt to assess the historical significance of the sustained demographic decline caused partly by the Black Death and recurrent plague epidemics in the Middle East. This assessment will be based both on the perceptible influence that depopulation exerted on the subsequent period of readjustment in Mamlūk Egypt and Syria, and on a comparison with the remarkable European Christian reaction to the same calamity.

[15] The Black Death in Europe has been recently analyzed in an attempt to judge the sources of and the limitations upon human society's ability to recover from a great catastrophe comparable to nuclear warfare (Jack Hirshleifer, *Disaster and Recovery: The Black Death in Western Europe*, RAND Corp., Santa Monica, 1966). The Black Death is similar to a nuclear explosion in its wide geographical extent, the abruptness of its onset, and the scale of casualties; however, the pandemic differs in its periodic recurrences and its non-destruction of material property. Earlier comparisons were drawn by historians between plague epidemics and conventional warfare; see, for example, James W. Thompson, "The Aftermath of the Black Death and the Aftermath of the Great War," *The American Journal of Sociology*, vol. 26 (1921), pp. 565-572, and G. G. Coulton, *The Black Death* (London, 1929), pp. 7, 74.

II

PLAGUE IN THE MIDDLE EAST

A. A HISTORY OF PLAGUE BEFORE THE BLACK DEATH[1]

Plague was well known to Middle Eastern peoples long before the Black Death; therefore, it was recognizable when it reappeared in the middle of the fourteenth century. Muslims of the fourteenth century could recall its macabre history, dating from the Muslim conquests of the Middle East in the seventh century. When plague ravaged the early Islamic Empire, the Muslims had responded to the danger; they sought both to explain it and to treat its victims. Subsequently, the early Muslim interpretations and social responses to plague gained authority with later generations when they were faced with plague epidemics. Thus, the initial encounters with it by the nascent Muslim community, which held special religious sanctity because of its association with the Prophet, came to determine the cultural attitudes and practices of traditional Muslim society. It is exactly this reliance on tradition that is so characteristic of medieval Islamic society and religion. In addition, the first historical pandemic of plague is comparable to the Black Death in its transmission, social and economic consequences, and cyclical reappearances. Its cyclical nature raises the medical and historical question of whether plague was endemic to the Middle East before the introduction of the Black Death in the mid-fourteenth century.

The origin of these early medieval recurrences of plague and

[1] For a fuller discussion of this topic, see "Ueber die grossen Seuchen," pp. 69-143; H.P.J. Renaud, "Les Maladies pestilentielles dans l'Orthodoxie Islamique," *Bulletin d'Institut d'Hygiène de Maroc*, vol. 3 (Rabat, 1934), pp. 5-16; and my "Plague in Early Islamic History," *JAOS*, vol. 94, no. 3 (1974), pp. 371-383.

of the Muslim traditions concerning the disease was the "Plague of Justinian," the first plague pandemic that can be fully documented in human history.[2] The Plague of Justinian derives its name from the fact that the pandemic spread throughout the Mediterranean world during the reign of the Byzantine Emperor Justinian (527-565). Beginning in 541 at Pelusium, an Egyptian port where the eastern effluent (the Pelusic channel) of the Nile entered the Mediterranean, plague moved westward to Alexandria and the rest of Egypt and eastward through Palestine and Syria. Evagrius Scholasticus describes a plague epidemic that appeared in Antioch, his home, in 542 and states that it had originated in Ethiopia.[3]

Evagrius may have been imitating the account of plague by Thucydides, who placed the origin of the famous "Athenian Plague" in Ethiopia. The precise origin of the Plague of

[2] Procopius, *History of the Wars*, ed. and trans. by H. B. Dewing, vol. 1 (New York, 1914), pp. 450-455. See also V. Seibel, *Die Grosse Pest zur Zeit Justinians* (Dillingen, 1857). The best modern introduction to the problem of the Plague of Justinian is J.-N. Biraben and J. Le Goff, "La Peste dans le haut moyen âge," *Annales*, vol. 24, part 6 (Paris, 1969), pp. 1484-1510, which attempts to outline the chronology and geographical distribution of the pandemic in Europe and the Middle East. Dr. Biraben has promised a more detailed study of plague in Byzantium and the Orient (*ibid.*, p. 1485, n. 1). Josiah Russell has also investigated the Plague of Justinian within the scope of his pioneering work on medieval demographic history; however, there is need for caution toward many of the author's hazardous assertions. At least for Middle Eastern demography, many statements are not based on primary sources for the period but rely heavily on very questionable comparisons with European population. (See Russell, "That Earlier Plague," *Demography*, vol. 5, part 1 [1968], pp. 174-184; also, "Late Ancient and Medieval Population," *Transactions of the American Philosophical Society*, Philadelphia, n.s., vol. 48, part 3 [1958]; "The Population of Medieval Egypt," *Journal of the American Research Center in Egypt*, vol. 5 [1966], pp. 69-82; "Recent Advances in Mediaeval Demography," *Speculum*, vol. 40 [1965], pp. 84-101; and *Population in Europe 500-1500* [London, 1969].)

[3] *The Ecclesiastical History*, book 4, section 29, ed. by J. Bider and L. Parmentier (London, 1898), pp. 177-179.

Justinian is uncertain, but it probably began in an endemic focus of plague in central or eastern Africa. Among the Arabic sources, the early medical compendium (235/850) of 'Alī ibn Rabban aṭ-Ṭabarī places the origin of plagues in the Sudan.[4] We know that plague epidemics since the sixteenth century have customarily been spread from East Africa through the Sudan by the caravan traffic to Egypt and North Africa. Beyond the Sudan, we have the testimony of the distinguished thirteenth-century Egyptian physician, Ibn an-Nafīs,[5] who identified the distinctive plague buboes with plague infection, in his influential commentary on Ibn Sīnā's famous medical encyclopaedia, *al-Qānūn fī ṭ-ṭibb*. More importantly, Ibn an-Nafīs mentions that he was told that plague often occurred in Ethiopia, where it was called *jaghalah*.[6] It appears, therefore, that it was endemic to Ethiopia during the early Middle Ages and that Ethiopia may have served initially as the center of transmission from Africa to the Mediterranean littoral by trade.[7]

There is no indication in the historical accounts, either oriental or occidental, that the Plague of Justinian originated in Central Asia, as it did in the two later pandemics.[8] Un-

[4] *Firdausu l-Ḥikmat or Paradise of Wisdom* (Berlin, 1928), p. 330.

[5] *EI*[2]: "Ibn an-Nafīs" (Meyerhof-Schacht).

[6] Quoted in *Kitāb aṭ-ṭibb*, fols. 145a-145b. Ibn Abī Hajalah states that this account was related to Ibn an-Nafīs by Shams ad-Dīn al-Ma'rūf, who had lived in Ethiopia. Also, the same story was related by Quṭb ad-Dīn ash-Shirāzī in his commentary on the *Qānūn*; he was reported to have heard the account from Ibn an-Nafīs along with the symptoms of plague (see *GAL*, vol. 2, pp. 211-212).

[7] Sticker, *Abhandlungen*, vol. 1, pp. 25-26; see also Major Greenwood, *Epidemics and Crowd-Diseases* (London, 1935), p. 290; Wu Lien-Teh, "The Original Home of Plague," *Far Eastern Association of Tropical Medicine: Transactions of the Fifth Biennial Congress* (Singapore, 1923), ed. by A. L. Hoops and J. W. Scharff (London, 1924), pp. 288-291.

[8] Sticker, *Abhandlungen*, vol. 2, p. 87. The thorough investigation of Chinese sources for plague epidemics in the sixth and seventh centuries would be highly desirable.

accountably, Professor Russell and others have assumed an Asiatic source for the Plague of Justinian.[9] On the contrary, the Byzantine historian Theophylact Simocattes, who continued the history of Procopius for the reign of the Emperor Maurice (582-602), mentions an embassy of western Turks to the emperor in 598. In describing these people, Theophylact refers to Mogholistan, the Issyk Kul region, where we have the earliest evidence of the Black Death. Theophylact states that in the late sixth century, "The Turks boast about two very important things: they say that in this region they have never seen the occurrence of any contagious disease since the most ancient times and that earthquakes are rare."[10]

Wherever the Plague of Justinian may have originated, its description by Procopius is important because it is the first unequivocal account of a bubonic plague epidemic.[11] Procopius observed the distinct symptoms of plague when it ravaged the Byzantine capital of Constantinople. Plague had probably reached the city in the spring of 542, or possibly as early as the autumn of 541, engulfing the lands and peoples of the known world: the Byzantine Empire and the rest of Europe, Persia and the barbarian hinterland.[12] Asia Minor and Egypt particularly were reported to have suffered severely.[13]

[9] Russell, *Medieval Regions and Their Cities* (Bloomington, 1972), pp. 227-229.

[10] Quoted in Édouard Chavannes, *Documents sur les Tou-Kiue (Turcs) Occidentaux* (Paris, 1942), p. 248.

[11] A controversy exists over the determination of true plague epidemics before the Plague of Justinian, such as the Biblical "plagues" of the Philistines (1 Sam. 5 and 6), the "Athenian Plague" described by Thucydides, and the fragmentary evidence of bubonic plague in North Africa and the Levant recorded by Rufus of Ephesus, which was preserved by Oribasius. For a summary of the literature on this topic, see Hirst, pp. 6-10; Pollitzer, *Plague* (Geneva, 1954), pp. 11-13; George Sarton, *An Introduction to the History of Science* (Baltimore, 1927-1948), vol. 3, part 2, p. 1650; Sticker, *Abhandlungen*, vol. 1, pp. 17-23.

[12] *History of the Wars*, vol. 1, pp. 450-473. Other Western sources mention the dissemination of plague in the Orient (see Russell, "That Earlier Plague," p. 179, n. 37).

[13] Russell, "That Earlier Plague," p. 180; "Recent Advances in Mediaeval Demography," pp. 98-101; and "The Population of Medieval Egypt," p. 71.

The Plague of Justinian may have played a crucial role in the history of the early Middle Ages.[14] Although there is considerable uncertainty about the demographic history of this period, it is fairly certain that the pandemic contributed to the perceptible contraction of Mediterranean population. Professor Russell estimates that the initial plague epidemic of 541-544 reduced the European-Mediterranean population by 20-25 percent and that there was a total decline of about 50-60 percent of the pre-plague population for the period 541-700.[15]

Despite the slight investigation of the demographic data for the Plague of Justinian, there has been dramatic speculation that the pandemic and its recurrent epidemics were the solvents of classical Mediterranean civilization and were largely responsible for the formation of new political, social, and economic patterns characteristic of the European Middle Ages. According to such speculation, political power gradually shifted to the peoples of northern Europe, who were relatively unaffected by the epidemics, and, conversely, plague greatly weakened the Byzantine Empire. Justinian's plan for re-establishing the Roman Empire was wrecked, and the diminished Byzantine armies were unable to defend the extensive fron-

[14] Russell, *Population in Europe 500-1500*, pp. 20-21, and "That Earlier Plague," pp. 175-178; Biraben and Le Goff, "La Peste," p. 1499.

[15] "That Earlier Plague," p. 180. These estimates raise a number of questions about the nature of the pandemic itself. Russell's assertions are based on the assumption that the demographic effect of the Plague of Justinian and its recurrences are comparable to that of the Black Death and its subsequent epidemics in Europe. This is highly questionable because it is doubtful that the second pandemic was responsible for a continued decline in European population. Moreover, it has not been proved that the pneumonic form of plague was present in this first pandemic and its recurrences (see chap. II). In addition, there is the debated issue of whether or not commensal rodents played a significant part in the causation of bubonic plague in Europe during this first pandemic. It has been suggested that the plague rat (*Rattus rattus*) was not present in Europe before the twelfth century, when it was transported to Europe by the returning Crusader ships, and could not have served as the efficient vehicle of plague (Pollitzer, *Plague*, pp. 13, 283; M.A.C. Hinton, *Rats and Mice as Enemies of Mankind* [London, 1918], p. 4; cf. Christopher Morris, "The Plague in Britain," *The Historical Journal*, vol. 14, no. 1 [1971], pp. 213-214).

tiers. Hence, there was the successful resurgence of barbarian invasions—the Slavic migrations into the Balkans and Greece, the Lombardic invasion into Italy, and the Berber incursions into Byzantine North Africa. In addition, the pandemic may have had significant economic repercussions comparable to those of the Black Death eight centuries later. The Pirenne Thesis that the advent of Islam produced a rupture in the commerce of the ancient Mediterranean world has been seriously questioned; the discussion of this historical problem should also take into account the consequences of the concomitant drastic decline in Mediterranean population.

With regard to the Middle East, the Plague of Justinian may have sapped the military strength of the Byzantine and Persian Empires, already weakened by heavy losses sustained in warfare before the Arab conquests. Professor Russell suggests that an additional advantage was given to the nomadic and semi-nomadic peoples adjacent to these empires because the nomads suffered a lower mortality, as a result of an environment unfavorable to plague. Conditions were therefore optimal, in Professor Russell's opinion, for the migration of Arab tribesmen from Arabia and their successful conquests of the Middle East and North Africa.[16]

It is particularly significant, with a view to the Black Death, that the Plague of Justinian recurred in discernible cycles of about nine to twelve years, according to the occidental sources.[17] Most of the plague treatises written by Arabic authors after the Black Death include a history of these early recurrences in the Middle East because they struck the incipient Muslim community.[18] The short histories usually begin

[16] "That Earlier Plague," pp. 181-184, and "The Population of Medieval Egypt," p. 82; Biraben and Le Goff, "La Peste," pp. 1499, 1508.

[17] Biraben and Le Goff, "La Peste," p. 1493; Sticker, *Abhandlungen*, vol. 1, pp. 24-41.

[18] The early Muslim discussion and enumeration of plague epidemics is to be found in the *ḥadīth* literature and can be reconstructed from their citation in the plague treatises posterior to the Black Death. From this late medieval material it is clear that the earliest and most important history of plague epidemics and their related *ḥadīths* was

with the Old Testament "plagues" and include the enumeration of possible plague epidemics up to the time of the Black Death. The result of the compilation of the early accounts by the Muslim writers of the later Middle Ages gives us a fairly uniform chronology of plague epidemics in early Islamic history, in which the Black Death was considered to be the sixth major epidemic.[19]

---

composed by al-Madā'inī (d. 225/840 or 231/845; see *EI*[1]: "al-Madā'inī" [C. Brockelmann]), who was an important Arab historian and a major source for the *History* of aṭ-Ṭabarī. Al-Madā'inī's work on plagues appears to be lost, along with most of his other compositions. Yet the majority of the later writers take their history of the early plagues in Islam from al-Madā'inī, for his work was incorporated into the writings of Ibn Abī d-Dunyā (d. 281/894; see *EI*[2]: "Ibn Abī d-Dunyā" [A. Dietrich]). The latter's *Kitāb al-i'tibār* (*GAL, Supplement*, vol. 1, p. 248, no. 41; I have been unable to locate a copy of this work) is the primary source for the plague treatise writers after the Black Death. Ibn Ḥajar also cites Ibn Abī d-Dunyā's *Kitāb at-tawā'īn* as the basis for a number of *ḥadīths* relating to plague (*Badhl*, fols. 86a, 120b-123b); the *Kitāb at-tawā'īn* is listed in *The Fihrist of al-Nadīm*, trans. by Bayard Dodge (New York, 1970), vol. 1, p. 185, but I have been unable to locate a copy of this treatise also. Another important source of *ḥadīths* was the great *Sunnī* polygraph, Ibn Qutaybah (d. 276/889; see *EI*[2]: "Ibn Ḳutayba" [G. Lecomte]), who discusses the difficulties arising from these traditions in his *Kitāb ta'wīl mukhtalif al-ḥadīth* (Cairo, A.H. 1326, pp. 125-126; French trans. by G. Lecomte, *Le Traité des divergences du ḥadīth d'Ibn Qutayba* [Damascus, 1962], p. 116). In his *Kitāb ma'ārif*, Ibn Qutaybah gives the history of plagues in early Islam (Cairo, 1960, pp. 601-602). All three early authors are quoted extensively in the treatises of Ibn Ḥajar and Ibn Abī Ḥajalah.

[19] The first full enumeration of epidemics, including plague, was written by Ibn Abī Hajalah in 764/1362 (*Daf' an-niqmah*, fols. 59b-76b). (Slightly earlier, a *Qaṣīdah fī ṭ-ṭā'ūn* by Bahā' ad-Dīn as-Subkī [d. 756/1355] mentions very briefly the plagues in early Islam [Dār al-Kutub al-Miṣrīyah MS no. 102 *majāmī' m*, fol. 198a]. Similarly, Ibn al-Wardī refers briefly to the early plagues in his *Risālat an-naba'*, p. 186.) The long historical account of Ibn Abī Hajalah was incorporated with modifications into the epilogue of Ibn Hajar's important treatise (*Badhl*, fols. 120b-131b). These two historical summaries of plague epidemics in early Islam—by Ibn Abī Ḥajalah and Ibn Hajar—were condensed by as-Suyūṭī (d. 910/1505) in his *Mā rawāhu l-wā'ūn*, pp. 144-156. As-Suyūṭī supplements this account with historical data from

The later chroniclers quote al-Madā'īnī to the effect that there were five great plagues in Islamic history before the Black Death.[20] The Muslim historians cite the "plague of Shīrawayh" as the first plague epidemic in the Muslim era. It occurred in 6/627-628 at Ctesiphon (Madā'in),[21] whose name is derived from Siroes (Kobad II), who succeeded Chosroes II in 628 as the Sassanian king of Persia.[22] Siroes himself died of plague in 629.[23] Comparing this epidemic to others, as-Suyūṭī quotes Ibn 'Asākir's history of Damascus about a "plague of Yezdigird,"[24] which must refer to a later appearance of plague during the reign of the last Sassanian king, Yezdigird II (634-642). Ibn Qutaybah does not mention

---

other chronicles, which add little to the information found in the earlier histories, but he brings the list of plagues up to his own time. The compendium of as-Suyūṭī forms the basis of Alfred von Kremer's important study of epidemics in an extensive introduction to his edition of the text ("Ueber die grossen Seuchen," pp. 69-143). See note 47 below.

[20] See *Mā rawāhu l-wā'ūn*, p. 144; *Badhl*, fol. 120b. Ibn Abī Ḥajalah also draws his information from al-Madā'inī and others but does not follow the same *five* plagues; he indiscriminately lists thirty "plagues" from early Islam to 749/1349 (*Daf' an-niqmah*, fols. 59b-76b). The determination of plague in Islamic history raises a difficult problem: Does the *sūrat al-fīl* (Qur'ān 105) refer to a plague outbreak? For a discussion of this point, see my "Plague in Early Islamic History," p. 375. See as well the discussion of Karl Opitz, *Die Medizin im Koran* (Stuttgart, 1906), pp. 43-44; Opitz points out that the description of a possible epidemic in this case, which he believes was smallpox, is similar to the description in the Qur'ān of the destruction of Sodom (Qur'ān 15: 73-74; 11: 84; 51: 32-34).

[21] *Mā rawāhu l-wā'ūn*, p. 144; *Badhl*, fol. 120b; *Daf' an-niqmah*, fol. 61b.

[22] Ibn Qutaybah, *Kitāb al-ma'ārif*, p. 601, l. 5: "ṭā'ūn Shīrawayh ibn Kisrā bil-'Irāq."

[23] At this time there is a brief mention in the Chinese sources of a "plague" in Hami (Camul), an important city on the famous Silk Route. The epidemic is recorded in Stanislas Julien, "Documents historiques sur les Tou-Kioue (Turcs), extraits du Pien-i-tien, et traduits du Chinois," *JA*, series 6, vol. 4 (1864), p. 231.

[24] *Mā rawāhu l-wā'ūn*, p. 144.

the plague of Yezdigird, but merely says that there was a long period between the plague of Shīrawayh and the "Syrian plague."[25] The plague of Yezdigird may simply be another name for the important epidemic in Syria.

The epidemic in Syria is known as the "plague of 'Amwās (or 'Amawās)"[26] because it struck severely the Arab army at 'Amwās, ancient Emmaus, in 17/638 or 18/639.[27] It is probable that as-Suyūṭī's suggestion that plague reappeared soon after its initial outbreak accounts for the two dates. Accordingly, Sayf ibn 'Umar related that the plague of 'Amwās occurred twice: it struck in Muḥarram and Ṣafar, disappeared, and returned again, and "many people died in it to the advantage of the enemy [the Byzantines]."[28] The historical accounts of the plague of 'Amwās state that about 25,000 Muslim soldiers died and that plague spread to the rest of Syria, as well as to

[25] *Kitāb al-ma'ārif*, p. 201.

[26] See the discussion of the name and etymology of "'Amwās" in *Badhl*, fols. 61b-62b.

[27] at-Ṭabarī, *Ta'rīkh*, Cairo ed. (1960-1969), vol. 3, p. 613, vol. 4, pp. 57-65, 96-97, 101; de Goeje ed. (Leiden, 1879-1901), series 1, vol. 5, pp. 2412, 2511-2521, 2570-2572, 2578. See also William Muir, *The Caliphate: Its Rise, Decline and Fall* (Beirut, 1963), pp. 164-167, based almost exclusively on the account of aṭ-Ṭabarī; *Mā rawāhu l-wā'ūn*, p. 144; *al-Bidāyah*, vol. 1, pp. 78-79; Ibn 'Asākir, *Ta'rīkh madīnat Dimashq* (Damascus, 1951-1963), vol. 1, pp. 554-555; and *EI*²: "'Amwās" (J. Sourdel-Thomine) for further bibliographical references. As for the dating, Ibn Ḥajar (*Badhl*, fol. 62a) reports both 17 and 18 A.H. for the epidemic but prefers 17 A.H.; Leone Caetani places the plague of 'Amwās in A.H. 18 (*Annali dell'Islām*, vol. 4 [Milan, 1911], pp. 4-6). Biraben and Le Goff refer to nearly contemporary plague epidemics in the West ("La Peste," p. 1497).

[28] *Mā rawāhu l-wā'ūn*, p. 145. Whether in 17 or in 18 A.H., this would have been in the months of January and February, and would suggest the probability of pneumonic plague. Another possible reference to pneumonic plague, in addition to bubonic plague, is made in A. E. Belyaev, *Arabs, Islam and the Arab Caliphate* (New York, 1969), p. 160. C. S. Bartsocas cites Byzantine sources for plague recurrences in 716-717 as well as for 695, 775, 1031, and 1056 ("Two Fourteenth Century Greek Descriptions of the 'Black Death,'" *Journal of the History of Medicine and Allied Sciences*, vol. 21, no. 4 [1966], p. 394).

Iraq and Egypt. The epidemic had been preceded by a severe famine in Syria-Palestine that may have predisposed the population to the disease. Famine is often associated with the appearance of plague epidemics, possibly as a result of lowered human resistance and the attraction of food reserves in human settlements, which brought the plague-infested rats into closer contact with men.

The Caliph 'Umar summoned Abū 'Ubaydah, the military commander in Syria, from 'Amwās to Medina in order to prevent his death from the plague epidemic in 18/639. Knowing Abū 'Ubaydah's courage and his loyalty to the army, the Caliph concealed his purpose and ordered him to return on an urgent matter. Abū 'Ubaydah realized the Caliph's intention and refused, preferring to stay with his army in Syria.[29] Therefore, the Caliph 'Umar set out for Syria and came to Sargh, where he met Abū 'Ubaydah and called a council of the military leaders. The council was divided on the issue and disagreed about what was to be done with regard to the plague epidemic. Finally, 'Umar accepted the advice of the leaders of the tribe of Quraysh (the tribe of the Prophet), to quit the region of the epidemic. Referring to the prohibition of the Prophet against a Muslim's either entering or fleeing a plague-stricken land, Abū 'Ubaydah protested that they were fleeing the decree of God. Not wishing to disagree with his military commander, 'Umar wisely replied with a parable: "Suppose that you come to a valley where one side is green with pasture and the other is bare and barren; whichever side you let loose your camels, it would be the will of God. But you would choose the side that was green."[30] According to another

[29] For the contents of the letters between Abū 'Ubaydah and 'Umar, see at-Tabarī, *Ta'rīkh*, Cairo ed., vol. 4, p. 61, de Goeje ed., vol. 5, pp. 2517-2518; *Badhl*, fols. 67b-72a, 79a-81b; and Muir, *The Caliphate*, pp. 164-167.

[30] *Badhl*, fols. 63a-77b; Muir, *The Caliphate*, p. 166, n. 1. There is considerable contradiction and ambiguity in the *ḥadīth* literature concerning the issue of flight from plague epidemics. The contradictions are clearly presented in Ibn Qutaybah's early discussion of contagion and plague; see his *Kitāb ta'wīl*, pp. 123-126 (Lecomte, trans., *Le Traité des divergences*, pp. 114-116 with a useful introduction, pp. xix-xxv).

version of this justification of flight, Muslims would be "fleeing from the decree of God to the decree of God."[31] The Caliph argued that in removing the people to a naturally more healthful region he was making no attempt to flee the command of God, thereby establishing a precedent for fleeing a plague epidemic. 'Umar then commanded Abū 'Ubaydah to take the army out of the infected area, while the Caliph felt justified in returning to Medina.

These events surrounding the plague of 'Amwās are very important because they demonstrate contemporary Muslim attitudes toward plague and directly affected later religio-legal explanations of the disease. Three principles, derived from the teaching of the Prophet, influenced the actions of the early Muslim community: (1) plague was a mercy and a martyrdom from God for the faithful Muslim and a punishment for the infidel; (2) a Muslim should neither enter nor flee a plague-stricken land; and (3) there was no contagion of plague, because disease came directly from God.[32] These three religio-legal tenets provoked sustained controversy, due to the constant reappearance of plague epidemics. As was evident during the plague of 'Amwās, disagreement with the principles was caused by the difficulty of accepting the horrible disease as a blessing and a martyrdom, the natural propensity to flee, and the empirical observations of contagion. It would be unreasonable to assume, therefore, that these tenets completely describe the Muslim response to plague at this time or during the later Middle Ages, but they do set the framework for normative communal behavior.[33]

With regard to the first principle, some men (motivated perhaps by natural human anxiety and native Christian and Jewish attitudes) considered the epidemic as a warning or punishment by God. In this manner, the plague epidemic was believed to be a divine punishment or warning for the moral laxity of the Muslims. For example, it was said that this plague occurred in Syria because the Muslims there drank

[31] *Badhl*, fols. 71a-71b; Muir, *The Caliphate*, p. 164.

[32] See Sublet, pp. 141-149.

[33] See chap. VIII.

wine, which Islam prohibits; therefore, by the order of Caliph 'Umar, Abū 'Ubaydah had the offenders lashed.[34] Nonetheless, the belief in plague as a mercy and a martyrdom is evident; it was contained in the speech of Abū 'Ubaydah to the army at 'Amwās and was expressed in the council held by the Caliph at Sargh.[35] This belief was popularly expressed in a poetic description of the plague of 'Amwās from Ibn 'Asākir's history of Damascus:

> How many brave horsemen and how many beautiful, chaste women were killed in the valley of 'Amwās.
> They had encountered the Lord, but He was not unjust to them.
> When they died, they were among the non-aggrieved people in paradise.
> We endure the plague as the Lord knows, and we were consoled in the hour of death.[36]

Apart from these views was the belief that God had sent the disease, and men should simply accept it. This belief is also found in discussions concerning the second principle. Whether one fled or remained in a plague-stricken region, God had already decreed one's death. This is the substance of the argument of Abū Mūsā al-Ash'arī regarding plague.[37] When some friends came to see him in Kūfah, he asked them not to stay, because someone in his home was ill with plague, and advised them to go out to the open spaces and gardens of the city. He states the popular belief that whoever left a plague-stricken land believed that if he stayed he would die, and

[34] *Mā rawāhu l-wā'ūn*, p. 145, which quotes at-Tabarī, *Ta'rīkh*, Cairo ed., vol. 4, pp. 96-97, de Goeje ed., vol. 5, pp. 2571-2572.

[35] Ibn 'Asākir, *at-Ta'rīkh al-kabīr* (Damascus, A.H. 1332), vol. 1, pp. 176-178.

[36] *Ibid.*, p. 175. The early plagues often served as a theme for Arabic poetry; see, for example, the poem of Abū Dhu'ayb al-Hudhalī translated by Omar S. Pound, *Arabic and Persian Poems* (New York, 1970), p. 35.

[37] *al-Bidāyah*, vol. 7, p. 78.

whoever stayed and was afflicted would think that if he had left he would not have been stricken. Implicit in this story is not only the common practice of fleeing the disease but the recognition of contagion, despite the fact that the Prophet had denied the pre-Islamic belief in contagion. In any case, a Muslim was not to be blamed for fleeing, according to Abū Mūsā, for God had already determined each man's fate. Abū Mūsā supported his argument for flight by citing the decision of 'Umar during the plague of 'Amwās when Abū Mūsā had been with Abū 'Ubaydah in Syria.

Following the Caliph's orders, Abū 'Ubaydah brought the army and its followers to the highlands of the Ḥaurān, but at al-Jābiyah he died of plague. Mu'ādh ibn Jabal was appointed to succeed Abū 'Ubaydah; however, he died almost immediately, along with his son, who was supposed to have assumed leadership after his father. It was left to 'Amr ibn al-'Āṣ, shortly to be the conqueror of Egypt, to lead the people to safety.[38] Thus, among the companions of the Prophet who died of the plague at this time were Abū 'Ubaydah, Yazīd ibn Abī Sufyān, Mu'ādh and his son.[39] Because of their deaths, 'Umar appointed Mu'āwiyah ibn Abī Sufyān commander in Syria and thereby provided the occasion for the foundation of Umayyad power.[40]

Besides the plagues of Shīrawayh and 'Amwās, there was the "violent plague" (*al-Jārif*) so named because it swept through Baṣrah "like a flood" about the year 69/688-689. The fourth major plague epidemic, called the "plague of the maidens" (*al-Fatayāt*) struck Baṣrah in 87/706. And the fifth

[38] aṭ-Tabarī, *Ta'rīkh*, Cairo ed., vol. 4, p. 62, de Goeje ed., vol. 5, p. 2519.

[39] Other prominent Muslims who died of plague included: Shuraḥbīl ibn Hasanah, al-Faḍl ibn al-'Abbās, Abū Mālik al-Ash'arī, al-Ḥārith ibn Hisham, Abū Janbal, Suhayl ibn 'Amr (aṭ-Ṭabarī, *Ta'rīkh*, Cairo ed., vol. 4, p. 60, de Goeje ed., vol. 5, p. 2516; *Mā rawāhu l-wā'ūn*, p. 145).

[40] aṭ-Ṭabarī, *Ta'rīkh*, Cairo ed., vol. 4, p. 62, de Goeje ed., vol. 5, p. 2520.

was the "plague of the notables" (*al-Ashrāf*) in 98/716-717 in Iraq and Syria.[41] Aside from the five important epidemics, there is evidence of other plague epidemics during the Umayyad Period (41-132/661-749).[42]

Unfortunately, the early Islamic Empire was literally plagued by this disease. We know that the Syrian and Iraqī populations suffered particularly from recurrent epidemics and famines during the Umayyad Period. Plague struck the governing élite as well as the common people, and expressly for this reason, when the plague season came during the summer, the Umayyad caliphs usually left the cities for their desert palaces.[43] Moreover, Arab commanders would remove their troops from their urban garrisons to the mountains or the desert until an epidemic had ceased.[44]

After the fall of the Umayyad dynasty, the Muslim chroniclers report that plague abated with the advent of the 'Abbāsid dynasty in 132/749.[45] There is a famous anecdote about an 'Abbāsid commander who came to Damascus, the former capital of the Umayyads, to make speeches on behalf of the new regime. The amir told the Damascenes that they should praise God, who had raised the plague from them since the 'Abbāsids had come to power. One courageous man in the crowd stood up and replied: "God is more just than to give you power over us and the plague at the same time!"[46]

Plague epidemics did recur, however, during the 'Abbāsid

[41] *Badhl*, fols. 62a, 121a; *Daf' an-niqmah*, fol. 63a; *Mā rawāhu l-wā'ūn*, pp. 150-152; Ibn Qutaybah, *Kitāb al-ma'ārif*, p. 201.

[42] See my "Plague in Early Islamic History," pp. 379-380.

[43] *Badhl*, fols. 62a, 121b; *Mā rawāhu l-wā'ūn*, p. 153; J. Wellhausen, *The Arab Kingdom and Its Fall* (Beirut, 1963 reprint), pp. 325-326. For a recent statement of the scholarship on the desert palaces, see Oleg Grabar, *The Formation of Islamic Art* (New Haven, 1973), pp. 15, 141-165, 225-226.

[44] von Kremer, *Culturgeschichte*, vol. 2, p. 493.

[45] *Mā rawāhu l-wā'ūn*, p. 153; C. E. Bosworth, *The Laṭā'if al-ma'ārif of Tha'ālibī* (Edinburgh, 1968), p. 153.

[46] *Badhl*, fol. 121b; *Mā rawāhu l-wā'ūn*, p. 153.

Period but with less frequency and severity.[47] In the previous period, it is clear that plague consistently reappeared in the Middle East, especially in Syria-Palestine and Iraq, following the outbreak of the pandemic in the mid-sixth century. Syria-Palestine experienced plague epidemics about every ten years from 69/688-689 to 127/744-745, but the epidemics in the major cities of lower Mesopotamia, Kūfah and Baṣrah, were more erratic.[48]

The first plague pandemic in the Middle East foreshadowed the second, the Black Death in the middle of the fourteenth

[47] For epidemics from the Umayyad Period to the Black Death in the mid-fourteenth century, where plague epidemics have yet to be clearly distinguished, see principally "Ueber die grossen Seuchen," pp. 110-135, and *Culturgeschichte*, vol. 2, pp. 490-492. Unfortunately, all later historians, including Sticker, Biraben, Le Goff *et al.* have relied heavily on von Kremer's work. Von Kremer limited himself to a very small number of primary sources, mainly the work of as-Suyūṭī, a highly abbreviated account, and, more seriously, von Kremer did not distinguish among epidemic diseases. He was greatly hampered in the determination of plague epidemics by his ignorance of the biological nature of plague. Von Kremer's erroneous belief in miasma as a cause of plague strongly influenced his historical interpretation of plague in the Middle East. However, his chronology, when emended, would suggest the *possible* incidents of plague recurrences. A close examination of the historical descriptions of these epidemics and their terminology may lead to a satisfactory account of plague and other epidemic diseases during the entire medieval period. Plague epidemics are also cited in the following works: Louis Hautecoeur and Gaston Wiet, *Les Mosquées du Caire* (Paris, 1932), vol. 1, pp. 81-82; Édouard Bloch, *La Peste en Tunisie* (*Aperçu historique et épidemiologique*) (diss., Faculty of Medicine, Paris), Tunis, 1929, pp. 1-3; J.-L.-G. Guyon, *Histoire chronologique des épidémies du Nord de l'Afrique* (Algiers, 1855), pp. 112-175; Sticker, *Abhandlungen*, vol. 1, pp. 24-77; Tholozan, *Histoire de la peste bubonique en Mésopotamie* (Paris, 1874), pp. 6-7, and *Histoire de la peste bubonique en Perse*, pp. 10-12; and C.-A. Julien, *History of North Africa* (New York, 1970), pp. 56, 59, 121.

[48] Within a reasonable margin of error in interpreting the imprecise historical accounts and allowing for failure to record small local epidemics, the calculations are based on the data collected in the plague treatises.

century. Due to the cyclical nature of plague, the repeated epidemics in the heartland of the Islamic Empire struck down the Arab conquerors as it had their Byzantine and Sassanian predecessors. The recurrences of plague may have continuously retarded natural population growth and served as a major factor in debilitating Umayyad strength, apart from the continual attrition of manpower in the Syrian army, which was extensively deployed throughout the empire. The constant infusion of Arab population, on the other hand, into the former Sassanian region of the empire during the Umayyad Period, and this region's apparent exemption from plague epidemics (outside lower Mesopotamia), would suggest an unbalanced growth of population in the empire that was reflected in the predominance and economic prosperity of the 'Abbāsid regime.

The geographical diffusion of these plague epidemics also followed the commercial routes in the Middle East and the Mediterranean littoral, promiscuously carrying the disease by trade from one urban center to another.[49] Although the direction of transmission differed in the Plague of Justinian and the Black Death—from East Africa in the first case and from Central Asia in the second—the epidemic outbreaks trace the principal commercial routes of the period and attest to significant trade throughout the Mediterranean world.[50]

With regard to early Islamic civilization in general, the plague recurrences evoked a medical interest, which resulted in the investigation and discussion of pre-Islamic medical works, especially the writings of Hippocrates and Galen,[51] as well as in personal observation.[52] In one instance the quotation from

[49] See the interesting essay on this historical phenomenon by André Siegfried, *Germs and Ideas: Routes of Epidemics and Ideologies* (London, 1965).

[50] For the Plague of Justinian, see Biraben and Le Goff, "La Peste," pp. 1493, 1499; for the Black Death, A. N. Poliak, "Le Caractère colonial de l'état mamelouk dans ses rapports avec le Horde d'Or," *REI* (Paris, 1935), pp. 231-248.

[51] *GAS*, vol. 3, pp. 23-47, 68-140.

[52] Medical discussions of plague in the Arabic sources anterior to the Black Death may be found in the following works, given in ap-

pre-Islamic medical works concerning plague is important. The famous physician ar-Rāzī quotes Ahrun the Priest, an Alexandrian doctor living about the time of the birth of Islam who wrote *The Medical Pandects*, the earliest medical work to

---

proximate chronological order: (1) 'Alī ibn Rabban at-Tabarī's early medical compendium, *Firdausu l-Hikmat*, pp. 328-331, which includes a discussion of plagues (*tawā'īn*) and quotations from Hippocrates' *Epidemics I and III* (see Max Meyerhof, "'Alī at-Ṭabarī's 'Paradise of Wisdom,' One of the Oldest Arabic Compendiums of Medicine," *Isis*, vol. 16 [1931], pp. 31, 51; and Ullmann, pp. 119-122, 244). (2) Al-Kindī (d. ca. 256/870) wrote two works on epidemics (see *GAS*, vol. 3, pp. 244-247) although not cited by the late medieval writers on plague. (3) Thābit ibn Qurrah (d. 288/901) devoted a chapter to plague in his work, *Kitāb adh-dhakhīrah* (Cairo, 1928), chapter 27 (see Max Meyerhof, "The 'Book of Treasure,' an early Arabic Treatise on Medicine," *Isis*, vol. 14 [1930], pp. 55-76). (4) There are two works by Qusṭā ibn Lūqā al-Ba'labakkī (d. ca. 300/912) concerning infection and epidemics: *Kitāb fī l-i'dā'* and *Kitāb fī l-wabā' wa asbābihi* (see *GAS*, vol. 3, pp. 270-271, and Ullmann, p. 244). (5) Ar-Rāzī (d. 313/925) discusses plagues after his famous chapter on smallpox and measles in *Kitāb al-hāwī fī ṭ-tibb* (Hyderabad, 1955-1968), vol. 17. It is uncertain whether the description of plague by ar-Rāzī was the product of personal observation of plague or was copied from earlier works (see Sticker, *Abhandlungen*, vol. 1, p. 36; Ernst Seidel, "Die Lehre von der Kontagion bei den Arabern," *AGM*, vol. 6 [Leipzig, 1913], p. 85; and Ullmann, pp. 128-136). (6) 'Alī ibn al-'Abbās al-Majūsī's (d. 384/994) *Kitāb al-Malakī* (Būlāq, 1294 A.H., vol. 1, pp. 168-170, vol. 2, pp. 62-65). (7) Muḥammad ibn Ahmad at-Tamīmī's (d. 370/890) plague treatise, *Kitāb māddat al-baqā' bi-iṣlāḥ fasād al-hawā' wat-taharruz min ḍarar al-awbā'* (see *GAS*, vol. 3, p. 317, and Ullmann, p. 245). (8) A treatise on the causes of plague in Egypt by the North African physician Ibn al-Jazzār (d. 369/979), *Kitāb fī na't al-asbāb al-muwallidah lil-wabā' fī Misr*, which is reported to be lost (*GAS*, vol. 3, pp. 304-307, and Ullmann, pp. 245-246). (9) Against this treatise of Ibn al-Jazzār, we have the very interesting work of 'Alī ibn Riḍwān entitled *Daf' maḍarr al-abdān bi-arḍ Miṣr* (Ullmann, pp. 159, 246). The latter reproaches Ibn al-Jazzār for his undemonstrable beliefs about plague in Egypt and offers a description of Fāṭimid Egypt; chapter fourteen gives advice against plague infection according to Yūsuf as-Sāhir (Ullmann, p. 124), ar-Rāzī, Ibn Māsawayh, and Ibn al-Jazzār. For a summary of this work of Ibn Riḍwān, see Max Meyerhof, "Climate and Health in Old Cairo according to 'Alī ibn Ridwān," *Comptes Rendus*

be translated into Arabic.[53] In the citation by ar-Rāzī, Ahrun describes the spitting of blood.[54] This is the earliest description, to my knowledge, of pneumonic plague and may also indicate the presence of this form of plague in the recurrences of the Plague of Justinian. Altogether, the massive translation of classical medical works into Arabic during the ninth and tenth centuries should be seen as part of an endeavor to understand the nature of recurrent disease and not as a purely academic exercise.

More importantly, the epidemics stimulated Muslim religious scholars to reach an acceptable interpretation of the meaning of this periodic scourge; such an explanation would dominate any understanding of the disease during the medi-

---

du congrès international de médicine tropicale et d'hygienè (Cairo, 1929), vol. 2, pp. 211-239; I am presently preparing the text and translation of this work based on the two manuscript copies (Dār al-Kutub al-Misrīyah MSS nos. 18 and 384 *tibb*). (10) Abū Sahl al-Masīḥī al-Jurjānī (d. 401/1010), who was the teacher of Ibn Sīnā, also wrote a medical work on plague (*Risālah fī taḥqīq amr al-wabā' wal-ihtirāz 'anhu wa-islahihī idhā waqa'a*) dedicated to the Khwarizmshāh, Abū l-'Abbās Ma'mūn ibn Ma'mūn (390-407 A.H.), according to Ferdinand Wüstenfeld (*Geschichte der Arabischen Aerzte und Naturforscher* [Göttingen, 1840], p. 60, no. 8; see also *GAS*, vol. 3, pp. 326-329, and Ullmann, p. 151). (11) By far the most influential medical discussion of plague was by Ibn Sīnā, see chap. IV. (12) Besides a commentary (*Mūjaz al-Qānūn*) on the important plague description of Ibn Sīnā (*GAL, Supplement*, vol. 1, p. 825, no. 82a), Ibn an-Nafīs wrote an exposition on Hippocrates' theory of epidemics, *Kitāb abīdhīmiya l-buqrāt wa tafsīruhu l-marad al-wāfid* (*GAS*, vol. 3, p. 35). (13) Ibn al-Quff (d. 685/1286) composed a work on surgery that contains a chapter on plague boils (*GAL*, vol. 1, p. 493; see also Otto Spies, "Zur Geschichte der Pocken in der Arabischen Literatur," *AGM, Supplement*, vol. 7 [Wiesbaden, 1966], pp. 187-188). A number of post-Black Death writers drew their medical information about plague from Ibn an-Nafīs' *Mūjaz al-Qānūn* and (14) Ibn al-Akfānī, another Cairene physician, who died in the Black Death (*GAL*, vol. 2, p. 137; *Supplement*, vol. 2, p. 169).

[53] Cyril Elgood, *A Medical History of Persia and the Eastern Caliphate* (Cambridge, 1951), pp. 99-100; Ullmann, pp. 87-89.

[54] *Kitāb hāwī fī t-ṭibb*, vol. 17, p. 4.

eval period. It was natural for them to turn first to the reported teachings of the Prophet, which we have already discussed in relation to the plague of 'Amwās. These teachings were supplemented by relevant material drawn from the Old and New Testaments, the Qur'ān, the traditions of the Prophet's companions and followers, the classical and medieval physicians, and native custom. A system of theological belief and a normative scheme of behavior with regard to plague were created in a manner characteristic of traditional Muslim law. The religious interpretation of plague was incorporated within the *ḥadīth* literature or corpus of pious traditions that make up Muslim law.[55] What is remarkable is that the early plagues came at a formative, eclectic period in Muslim legal scholarship, which gave plague a special status and uniqueness among other natural disasters. The pious traditions about plague influenced the thinking of the early Muslim community and continued to be operative in Muslim religious life until the twentieth century. Thus, the juristic literature and medical commentaries furnished the later medieval writers not only with religio-legal precedents, which set limits to intellectual discussion and to communal behavior, but also with an etiological explanation of plague, methods of prevention and treatment, and a precise Arabic terminology.[56]

The recurrences of plague in early Islamic history also raise the question of its prevalence before the Black Death in the middle of the fourteenth century. Was plague endemic to Egypt and Syria before the Black Death, as it seems to have been in Europe?[57]

[55] Sublet, pp. 141-149. See also Seidel, "Die Lehre von der Kontagion bei den Arabern," pp. 83-84.

[56] See "The Plague and Its Effects," p. 67, n. 2, and my additions to plague terminology in Appendix 2.

[57] Apparently, Europe witnessed a number of plague epidemics bebore the Black Death. Bubonic plague attacked the army of Frederick Barbarossa before Rome in 1167 and, later, the city itself. There are reports of plague in Rome in 1230, Florence in 1244, southern France and Spain in 1320 and 1333; the latter gave rise to the cult of the famous saint against plague, Saint Roch. The history of plague in Europe

According to Alfred von Kremer, no major epidemics appear to have occurred in Egypt and Syria from the mid-eighth century until the middle of the eleventh century.[58] In 448-449/1056-1057 there was an important epidemic throughout the Middle East that was probably plague.[59] Ibn Ḥajar states: "The epidemic occurred in Samarkand and Balkh and killed every day more than 6000 inhabitants. The people were busied night and day with washing, shrouding, and burying the bodies. Among the people whose hearts were split, blood welled up from their hearts and dropped from their mouths, and they would fall down dead." This gruesome account may be an accurate description of pneumonic plague. However, the chroniclers usually do not give adequate descriptions of the epidemics before the Black Death in order for us to determine satisfactorily the nature of the individual epidemics.[60]

After the plague epidemic of 448-449/1056-1057, there were a number of epidemics in Egypt and Syria whose nature is uncertain. In 455/1063 there occurred in Egypt an epidemic that may have been plague and is reported to have spread to Europe.[61] The evidence for this epidemic has been found in the plague treatises written after the Black Death and not in the general histories for the Fāṭimid Period. In 469/1076-1077 an indeterminable epidemic (*wabā' 'aẓīm*) took place in Syria.[62] Likewise, in 537/1142-1143 an uncertain epidemic (*wabā' 'aẓīm*) is reported by the major chroniclers to have attacked

---

before the Black Death has not been systematically studied; see, however, Raymond Crawfurd, *Plague and Pestilence in Literature and Art* (Oxford, 1914), pp. 104-106.

58 "Ueber die grossen Seuchen," pp. 115-121.

59 *Ibid.*, pp. 121, 124; *Badhl*, fols. 122a-123a; cf. Renaud, "Les Maladies pestilentielles," pp. 12-13, and Lane-Poole, *History*, p. 143.

60 *Daf' an-niqmah*, fols. 70a-74b uncritically refers to all the epidemics before the Black Death as "plague" (*ṭā'ūn*).

61 "Ueber die grossen Seuchen," pp. 121, 124; *Badhl*, fols. 122a, 123a.

62 "Ueber die grossen Seuchen," pp. 122, 124; *Badhl*, fol. 123a; Ibn al-Athīr, *al-Kāmil fī t-ta'rīkh* (Beirut, 1965-1967), vol. 10, p. 105.

the major cities of Egypt and Syria.[63] With somewhat greater certainty, there appears to have been a local outbreak of plague in the Ḥijāz and the Yemen in 552/1157 and to have spread to Egypt.[64] Shortly thereafter, a local epidemic (*wabā'*) occurred in Syria in the year 558/1163, but the nature of the disease cannot yet be established.[65]

At the beginning of the thirteenth century, a great famine and epidemic occurred in Egypt. Ibn al-Athīr records in his chronicle that in the years 597-598/1200-1202 there were high prices in Egypt because the Nile did not rise sufficiently and an ensuing epidemic (*wabā'*), a "great dying" (*maut ḳathīr*), annihilated the people.[66] This period of famine and disease is the subject of a long account by 'Abd al-Laṭīf, a Baghdad physician who was in Cairo at the time. There is a remarkable absence of medical description of the epidemic by him, and definitely no observation of plague symptoms, which would have been conspicuous if it had been a plague epidemic.[67] The fifteenth-century Egyptian historian, Ibn Ḥajar, states emphatically that this epidemic was other than plague.[68] The epidemic disease was more likely typhus or typhoid-paratyphoid.

The only evidence of plague during this period is found in a fragment of a letter dated 1217 among the documents of the Jewish community in Fusṭāṭ (Old Cairo): "May God spare

[63] "Ueber die grossen Seuchen," p. 125; Ibn al-Athīr, *al-Kāmil*, vol. 11, p. 92.

[64] "Ueber die grossen Seuchen," pp. 84, 123; see also Andrew S. Ehrenkreutz, *Saladin* (Albany, New York, 1972), p. 17.

[65] "Ueber die grossen Seuchen," p. 125.

[66] *al-Kāmil*, vol. 12, p. 170.

[67] *The Eastern Key (Kitāb al-ifādah wal-i'tibār)*, trans. by K. H. Zand, J. A. and I. E. Videan (London, 1964), pp. 223-263; A. I. Silvestre de Sacy, trans., *Relation de l'Égypte par Abd-Allatif, medicin arabe de Baghdad* (Paris, 1810), pp. 360-413. Cf. Lane-Poole, *History*, pp. 215-216, and S. D. Goitein, *A Mediterranean Society*, vol. 2 (Berkeley and Los Angeles, 1971), p. 141.

[68] *Badhl*, fol. 123b.

Israel from the plague ravaging in your parts (Fusṭāṭ)."[69] However, the Muslim historians fail to mention any epidemic at this time. Another epidemic in 633/1235-1236 occurred in Egypt, but is not designated as a "plague" (*ṭā'ūn*).[70] Al-Maqrīzī mentions an epidemic (*wabā'*) in 656/1258 in Syria without any details except to note the high prices of agricultural commodities.[71] The chronicler Abū l-Fidā', who is surprisingly uninformative about the epidemics of the eleventh, twelfth, and thirteenth centuries, states that a "plague" occurred in Syria in 656-657/1258-1259 and was particularly severe in Damascus.[72] In the year 672/1273-1274, there was an epidemic (*wabā'*) in Egypt, and many perished, especially women and children.[73] The years 694-696/1295-1297 were a time of great famine as a result of the Nile's failure to rise to the requisite level; consequently, there were high prices and pestilence (*wabā'*), which killed a considerable proportion of the population.[74]

[69] Goitein, *A Mediterranean Society*, vol. 2, p. 276.

[70] *Mā rawāhu l-wā'ūn*, p. 155 based on *Badhl*, fol. 123b; *Daf' an-niqmah*, fol. 73b: "waba' 'aẓīm."

[71] *as-Sulūk*, part 1, vol. 2, p. 410.

[72] *al-Mukhtaṣar fī akhbār al-bashar* (Cairo, 1907), vol. 3, pp. 195, 197.

[73] Ibn al-Furāt, *Ta'rīkh ad-duwal wal-mulūk* (Beirut, 1936-1942), vol. 7, p. 10.

[74] *as-Sulūk*, part 1, vol. 3, pp. 808-810, 813-815, 829-830; *Daf' an-niqmah*, fols. 74a-74b; *al-Bidāyah*, vol. 13, p. 340; Abū l-Fidā', *al-Mukhtaṣar*, vol. 4, p. 33, and Ibn al-Wardī, *Tatimmat al-mukhtaṣar fī akhbār al-bashar* (Cairo, 1295 A.H.), vol. 2, p. 241; *an-Nujūm*, Cairo ed., vol. 8, p. 79; *Beiträge zur Geschichte der Mamlūken-sultane in den Jahren 690-741 der Hegra*, ed. by K. V. Zetterstéen (Leiden, 1919), pp. 37-38; Ibn al-Furāt, *Ta'rīkh*, vol. 8, pp. 196-197, 199-200, 208-212; Mufaḍḍal ibn Abī al-Faḍā'il, *an-Nahj as-sadīd wad-durr al-farīd*, ed. and trans. by E. Blochet, "Histoire des Sultans Mamlouks," *Patrologia Orientalis*, vol. 14 (Paris, 1920), pp. 591-592; Gaston Wiet, trans., "Le Traite des famines de Maqrīzī," *JESHO*, vol. 5 (1962), pp. 32, n. 2, 33-41. Unavailable manuscript sources may contribute new data to the evaluation of this and other epidemics; see the historical manuscript sources cited in D. P. Little, *An Introduction to Mamlūk Historiography* (Wiesbaden, 1970). For Little's analysis of the year 694 A.H. in the sources, see pp. 6 (Baybars al-Manṣūrī), 56 (al-Jazarī), 62 (adh-Dhahabī), 82 (al-'Aynī). In addition, it would be interesting to learn

The reports of the numbers of dead and their burial in some of these epidemics (particularly 448-449/1056-1057, 597/1200-1201, and 694-696/1295-1297) are similar to the morbid depiction of the Black Death. Yet the epidemics are not usually designated as *ṭā'ūn*, "plague," which was the commonly accepted term used by many of the same chroniclers to describe the Black Death and its recurrences from the mid-fourteenth century. The common descriptive term used for most of the pestilences before the Black Death was *wabā'*, which may mean any epidemic disease such as typhus, smallpox, cholera, etc. Furthermore, none of these epidemics, with the exception of that of 448-449/1056-1057, are accompanied by observations of any of the distinguishing plague symptoms. There are no extant treatises on plague dating from this period, nor are there discernible cycles of plague recurrence. Plague epidemics dating from the time of the Plague of Justinian did occur, but plague does not appear to have been endemic to the Egypt and Syria immediately before the Black Death.

If we accept the slight evidence of Abū l-Fidā' for the Syrian epidemic of 656-657/1258-1259, it was at least a hundred years before plague violently reappeared in Egypt and Syria. The disease was recognized medically, and the people were informed of the established religious prescriptions, formulated during the earlier exposure of the Muslim community to plague. Like an invincible army—to borrow a medieval simile—the Black Death advanced westward, invading the entire Mediterranean world.

B. THE TRANSMISSION OF THE BLACK DEATH: CHRONOLOGY AND GEOGRAPHICAL DISTRIBUTION

1. Origin

The Black Death almost certainly originated in the Asiatic steppe, where a permanent reservoir of plague infection still

---

whether this dramatic epidemic is related to the great European famine and epidemic in 1315-1317 (see H. S. Lucas, "The Great European Famine of 1315, 1316, and 1317," *Speculum*, vol. 5 [1930], pp. 343-377).

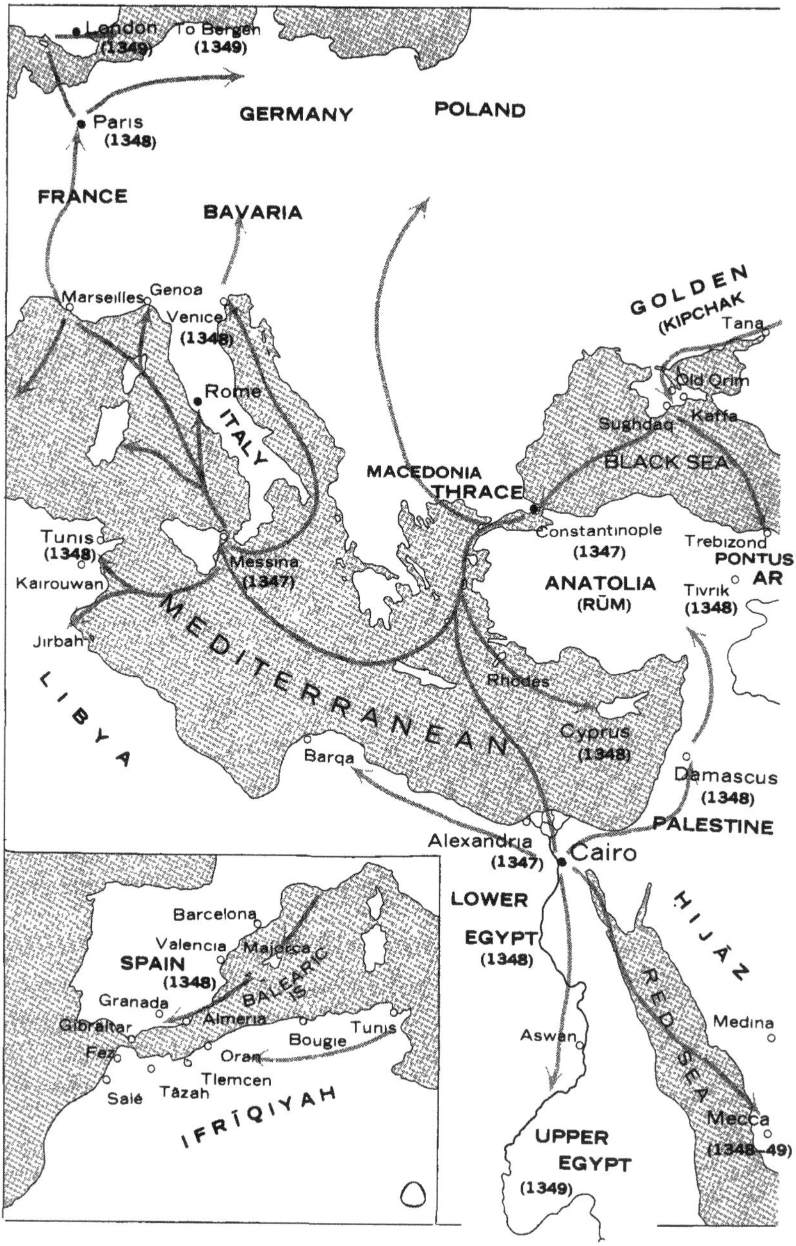
London
(1349)
To Bergen
(1349)
Paris
(1348)
GERMANY
POLAND
FRANCE
BAVARIA
Marseilles
Genoa
Venice
(1348)
Rome
ITALY
GOLDEN
(KIPCHAK
Tana
Old Qrim
Sughdaq
Kaffa
BLACK SEA
MACEDONIA
THRACE
Constantinople
(1347)
Trebizond
PONTUS
AR
Tunis
(1348)
Kairouwan
Messina
(1347)
ANATOLIA
(RŪM)
Tivrik
(1348)
Jirbah
MEDITERRANEAN
LIBYA
Rhodes
Cyprus
(1348)
Barqa
Damascus
(1348)
PALESTINE
Alexandria
(1347)
Cairo
LOWER
EGYPT
(1348)
HIJĀZ
RED SEA
Aswan
Medina
Mecca
(1348–49)
UPPER
EGYPT
(1349)
Barcelona
Valencia
Majorca
SPAIN
(1348)
BALEARIC IS.
Granada
Almeria
Gibraltar
Fez
Tunis
Bougie
Oran
Tlemcen
Salé
Tāzah
IFRĪQIYAH

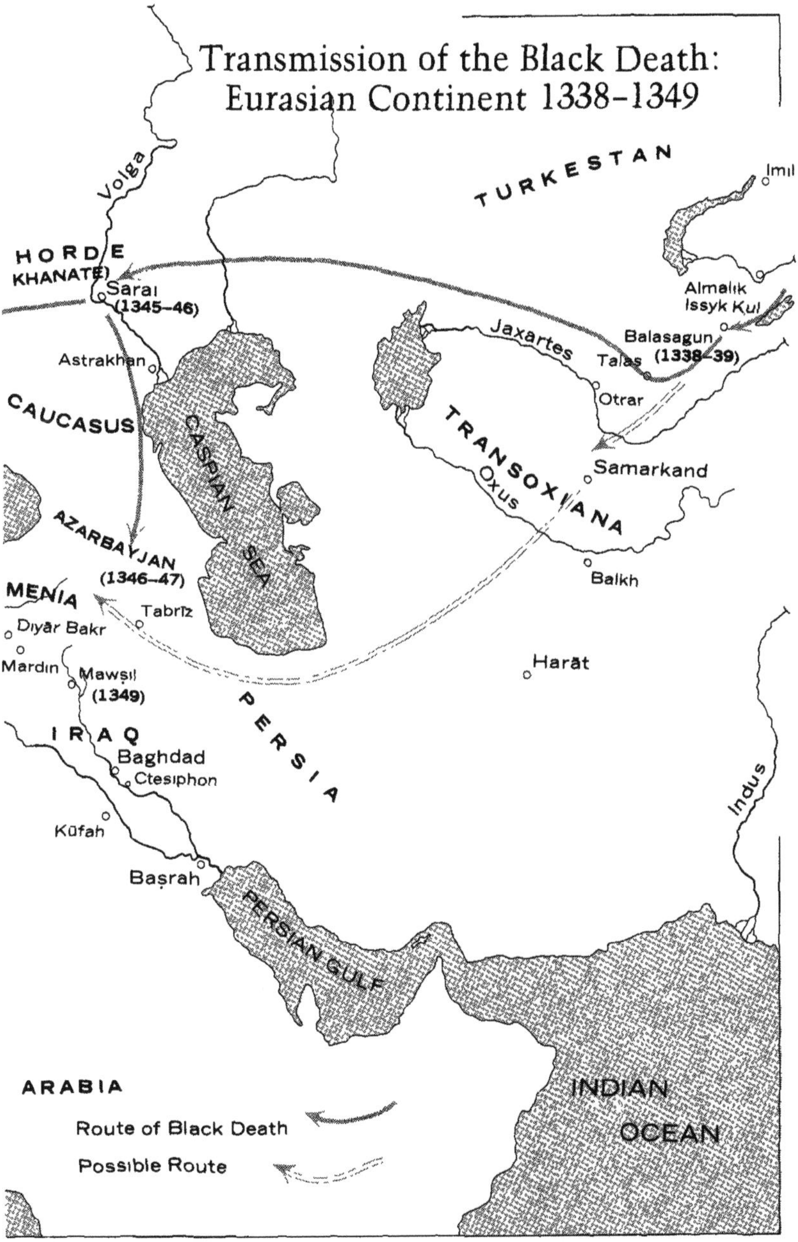

Transmission of the Black Death:
Eurasian Continent 1338–1349

TURKESTAN
Imıl

Volga

HORDE
KHANATE
Saraı
(1345–46)

Almalık
Issyk Kul

Jaxartes
Balasagun
Talas (1338–39)

Astrakhan

Otrar

CAUCASUS

CASPIAN SEA

TRANSOXIANA

Oxus

Samarkand

AZARBAYJAN
(1346–47)

Balkh

MENIA
Diyār Bakr

Tabrīz

Harāt

Mardın
Mawṣıl
(1349)

PERSIA

IRAQ
Baghdad
Ctesıphon

Indus

Kūfah

Baṣrah

PERSIAN GULF

ARABIA

INDIAN
OCEAN

Route of Black Death

Possible Route

exists among the wild rodents of the region: the whole of the Central Asiatic plateau has been called "one huge endemic area."[1] From the steppe, the pandemic spread outward, like the earlier Mongol invasions from this region, to the south and to the west. The Black Death descended on China and India[2] and moved westward to the lands of the Khiṭai[3] and the Uzbeks,[4] Transoxiana, Persia, and finally to the Crimea[5] and the Mediterranean world.

[1] Wu Lien-Teh, "The Original Home of Plague," p. 12; Pollitzer, *Plague*, p. 13.

[2] *Risālat an-nabā'*, p. 184. There is a danger in following Ibn al-Wardī's account of the dissemination of the Black Death too closely; in some cases, historical accuracy may have been sacrificed for the benefit of literary conceits and rhyme.

[3] *Ibid.* It is not altogether clear what peoples Ibn al-Wardī means by the "Khitai"; he seems to refer here to the Qara-Khitai, who established an empire in the twelfth and early thirteenth centuries in eastern Turkestan. This Mongol dynasty was conquered by the later Mongol invasion of Jenghiz Khan and in the fourteenth century was a part of the Khanate of Jagatai (René Grousset, *The Empire of the Steppes: A History of Central Asia*, trans. by N. Walford [New Brunswick, N.J., 1970], pp. 159-160, 164-166, 233-236, 341-346; *EI*[1]: "Ḳara Khitai" [Barthold]). All other references to Khiṭai refer to northeastern China. The Qara-Khiṭai were only a branch of the northern Mongol race that originated on the west bank of the Liao River and reigned at Peking from 936 to 1122. Like the Arabic chroniclers, Marco Polo and other Europeans designated northern China (or China in general) as "Cathay" from the name "Kitan" (in Chinese transcription) or "Khiṭai" (Arabo-Persian transcription). See Grousset, *The Empire of the Steppes*, pp. 127-134, 164, 307; Muḥammad Haidar, *Tarikh-i-Rashidi*, trans. by E. D. Ross (London, 1895), pp. 51-98, 152-153; Ibn Baṭṭūṭah, *Travels, A.D. 1325-1354*, trans. by Sir Hamilton Gibb (Cambridge, 1958-1971), vol. 3, p. 551, n. 44.

[4] *Risālat an-nabā'*, p. 184. "Uzbek" or "Özbeg" were Turko-Mongol tribes subject to the Mongol khanates of southern Russia. Howorth has very plausibly argued that the designation refers to the subjects of the Golden Horde after the name of the Khan, Ghiyāth ad-Dīn Muḥammad Uzbek (712-742/1312-1341); hence, Kipchak should be equated with Uzbek by the mid-fourteenth century when the latter term was commonly used in the Arabic sources (Sir Henry H. Howorth, *History of the Mongols* [London, 1876-1927], vol. 2, part 1, pp. 9-10). Grousset states: "About the middle of the fourteenth century, the hordes subject to the Shaybānids took the name of Özbeg or, in the

Both the Latin and Arabic sources emphasize the fact that the pandemic was initially accompanied in the Far East by violent ecological changes, such as flooding, famines, and earthquakes.[6] From the Chinese annals, it is clear that the second quarter of the fourteenth century witnessed an unusually large number of damaging environmental disturbances.[7] These natural disasters may have destroyed rodent shelters and food supplies and forced the rodents beyond their normally very restriced habitat into contact with domestic rodents and human settlements, carrying the epizootic with them.[8] By the

---

spelling now usual, Uzbek, by which they are known to history, although the origin of the name is still obscure." (*The Empire of the Steppes*, p. 479; see also *EI*[1]: "Shaibānids [Barthold].) Ibn Battūṭah uses the term in his journey through the Golden Horde in 1333 (*Travels*, A.D. *1325-1354*, vol. 3, pp. 541, 556).

[5] *Risālat an-naba'*, p. 184; cf. *'Iqd al-jumān*, chap. 24, part 1, p. 19.

[6] Deaux, *The Black Death 1347*, p. 2, and Ziegler, p. 13, are based on J.F.C. Hecker, *The Epidemics of the Middle Ages*, trans. by B. G. Babington (London, 1846), p. 11. Most of the information in these modern accounts of the Black Death in the Middle East rely on Hecker's work, which in turn was based on J. de Guignes, *Histoire générale des Huns, des Turcs, des Mongols, etc.* (Paris, 1758), vol. 4, pp. 223-226; this latter work contains large extracts from al-Maqrīzī's narrative in translation.

[7] Howorth, *History of the Mongols*, vol. 1, pp. 302-312.

[8] The central epidemiological problem of why epidemics begin is still unresolved. They may be directly related to major ecological changes that affect the plague micro-organism and its hosts. It is possible that there occurs a mutation of the micro-organism; such a change might produce a more virulent form of plague. A significant change would alter its pathological characteristics and differentiate it historically from other plague pandemics. For example, both the Latin and Arabic sources for the Black Death describe the massive destruction of a large variety of animals; this may be explained by large-scale plague infection, accompanying murrain diseases, or simply exaggeration. However, if some animals that are normally resistant to plague infection in modern experiments actually did contract plague at this time, it may indicate a change in the nature of the plague bacillus itself. While the leading medical authority on plague has stated that there have been no convincing modern observations of a mutation of plague (Pollitzer, *Plague*, pp. 91-93), new strains have been created for bacteriological warfare (see Hirshleifer, *Disaster and Recovery*, p. 2).

end of 1346, it was known, at least in the major Mediterranean seaports, that an unprecedented pestilence was sweeping the Orient.[9] Both the Latin and Arabic authors believed that a corruption of the air, a so-called miasma, had been produced, which was visible in the form of mist or smoke, and was spreading over the land, killing all living things.[10]

Among the Arabic writers on the pandemic, Ibn al-Wardī was an eyewitness to the Black Death in Aleppo and was himself to die of plague in 749/1349.[11] In his account of the Black Death, he states that the disease had begun in the "land of darkness." This region should be interpreted as inner Asia or Mongolia, and not as China.[12] The pandemic, according to Ibn al-Wardī, had been raging there for fifteen years, which is not an inordinate length of time for the dissemination of the Black Death from its source, considering the slow development of the third pandemic within Asia in the late nineteenth century.[13] If we date the appearance of plague in the Asiatic hinterland from its outbreak in the Crimea in 747/1346, plague would have reached significant epidemic proportions in Central Asia about the year 732/1331-1332.

Al-Maqrīzī, the famous Egyptian historian of the Mamlūk Empire, wrote the most important account of the Black Death in the Middle East, although he was not a contemporary of the event. In a disjointed description of the origins of the pandemic,[14] al-Maqrīzī tells us that before the disease reached

[9] Ziegler, pp. 14-15.

[10] *Ibid.*, and *as-Sulūk*, part 2, vol. 3, p. 773. See the discussion of plague etiology below.

[11] *EI*²: "Ibn al-Wardī" (G. el-Din el-Shayyal); *GAL*, vol. 2, pp. 140-141, *Supplement*, vol. 2, pp. 174-175.

[12] *Risālat an-naba'*, p. 184. Cf. Wu Lien-Teh, "The Original Home of Plague," p. 301; "Ueber die grossen Seuchen," p. 136, n. 1; *Kunūz adh-dhahab*, vol. 2, p. 10; and Ibn Baṭṭūtah, *Voyages d'Ibn Batoutah*, ed. and trans. by C. Defrémery and B. R. Sanguinetti (Paris, 1853-1858), vol. 2, pp. 399-402.

[13] See Hirst, pp. 101-102, for the chronology of the third pandemic.

[14] *as-Sulūk*, part 2, vol. 3, pp. 772-791; copied by Ibn Taghrī Birdī (*an-Nujūm*, Cairo ed., vol. 10, pp. 195-213). As Gaston Wiet has suggested, this disjointed narrative may be due to the random collection of lecture notes drawn from various sources by al-Maqrīzī. The nature

Egypt it had begun in the lands of the Great Khan—"a six months' journey from Tabrīz"—a country inhabited by the Khiṭai and the Mongols, presumably Mongolia and northern China. These pagan peoples, according to al-Maqrīzī, numbered more than three hundred tribes, and all perished without apparent reason in their summer and winter encampments, in the course of pasturing their flocks and during their seasonal migrations. Their mounts died, and beasts and men were abandoned where they fell. Al-Maqrīzī reports as well that exceptionally heavy rains fell at an unaccustomed time in the land of the Khiṭai, destroying pack animals and cattle. The land of the Khiṭai, between Yen-King and Korea, became deserted; in three months, sixteen princes died. The soldiers of the Mongol Great Khan perished in considerable numbers; ultimately, the Khan himself and six of his children succumbed to the disease. Subsequently, China was depopulated by the pandemic, while India was damaged to a lesser extent.[15]

This account of al-Maqrīzī may correctly depict the events in the Great Mongol Khanate of Mongolia and northern China, known as the Yüan Dynasty in Chinese history. If plague was epidemic in Asia about 732/1331-1332, as Ibn al-Wardī suggests, it would explain the premature deaths of the Great Khan Jijaghatu Toq-Temür (Wen-Tsong) and his sons. Toq-Temür died on October 2, 1332, at the age of twenty-eight, at Shangtu; his death is chronicled in the Chinese annals among reports of natural disasters that correspond to the Latin tales about the Far East and to al-Maqrīzī's statements about torrential rains.[16]

---

of his notes may be seen in his autographed copy of the *Muqaffā* (Paris MS no. 2144). See "La Grande Peste Noire," pp. 267-268, and "Kindī et Maqrīzī," *BIFAO*, vol. 12 (1916), pp. 61-73, especially p. 62. There does not appear to be a single parent source for the plague accounts in al-Maqrīzī and Ibn Taghrī Birdī.

[15] *as-Sulūk*, part 2, vol. 3, pp. 773-774.

[16] Howorth, *History of the Mongols*, vol. 1, pp. 308-310; L. Hambis, "Le chapitre cvii du Yuan Che, les généologies impériales mongoles dans l'histoire chinoise officielle de la dynastie mongole," *Supplement*

Two contemporary Arabic descriptions of the Black Death that are entirely independent of the Middle Eastern accounts express opinions about the origins of the pandemic. Ibn Khātimah wrote a plague treatise in Almería in the year 749/1349. The author states that he learned from Christian merchants that plague had started in the land of the Khiṭai, which he interpreted as China. From there, it had spread to the regions inhabited by the Turks and to Iraq, but particularly to the Crimea, Pera (the settlement of the foreign community outside Constantinople), and Constantinople.[17] Ibn al-Khaṭīb, the second Andalusian writer, remarks that the pandemic began in the land of the Khiṭai and Sind (the Indus Valley) in 734/1333-1334 and that he had learned this from credible men.[18]

As before, during the "Athenian Plague" and the Plague of Justinian, there was also a belief, notably in Europe, that this plague pandemic orginated in Ethiopia or the Upper Nile. The genesis of plague in Ethiopia is proposed in the earliest datable Christian plague treatise (April 24, 1348) by the Catalan physician, Jacme d'Agramont.[19] In the Arabic sources, this opinion is offered only by the Andalusian author, Ibn Khātimah, as an alternative to the Asiatic origin for the Black Death mentioned above.[20] The Egyptian chroniclers, who would have been best informed, make no mention of an Ethiopian source for the Black Death.

2. Transmission

From the history of communicable diseases, we know that epidemics usually follow very closely the commercial trade

---

to *T'oung Pao*, vol. 38 (Leiden, 1945), pp. 139-142; Grousset, *The Empire of the Steppes*, p. 321 and map (p. 322). There is the possibility that plague may have been the cause of death of Toq-Temür's predecessor, Yesün Temür (d. August 15, 1328), whose four sons all died without issue. The final solution of this matter must await a thorough study of the Chinese sources for the Black Death.

17 *Tahṣīl*, fols. 57b-58a.

18 *Muqni'at*, fol. 43b.

19 Sarton, *Introduction*, vol. 3, part 1, p. 862.

20 *Taṣḥīl*, fol. 57b.

routes.[21] It is logical, therefore, to investigate the occurrences of plague along the major routes from Asia to the Middle East, in order to establish its probable means of transmission.[22] There were three important routes in the middle of the fourteenth century: (1) the overland route from Mongolia and northern China through Turkestan to the Black Sea region;[23] (2) the combined overland and sea route from India and China through the Indian Ocean and the Persian Gulf to the Fertile Crescent, where the commodities were dispersed among the major commercial centers of the Middle East;[24] and (3) the sea route from the Far East through the Indian Ocean and the Red Sea to Egypt.[25]

Transmission of the Black Death along the second and third routes appears unlikely. There is no evidence in the Arabic sources of the occurrence of plague in Mesopotamia, Arabia, and Egypt before its appearance in the Crimea or the Mediterranean littoral. Furthermore, these two routes would have carried plague to India beforehand, but there is no concrete evidence that plague infected India before its introduction into the Middle East.

Only the great medieval Muslim traveler, Ibn Baṭṭūṭah, who later witnessed the plague epidemic (*ṭāʿūn*) in Damascus in Rabīʿ II, 749/July 1348,[26] mentions an epidemic (*wabāʾ*) of

[21] Bertold Spuler, *Die Goldene Horde* (Wiesbaden, 1965), p. 103.

[22] See the misleading discussion on plague transmission in Gasquet, *The Black Death of 1348 and 1349*, pp. 3-4.

[23] S. Y. Labib, *Handelsgeschichte Ägyptens im Spätmittelalter (1171-1517)*, (Wiesbaden, 1965), pp. 67-73, 122, chart 1 (showing the major trade routes); S. A. Huzayyin, *Arabia and the Far East* (Cairo, 1942), pp. 169-180; E. Powers, "The Opening of the Land Routes to Cathay," *Travel and Travellers of the Middle Ages*, ed. by A. P. Newton (London, 1926), pp. 124-158; W. Heyd, *Histoire du commerce du Levant au moyen âge* (Leipzig, 1936), vol. 2, pp. 57-253, particularly for the northern land route.

[24] Labib, *Handelsgeschichte*, pp. 69-70, 122; Huzayyin, *Arabia and the Far East*, pp. 172-173.

[25] Labib, *Handelsgeschichte*, pp. 122-131.

[26] *Voyages*, vol. 1, pp. 227-229 and *Travels*, A.D. *1325-1354*, vol. 1, pp. 143-144.

an undetermined disease in Mutrah (Madurai, southern India) about the years 744-745/1344.[27] The Mutrah epidemic may have been plague, but there can be little certainty because the author fails to describe the disease, which he himself contracted; nor does the author use the accepted term for plague, *ṭā'ūn*. Ibn Baṭṭūṭah did not even connect the two events—in Mutrah and Damascus—when he later composed his work, as would have been likely if the striking symptoms of plague had been the same. Neither does Ibn al-Khaṭīb, who relates information he received from Ibn Baṭṭūṭah and others, mention Mutrah as a source of the Black Death. Yet there have been repeated, unwarranted assertions by modern historians that Ibn Baṭṭūṭah saw plague in India and, consequently, that plague originated in the Indian sub-continent.[28] Regrettably for our determination of plague transmission, there is no satisfactory evidence for the Black Death in India.[29]

There is a dearth of information concerning the trade route through the Persian Gulf[30] and Mesopotamia primarily to

[27] *Voyages*, vol. 4, pp. 200-202.

[28] Sarton, *Introduction*, vol. 3, part 2, p. 1651; Shrewsbury, *A History of Bubonic Plague*, pp. 37 ff. The earliest statement of this claim, which I have been able to locate, is in Sticker's history of plague (*Abhandlungen*, vol. 1, pp. 41-42; Sticker drew his knowledge of Ibn Battūtah from Samuel Lee's translation of Ibn Baṭṭūtah [London, 1829]). Ibn Baṭṭūṭah was supposed to have witnessed plague in India during 1332 according to Sticker—the origin of the pandemic thus being Indian—and again in 1344. As for the first date, Ibn Baṭṭūtah did not even enter India until 1 Muharram 734/12 September 1333 (*EI*[2]: "Ibn Battūṭa [A. Miquel]"). Sticker's early "plague" of 1332 may have been mistakenly taken from the mention of an uncertain epidemic that befell the sultan's army at an undetermined date (*The Travels of Ibn Batūta*, trans. by Lee, pp. 147-148, *Voyages*, vol. 3, p. 334, and *Travels*, A.D. *1325-1354*, vol. 3, pp. 717 and 718, where *wabā'* is translated as "plague").

[29] See Sir Wolseley Haig, ed., *The Cambridge History of India*, vol. 3 (Cambridge, 1928), pp. 148-150.

[30] See Jean Aubin, "Les Princes d'Ormuz du XIII au XV siècle," *JA*, vol. 241 (1953), pp. 77-137; there is no indication of a plague epidemic.

Trebizond and Lesser Armenia at this time. Virtual anarchy prevailed from the end of the Mongol dynasty of Hūlāgū Khan in Persia and Mesopotamia to the invasion of Timūr at the end of the fourteenth century. A Persian source for the Jalāyirid dynasty,[31] which contended for power in Iraq during this period, mentions a serious plague in nearby Azarbayjan in 747/1346-1347[32] while one of the contestants for leadership, Malik Ashrāf, was attacking Tabrīz. Malik Ashrāf then turned to Baghdad in the year 748/1347 and besieged Shaykh Ḥasan Buzurg in that city.[33] The Jalāyirid source claims that the siege was terminated because of a lack of provisions and the summer heat. However, al-Maqrīzī relates that plague broke out in the army besieging Shaykh Ḥasan, and the siege had to be lifted. Plague also reached within the city; Shaykh Ḥasan wrote an account of this epidemic and sent it to the mamlūk sultan in Egypt.[34] It would appear, therefore, that the army of Malik Ashrāf brought plague to Baghdad from the north.[35]

31 *EI²*: "Djalāyir" (J. M. Smith).

32 Abū Bakr al-Quṭbī al-Ahrī, *Ta'rīkh ash-Shaykh Uwais*, partially trans. by J. B. van Loon (The Hague, 1954), p. 73.

33 *Ibid.*, pp. 11, 73.

34 *as-Sulūk*, part 2, vol. 3, p. 774.

35 Subsequently, Janibeg, Khan of the Golden Horde, took advantage of the anarchy in Azarbayjan to launch a large-scale attack. He succeeded in taking Tabrīz in 1357. "Jānī Beg, however, did not exploit his victory. He left Tabrīz almost immediately and entrusted the government of the area to his son." There is reason to believe that he did so in order to escape from a new epidemic of plague that had already claimed large numbers of victims in the Crimea. Directly after his return to Sarai, Janibeg died, having probably brought the fatal infection with him from Azarbayjan (see Spuler, *The Muslim World*, vol. 2, pp. 54-55, and *Die Goldene Horde*, p. 102). Tabrīz was apparently a common victim of plague epidemics; there is evidence for plague in 892/1487, 893/1488, and 895/1490 (see Vladimir Minorsky, *Persia in* A.D. *1478-1490*, Royal Asiatic Society, vol. 26 [London, 1957], pp. 56, 87, 107-109 respectively). The recurrence of plague epidemics in Tabrīz may indirectly account for the change in miniature painting of the Tabrīz School that is perceptible in the later fourteenth century.

Plague was in Mawṣil in 750/1349,[36] as well as in Baghdad.[37] This chronology reinforces the contention that it was diffused southward from the Caucasus, rather than north and westward from the Persian Gulf and the southern trade route. According to Professor Tholozan, who has studied the history of plague with special attention to the plague epidemics of the nineteenth century in Iraq, the great epidemics in the central Middle East usually originated outside of Mesopotamia. They customarily spread from the Caucasus region southward, following the riverine commercial routes.[38] Furthermore, the earliest mention of plague in the Armenian sources is September 10, 1348, from the monastery records of Tivrik (Divrigi)[39] in eastern Anatolia.[40] In the following year, there was evidently widespread famine and plague among the Armenians.[41] Thus, there is no convincing evidence for the common European view that plague began in India and was transmitted up the Tigris to the Crimea.[42] As for the possibility that it was brought overland from India or China across the Iranian plateau, there is no documentation for its appearance in Persia before or during the Black Death.[43]

[36] 'Abbās al-'Azzāwī, *Ta'rīkh al-'Irāq bayn iḥtilālayn* (Baghdad, 1935-1956), vol. 2, p. 60.

[37] *Ibid.*; *as-Sulūk*, part 2, vol. 3, p. 774.

[38] Tholozan, *Histoire de la peste bubonique en Mésopotamie*, pp. 2, 89. Through the nineteenth century, Kurdistan was the chief endemic focus for a large area of western Asia; it was partly responsible for plague invasions of Syria and Palestine, which were also vulnerable to the inroads of plague by the sea routes (Pollitzer, *Plague*, p. 28).

[39] Arabic: "al-Abrīk" or "al-Abrūk."

[40] A. K. Sanjian, *Colophons of Armenian Manuscripts 1301-1480* (Cambridge, Mass., 1969), p. 86.

[41] *Ibid.*, p. 87.

[42] Ziegler, p. 16; Deaux, *The Black Death 1347*, p. 46; and Muir, *The Mameloukе or Slave Dynasty of Egypt*, p. 94, who uncritically assumes that the pandemic passed from India through Persia and Mesopotamia to Syria and Egypt.

[43] There is very little documentation for this period of pre-Timūrid Persia and Iraq because of the unstable political conditions, which would also have limited trade and diverted commercial traffic to the more northernly route. Added to this political instability was the hostile

When we turn to the Red Sea route, we find it reasonable that there would be some evidence for plague in the Yemen, which was an important stopping-point of commercial traffic bound for Egypt.[44] However, an examination of the Yemenī sources does not provide us with any early incidence of the Black Death.[45] On the contrary, plague occurred in 752/1351 when Mujāhid, the king of the Yemen, was returning to his country after his imprisonment in Cairo.[46] Evidently plague reached the Yemen from its dissemination along the Mediterranean coast or by its later introduction from the Far East. Moreover, the Red Sea route in the mid-fourteenth century

---

division of the Khanate of Jagatai between Transoxiana and Mogholistan in the middle of the fourteenth century, which would also have impeded trade (see Grousset, *The Empire of the Steppes*, pp. 341-343; the *Zafer-name*, trans. by A.L.M. Pétis de la Croix, *Histoire de Timur-Bec* [Paris, 1722], pp. 1-19; and Tholozan, *Histoire de la peste bubonique en Perse*, p. 12). Incidentally, the only Arabic inscription related directly to plague in the late medieval period, to my knowledge, comes from the town of Demavand, north of Teheran. The inscription is engraved on wood at the door of a mosque with several Qur'ānic verses, dated 1097/1686: "Ibn-Mahmoud-momem charpentier, par un sentiment, avec un coeur religieux, a renouvelé cette grande porte afin de gagner le Paradis. L'année où fut placée cette porte est l'année de la peste (*ṭā'ūn*) en 1097 de l'Hégire." (Quoted in Tholozan, *Histoire de la peste bubonique en Perse*, p. 10.)

44 Huzayyin, *Arabia and the Far East*, pp. 175-176, argues that the eastern trade through the Red Sea was far less important at this time than the Persian Gulf route because of the heavy taxation imposed by the mamlūk regime in Egypt; cf. Labib, *Handelsgeschichte*, pp. 82-86.

45 I have consulted the following: al-Waṣṣābī, *Kitāb al-i'tibār fī t-tawārīkh wal-'āthār* (Dār al-Kutub al-Misrīyah microfilm no. 85) and al-Khazrajī, *Kifāyah wal-i'lam fīman waliya al-Yaman* (Dār al-Kutub al-Miṣrīyah microfilm no. 2206). The published work of al-Yāfi'ī (d. 768 A.H.), *Mir'āt al-jinān wa 'ibrat al-yaqẓān* (Beirut, 1970) is a history of Yemen, comprising mostly biographies; there is no mention of plague by al-Yāfi'ī in the last ten years (A.H. 740-750) of his history.

46 al-Waṣṣābī, *Kitāb al-i'tibār*, fol. 43b; al-Khazrajī, *Kifāyah*, fols. 175b-176a, and *Kitāb al-'uqūd al-lu'lu'īyah* (Cairo, 1914), vol. 2, p. 89. On the imprisonment of Mujāhid, see *al-Khiṭaṭ*, vol. 2, p. 316; al-Mu'minī, *Kitāb futūḥ an-nasr*, vol. 2, p. 297.

had relinquished its commercial importance to the northern land route.

The northern itinerary from the Black Sea to the Asian markets served as the major artery of international trade in the thirteenth and fourteenth centuries, and is the most plausible path of the Black Death. The westward march of Jenghiz Khan in 616/1219 had established this overland route as far as Otrar on the Jaxartes River (Syr Darya). The one great beneficial result of the Mongol conquests had been to draw China, Turkestan, Persia, and southern Russia into one huge empire, bridging traditional boundaries and ensuring freedom of passage for men and merchandise. By the fourteenth century, the northern transcontinental route ran from the Genoese and Venetian countinghouses of the Crimea to Peking. The principal stages were Sarai on the Lower Volga, Otrar, Talas, and Balasagun,[47] west of Lake Issyk Kul. From Issyk Kul, one path led north of the T'ien Shan mountain range into Mongolia by way of Imil, the Black Irtysh and the Urungu Rivers to Karakorum (the Mongol capital) on the Upper Orkhon River, where it descended to Peking. Another trail from the western Issyk Kul led to Almalik (near Kuldja)[48] on the Upper Ili River, Beshbaligh (present-day Dzimsa), Hami, and Suchow in Kansu, and thence into China proper.[49]

The security and extensive international trade of the route to Karakorum and Peking are attested by numerous European merchants and missionaries. Piano Carpini, who journeyed to Karakorum in 1246-1247, has left us a valuable description of the Mongol court;[50] William of Rubruck followed the same path to Karakorum in 1253-1254;[51] Niccolò and Maffeo Polo

[47] *EI*²: "Balāsāghūn" (Barthold-Boyle).

[48] *EI*²: "Almaligh" (Barthold, Spuler, and Pritsak).

[49] Grousset, *The Empire of the Steppes*, p. 312. At certain periods, the overland route from China bifurcated at Otrar in Transoxiana; one route led north of the Caspian, as has been outlined, and the second crossed Khurasan, the southern coast of the Caspian, and then via Tabrīz to the Black Sea. It is possible, although it cannot yet be verified, that the second route may have served as an avenue for the western advance of the pandemic.

[50] *Ibid.*, pp. 270-271.

[51] *Ibid.*, pp. 276-281.

traveled to Peking in 1260-1266 along this route;[52] and Giovanni da Marignolli, a missionary sent by Pope Benedict XII, traced their paths and arrived in Peking in 1342.[53] The Italian merchant Pegolotti wrote in his *Pratica della mercatura*, which was compiled in Florence between 1335 and 1343,[54] about the northern Caspian route to the Far East under the Mongols in the following manner: "The road you travel from Tana to Cathay is perfectly safe, whether by day or by night, according to what merchants say who use it."[55] It flourished until it was destroyed by Timūr at the end of the century.

All the historical sources corroborate the thesis that the Black Death followed this overland route from Central Asia to the Black Sea region, attacking the inhabitants along its path. The most convincing proof for the pandemic in Central Asia is the investigation by the Russian archeologist Chwolson near Lake Issyk Kul, which occupied a pivotal position on the long-distance journey. Professor Chwolson has shown that there was an abnormally high mortality in 1338 and 1339; inscriptions on three Nestorian headstones state that the persons interred had died of plague.[56] These dates are consistent with the suggested genesis of the pandemic in Mongolia in

[52] *Ibid.*, pp. 304-305.

[53] *Ibid.*, p. 319; A. C. Moule, *Christians in China Before the Year 1550* (New York, 1930), pp. 255-257. For the routes of a number of these travelers, see W. R. Shepherd, *Historical Atlas* (9th ed., New York, 1964), map no. 104b-c, or Spuler, *The Muslim World*, vol. 2, map facing p. 68.

[54] Cf. Heyd, *Histoire du commerce du Levant*, vol. 1, p. xviii.

[55] Sir Henry Yule, ed. and trans., *Cathay and the Way Thither*, rev. ed. by Henri Cordier (London, 1913-1916), vol. 3, pp. 152-155. See the interesting article by V. N. Fedorov, "Plague in Camels and its Prevention in the USSR," *Bulletin of the World Health Organization*, vol. 23, nos. 2-3 (1960), pp. 275-282, regarding camels as possible carriers of plague.

[56] J. Stewart, *The Nestorian Missionary Enterprise* (Edinburgh, 1928), p. 209; *Encyclopaedia Britannica* (1956): "Plague" (K. F. Meyer); Grousset, *The Empire of the Steppes*, pp. 341-342. The only precise mention of plague in Central Asia known to me, which would suggest an endemic focus of plague, is found in a sixteenth-century plague treatise that refers to the magical practices in Kāshgār (Shufu) during plague epidemics (Ṭāshkóprüzāde, fols. 54a-54b).

732/1331-1332. The pandemic appears to have advanced gradually westward with merchants and their cargoes, travelers, and tribal migrations.

Most importantly, plague spread throughout the domain of the Golden Horde, which encompassed this trade artery. The Golden Horde or Kipchak Khanate included the vast domain of the steppe of southern Russia—the whole of ancient European Scythia. This domain had been conquered by the armies of Jenghiz Khan's grandson in 1236-1239. The center of this Mongol khanate lay along the Volga River, and it was on the Lower Volga that the capital, the Great Sarai, was founded about 1253 and lasted until 1395, when it was destroyed by Timūr. The capital quickly became a cosmopolitan city under the Mongols—the center for Islamic learning and an important stage for the brisk international trade bound for Central Asia and the Far East. Thus, at approximately the same time that the Mamlūk Sultanate was established in the Middle East, the Golden Horde was created by a comparatively small Mongol military élite, officering native Turkish troops.

Plague clearly struck the major cities of the Golden Horde; in 745-746/1345-1346, it was reported in Sarai, Astrakhan, and other cities of southern Russia.[57] From Astrakhan, it reached southward through the Caucasus to attack Azarbayjan and Greater Armenia, which is consonant with the dating of the plague epidemics in the Jalāyirid and Armenian sources.

Unaware of the remote Asiatic background of the pandemic, the contemporary Byzantine historian Nicephoros Gregoras (d. 1360) reported that plague arose in Scythia and Maeotis in the springtime of 1346.[58] In addition, the Byzantine Emper-

[57] Joseph, Freiherr von Hammer-Purgstall, *Geschichte der Goldenen Horde in Kiptschak* (Pest, 1840), p. 308; Howorth, *History of the Mongols*, vol. 2, part 1, p. 175; B. Grekov and A. Iakoubovski, *La Horde d'Or*, trans. by F. Thuret (Paris, 1939), p. 94; Spuler, *Die Goldene Horde*, p. 102 (the Russian sources state mistakenly that the Black Death came from Egypt [p. 102, n. 10]).

[58] Bartosocas, "Two Fourteenth Century Greek Descriptions of the 'Black Death,'" p. 395.

or, Ioannes Cantacuzenos (John VI, d. 1383), who abdicated his throne in 1355 in order to write a history of the Byzantine Empire, agreed that the pandemic's source was in southern Russia (Scythia); he refers to the plague victims of the steppe as "Hyperborean Scythians."[59] Notwithstanding their misconceptions concerning the beginnings of the Black Death, the two historians confirm the transmission of the pandemic to the west through the Golden Horde.

From Ibn al-Wardī's *History* we learn that he gathered his information about the course of the Black Death from Muslim merchants returning from the Crimea to Syria.[60] The Black Sea region, as the western terminus of the Asiatic trade route, was an important commercial center for Muslims, as well as for European Christians. The Muslim merchants related to Ibn al-Wardī that the epidemic occurred in Rajab 747/October-November 1346, in the land of the Uzbeks—the Golden Horde—and emptied the villages and towns of their inhabitants. Then it spread to the Crimea and to Byzantium (Rūm). A *qāḍī* or Muslim judge in the Crimea, probably in Kaffa (Fedosia), is reported to have said that they counted the dead

[59] *Ibid.*, p. 398. The modern epizootic foci of plague in southern Russia (the Ural-Volga region, the Ust-Urt plateau, and Turkestan) have been the subject of considerable study; see Y. M. Rall, "The Geography and Some Pecularities of the Natural Foci of Rodent Plague" (in Russian) *Zhournal Mikrobiologii*, vol. 29, no. 2 (Moscow, 1958), pp. 74-78; B. K. Fenyuk, "Experience in the Eradication of Enzootic Plague in the North-West Part of the Caspian Region of the USSR," *Bulletin of the World Health Organization*, vol. 23, nos. 2-3 (1960), pp. 263-274, and "The Epizootic and Epidemic Situation in the Natural Foci of Plague in the USSR and the Prophylactic Measures Taken," *ibid.*, pp. 401-404; R. Pollitzer, *Plague and Plague Control in the Soviet Union* (Bronx, New York, 1966).

[60] *Tatimmat al-mukhtaṣar*, vol. 2, pp. 350-358. The work is an abridgment of the chronicle of Abū l-Fidā' with a continuation from 729 to 749/1329 to 1349. (There is a recent Baghdad edition [1969], vol. 2, pp. 501-506.) Russian scholars have used the translation of Ibn al-Wardī in vol. 1 of W. Tiesenhausen, *Documents Concerning the History of the Golden Horde* (in Russian), St. Petersburg, 1884.

who were struck by plague, and the number known to them was 85,000.[61] Thus, the account of Ibn al-Wardī concurs with the standard European narrative for the westward dissemination of the pandemic through the Crimea.

It is precisely from the Genoese factory at Kaffa that western scholars have traced the transmission of the Black Death to Europe. The basic European source for the westward progress of the pandemic is the account of the transportation of plague by Genoese galleys from the Crimea written by Gabriele de' Mussi.[62] Although the author never left his native town of Piacenza, he must have obtained his information concerning the East—like Ibn al-Wardī—from his compatriots who were trading in the Crimea. The Golden Horde fostered trade with the Genoese and Venetians by allowing the establishment of trading agencies in the Crimea; as was true in Byzantium and the Mamlūk Sultanate, hostility to the western European states did not prevent active commercial relations. The Crimean trading stations dated from about 1266, when the Mongols ceded land to the Genoese at Kaffa and later at Tana on which to build a consulate and warehouses. However, the Italian merchants had been expelled from Tana in 1343 by the Mongols and were besieged in their fortified city of Kaffa in 1343 and 1345-1346. During the latter siege, plague appeared among the Mongol army, as well as throughout the Golden Horde in 1346.[63] The Kipchak Khan Janibeg (742-758/1341-1357) had corpses of his plague-stricken men catapulted over

[61] Ibn al-Wardī. *Ta'rīkh* (Baghdad, 1969), vol. 2, p. 492; also reported in *al-Bidāyah*, vol. 14, p. 225.

[62] *Historia de Morbo s. Mortalitate quae fuit Anno Dni MCCCXLVII*, ed. by Henschel in H. Haeser, *Archiv für die gesammte Medizin*, vol. 2 (Jena, 1842), pp. 26-59; text reprinted in Haeser, *Lehrbuch der Geschichte der Medizin und der epidemischen Krankheiten*, 3rd ed., vol. 3 (Jena, 1882), pp. 157-161. The text is also found in A. C. Tononi, "La peste dell 'anno 1348," *Giornale Ligustico*, vol. 11 (Genoa, 1884), pp. 144-152. For secondary material, see Ziegler, pp. 15-16; A. A. Vasiliev, *The Goths in the Crimea* (Cambridge, 1936), p. 175; and Heyd, *Histoire du commerce du Levant*, vol. 2, p. 196.

[63] Vasiliev, *The Goths in the Crimea*, p. 176; Howorth, *History of the Mongols*, vol. 2, part 1, p. 175.

the walls of the city. The Christian defenders hauled the bodies back over the walls and dumped them into the sea. Nevertheless, the infection spread within the city, a fact that de' Mussi attributed to the corrupted air and the poisoned well-water. The Genoese colony was able to put up a stout resistance and compel Janibeg to raise the siege, which was followed by a successful blockade of the Mongol coasts of the Black Sea by the Genoese and Venetian navies. Some of the Genoese, however, fled in their ships to Constantinople and brought plague with them.[64]

Like Procopius, who witnessed and fully described the Plague of Justinian, Nicephoros Gregoras and the Emperor Ioannes Cantacuzenos have left us good accounts of the plague's ravages in the Byzantine capital in 1347. Certain elements of the description by the Emperor, however, imitate the depiction of the "Athenian Plague" by Thucydides; for example, the Byzantine ruler lost his son Andronicus in the pandemic, as Pericles lost his son Paralus. Moreover, there is a comparable description of the demoralization of the people of Constantinople, their suffering and sense of futility.[65] Yet the Emperor, relying perhaps on personal experience, described the various forms of plague and noted the contagious nature of the epidemic. Cantacuzenos believed that it was a special punishment from God on his people and the Genoese for their previously helping the Muslims capture the city of Romanais from fellow Christians.[66]

The Emperor also observed the spread of the pandemic throughout the Mediterranean world:

> The plague attacked almost all the sea-coasts of the world and killed most of their people. For it swept not only

[64] A. A. Vasiliev, *History of the Byzantine Empire* (Madison, 1964), vol. 2, p. 626. The plague epidemic in Constantinople ("Istanbul") was noted by the Arabic authors: *as-Sulūk*, part 2, vol. 3, p. 773; Ibn al-Wardī, *Ta'rīkh*, vol. 2, p. 501; and *Taḥṣīl*, fol. 58a.

[65] Bartsocas, "Two Fourteenth Century Greek Descriptions of the 'Black Death,'" pp. 396-398.

[66] Ziegler, p. 16.

> through Pontus, Thrace and Macedonia, but even Greece, Italy and all the Islands, Egypt, Libya, Judea, Syria, and spread throughout almost the entire world.[67]

The Black Death arrived in Sicily early in October, 1347. According to Michael of Piazza, a Franciscan chronicler, it was brought by twelve Genoese galleys, probably from the Crimea or Constantinople, to the port of Messina, and radiated out to the rest of the island.[68] The Messinese drove the ships that brought them the disastrous cargo from their port and, in so doing, ensured that it spread more rapidly throughout the western Mediterranean. Following the main trade-routes, the Black Death spread apparently to North Africa by way of Tunis, to Corsica and Sardinia, to the Balearics, Almería, Valencia, and Barcelona on the Iberian peninsula, and to southern Italy.

The three major centers for the dissemination of the Black Death in southern Europe were Sicily, Genoa, and Venice. In January, 1348, about three months after its arrival in Sicily, plague was introduced into Genoa and Venice. Slightly later, Pisa was struck and served as the point of entry to central and northern Italy. Florence is most closely associated with the Black Death because it was the first great European city to be struck, but also because of the great mortality in the city and the brilliant description of the Black Death by Boccaccio in his preamble to the *Decameron*. The epidemic began to subside by the winter of 1348 in most of Italy but only after having caused an astonishing number of deaths. Despite a multitude of qualifications, Philip Ziegler has proposed a decline of a third or slightly more for Italy's total population.

Only a month or two after the arrival of the Black Death on the mainland of Italy, it was brought to Marseilles by a galley that had been expelled from Italy. Driven out, in turn,

[67] Bartsocas, "Two *Fourteenth Century Greek Descriptions of the* 'Black Death,'" p. 395.

[68] The following survey of the Black Death in Europe is based primarily on Ziegler, pp. 40-201.

from Marseilles, the galley contaminated the coast of Languedoc and Spain. The Black Death swept through Marseilles and then began its journey into the hinterland along two main paths. Moving westward, it reached Bordeaux by August, 1348. To the north, it attacked Avignon and Lyons, and reached Paris in June and Burgundy in July and August. The plague in Paris did not abate until the winter of 1349.

From Paris the Black Death advanced northward to the coast in August, 1348. The king of France and the court fled from Paris to Normandy but could not escape; the plague pursued them. By the end of the year, the Black Death had crossed the English Channel and had struck southern England. Having penetrated most of France, it broadened outward, slowly moving through England, Ireland, and Scotland, through Flanders and the Low Countries, and through Germany in 1349.

By June, 1348, the Black Death had crossed the Tyrolese Alps and had entered Bavaria. It had also travelled through the Balkans into Hungary and Poland, so that central Europe was apparently attacked from three sides. Scandinavia was contaminated from England; plague was reported to have been transmitted by one of the wool ships that sailed from London to Bergen in May, 1349.

With fateful caprice, the Black Death struck the peoples of Europe with varying degrees of intensity, but virtually nowhere was left inviolate. It is our purpose here, not to retell the well-known story of the Black Death in Europe, but to stress the fact that European and Middle Eastern societies shared the same plight.[69] The general degree of depopulation in the West is as uncertain as it is in the Middle East, but the current opinion is that the mortality was at least a quarter of the entire population.[70] It may not be greatly mistaken to

[69] A number of the Arabic sources do note the extension of plague to Europe: *'Iqd al-jumān*, chap. 24, part 1, p. 85; *Taḥṣīl*, fol. 38a; *al-Bidāyah*, vol. 14, p. 225; *as-Sulūk*, part 2, vol. 3, pp. 773, 775-776; Ibn Iyās, vol. 1, p. 191.

[70] Langer, "The Black Death," p. 114.

estimate that a third of the population of Europe perished from 1348 to 1350.[71]

The same Italian merchants, who seem initially to have brought the Black Death, along with Far Eastern luxuries, to Sicily and the coastal ports of Italy, also carried the disease to the eastern Mediterranean. The Genoese and Venetian traders conveyed similar merchandise to the Middle East; in addition, they were especially instrumental in the valuable slave trade from the Golden Horde to Mamlūk Egypt.[72] We are well informed about the lively commerce between the Mongols at Sarai and the Mamlūk Empire, which included other commodities of the steppe besides Kipchak and Russian slaves, such as horses, furs, hides, and wax. These articles were customarily shipped through the trading stations of the Italian merchants at Kaffa and Tana or the Mongol entrepôts at Sughdaq and Old Qrim (Solkhat). Transported across the Black Sea, the trade went either overland across Anatolia or, more frequently at this time, by sea through the Bosporus. The mamlūk sultans of Egypt consistently sought cordial relations with both the Byzantine Empire and the Golden Horde to ensure this important commerce with the Eurasian steppe, in addition to securing alliances against the hostile Mongol Khanate in Persia.[73] To facilitate the maritime trade between

[71] Ziegler, pp. 230-231.

[72] Labib, *Handelsgeschichte*, pp. 103-119; Spuler, *The Muslim World*, vol. 2, pp. 50-53; Wiet, *L'Égypte Arabe*, p. 241; Hautecoeur and Wiet, *Les Mosquées du Caire*, vol. 1, p. 48; E. Ashtor, *Les Métaux précieux et la balance des payments du Proche-Orient à la basse époque* (Paris, 1971), pp. 89ff; C. E. Bosworth, "Christian and Jewish Religious Dignitaries in Mamlūk Egypt and Syria," *IJMES*, vol. 3, no. 1 (1972), p. 62, n. 4. On relations between the Golden Horde and Egypt, see the monograph of S. Zakirov, *Diplomaticheskie otnosheniya Zolotoy Ordy s Egiptom* (XIII-XIV *vv.*), Moscow, 1966.

[73] The Byzantine emperor, who was re-established in Constantinople at approximately the same time that the mamlūk regime assumed control in Egypt, was initially on good terms with the Mongol Khanate of Persia because of the pressure that the Mongols in Persia could bring against their common enemy, the Turkish Sultanate in Anatolia. But the devastating campaigns into the Balkan possessions of Byzantium

the Golden Horde and Egypt, a Mongol *funduq* or entrepôt existed in Alexandria, primarily for slaves.[74]

It is reasonable to assume that plague-carrying rats may have been transported by the merchant fleets coming from the Black Sea region to Egypt. Equally important, perhaps, was the effective transportation of infected fleas in merchandise and foodstuffs, which have been proven by modern studies to be efficient means of plague transmission.[75] Furs were a particularly popular fashion in Mamlūk Egypt, and the active trade in furs from southern Russia may have been a favorable means for transporting infected fleas.[76] Far less emphasis should be placed on men, in this case merchants and slaves, as passive porters of infected fleas, because human fleas are generally poor transmitters of plague. In whatever manner, plague was able to follow trade to Egypt as easily as it did to Sicily and Italy.[77] Conversely, it has been argued that the itinerary of the Black Death makes possible our re-establishing the map of the principal trade routes in the Near East in the fourteenth century,[78] particularly the so-called "Sarai-Cairo axis."[79]

Al-Maqrīzī informs us that the Black Death reached Egypt in the early autumn of 748/1347—about the same time that it arrived in Sicily.[80] It may have been spread simultaneously to

---

by the Mongols of the Golden Horde, together with the Bulgars, in 1264 and 1271 induced Michael VIII Palaeologus to ally himself with the Golden Horde (1272) and the Mamlūk Sultanate—a virtual "Triple Alliance" against the Mongol Khanate of Persia and the Latin states in Syria-Palestine.

[74] Labib, *Handelsgeschichte*, pp. 67-73, 108-111.

[75] Hirst, p. 308.

[76] Labib, *Handelsgeschichte*, p. 294; "England to Egypt," pp. 126-127; L. A. Mayer, *Mamlūk Costume* (Geneva, 1952), pp. 23-25.

[77] Grekov and Iakoubovski, *La Horde d'Or*, p. 94.

[78] Poliak, "Le Caractère colonial de l'état Mamelouk," p. 232.

[79] Spuler, *Die Goldene Horde*, pp. 4-5, 46-47, 371-372, 391-408.

[80] *as-Sulūk*, part 2, vol. 3, pp. 772, 780. Generally, this chronology agrees with the information from all the other available sources: Ibn al-Furāt quoted in *Badhl*, fol. 130b; *'Iqd al-jumān*, chap. 24, part 1,

Asia Minor and the Levant by merchant ships. Ibn Khātimah relates that after attacking Kaffa and Constantinople, plague came to Cilicia.[81] However, when Ibn al-Wardī composed his essay on the epidemic in Aleppo in early 749/1348, Sīs (the capital of Cilicia or Lesser Armenia) had not yet been struck.[82] Because Sīs was only later subjected to a severe epidemic,[83] plague may have been communicated not by maritime trade but overland or by contact with the pandemic in Syria.

In any case, it is evident that plague raged among the merchant fleets of the eastern Mediterranean and was carried from one port to another. In Spain, Ibn al-Khaṭīb recognized the fact that epidemics coincided with the arrival of contaminated merchants and goods from foreign lands where plague was raging.[84] The communication of the disease by ship in the eastern Mediterranean is clear from the account of Cyprus.

The Black Death struck Cyprus in 1348[85] and was particularly devastating, according to Latin and Arabic sources.[86] Al-Maqrīzī tells us that plague struck first the beasts and then the infants and adolescents. Confronted by this calamity, the Cypriots assembled all the Muslim slaves and prisoners

---

p. 85 states that plague lasted in Syria and Egypt from the beginning of Jumādā II, A.H. 748 until 750. Unfortunately, the pilgrimage account of Niccolò da Poggibonsi, who travelled through the Near East from 1346 to 1350, makes no mention of the Black Death whatsoever (*A Voyage Beyond the Seas*, trans. by Bellorini and Hoade, Jerusalem, 1946).

[81] *Taḥṣīl*, fol. 58a.

[82] *Risālat an-naba'*, p. 187.

[83] *EI*[1]: "Sīs" (V. F. Büchner); *as-Sulūk*, part 2, vol. 3, p. 774 (no date); N. Jorga, *Brève histoire de la Petite Arménie* (Paris, 1930), p. 144.

[84] *Muqni'at*, fol. 42b.

[85] Bartsocas, "Two Fourteenth Century Greek Descriptions of the 'Black Death,'" p. 395. Plague may have reached Cyprus in the late summer of 1347 (see Ziegler, p. 111).

[86] Leontios Makhairos, *Recital Concerning the Sweet Land of Cyprus*, ed. and trans. by R. M. Dawkins (Oxford, 1932), vol. 1, pp. 60-61; Sir George Hill, *A History of Cyprus* (Cambridge, 1948), vol. 2, p. 307; *al-Bidāyah*, vol. 14, p. 225; Ibn al-Wardī, *Ta'rīkh*, vol. 2, p. 492; *as-Sulūk*, part 2, vol. 3, p. 776.

together and devoted one entire afternoon until sundown massacring them because of their fear that the Muslims would gain control of the island when so many of the Christians were dying and fleeing in panic. Panic was induced by an accompanying earthquake and tidal wave that destroyed the navy, the fishing fleet, and the olive groves. During one week, three of the Cypriot princes reportedly perished, and the fourth fled the island, possibly to Rhodes. Within twenty-four hours of their sailing, plague struck the ship, and the few who reached the neighboring island died.

Somewhat later, a ship of merchants appeared in Rhodes; all had died except for thirteen merchants. The merchants went on to Cyprus, but by the time they arrived only four had survived. They found no one in the Cypriot port and made sail for Tripoli (in Syria), where they recounted their odyssey. Shortly thereafter, the surviving merchants died and may have communicated the disease still further.[87] Thus, the Black Death appears to have been widespread among the Christian islands. When the traders met someone in the seaports, it was said that they were allowed to carry away all the merchandise that they wanted without making the customary cash payment. The mortality in the ports was so great that bodies were thrown directly into the sea.[88]

The fact that the Black Death arrived in Egypt at approximately the same time that it reached Sicily would strongly

[87] *as-Sulūk*, part 2, vol. 3, p. 776.

[88] *Ibid.* Later in the century, we have an accidental (and rare) reference to the abundance of fleas in Cyprus, which are extremely important in the etiology of plague but were understandably not associated with plague by the medieval observers. This mundane nuisance is mentioned by Nicolai de Martoni on his journey from Famagusta in 1394: ". . . I travelled all day to a village where I slept that night on a rug on the ground, for in those parts beds are not to be found for money, and nearly everyone sleeps on the ground; and throughout the island there are so many fleas that a man cannot sleep at night, and this on account of the pigs which they keep in their houses." (C. D. Cobham, ed. and trans., *Excerpta Cypria* [Cambridge, 1908, reprint 1969], pp. 25-26.)

suggest its transmission by the brisk Christian maritime trade from the Black Sea and Constantinople.[89] Al-Maqrīzī gives an interesting example of this probable transmission in his description of Alexandria during the Black Death. A slave ship carrying thirty-two merchants and three hundred men, including crew and slaves, sailed into the harbor of Alexandria. At its arrival, only four merchants, one slave, and about forty sailors were still alive, and these survivors died in the port.[90] This account of the slave trade may refer precisely to the important commerce of the Mamlūk Empire with the Golden Horde.

Introduced by maritime trade in 748/1347, the Black Death spread from Alexandria throughout Egypt; the lower Nile Valley was subjected to the disease from the beginning of 749/April 1348. The Black Death moved southward to Upper Egypt, which it entered at the end of 749/1349.[91] It appears that at the same time the plague advanced westward to Barqa and eastward to Qaṭyā[92] and Gaza. Gaza was seriously assailed by plague from 2 Muḥarram to 4 Ṣafar/2 April to 4 May 1348, when many died and the markets were closed.[93] Plague may have followed the Syrian coast northward, in one manner or

[89] Cf. Volney's observations about plague epidemics in the late eighteenth century: *Voyage en Égypte et en Syrie*, ed. by Jean Gaulmier (Paris, 1959), pp. 142-144.

[90] *as-Sulūk*, part 2, vol. 3, p. 776.

[91] aṣ-Ṣafadī quoted in *ibid.*, pp. 775, 788.

[92] *Ibid.*, p. 784. The dissemination of plague in Egypt in the fourteenth century follows closely that of the third pandemic at the end of the nineteenth century; see A. W. Wakil, *The Third Pandemic of Plague in Egypt*, Egyptian University, Faculty of Medicine, no. 3 (Cairo, 1932) and A. Makar, *Contribution à l'étude de l'épidémiologie de la peste*, diss., Faculty of Medicine, University of Lausanne, 1938. If the recent pandemic (1899-1930) is any indication, the incidence of plague was greater in Upper Egypt, where the province of Asyūṭ became the chief focus, than in Lower Egypt and the ports; pneumonic plague was far more frequent in the south than in the north.

[93] *as-Sulūk*, part 2, vol. 3, p. 775. For Gaza, see also Ṣāliḥ ibn Yaḥyā, *Ta'rīkh Bayrūt*, vol. 14, p. 225, which gives a similar account of the official report from the governor of Gaza to the governor of Damascus but states that 10,000 died during the period 10 Muharram to 10 Safar/10 April to 10 May 1348.

another, as Ibn al-Wardī has suggested. He naturally devoted most of his attention to Aleppo, where he witnessed the Black Death that began there in Rajab 749/October 1348.[94] In the same month, plague was most severe in Damascus.[95]

Accordingly, Ibn Baṭṭūṭah states that while he was in Aleppo in Rabī‘ I, 749/June 1348 he heard that plague had occurred in Gaza and had caused great destruction. Going south to Ḥomṣ, he found plague there. He went on to Damascus and arrived on a Thursday when fasting and processions for the raising of the plague epidemic were taking place.[96] He then journeyed to ‘Ajlūn and Jerusalem; in the latter city, plague had apparently already subsided. He tells us that he met in Jerusalem the preacher ‘Izz ad-Dīn ibn Jamā‘ah, a relative of the chief judge of Cairo, who had arranged a feast that Ibn Baṭṭūṭah was invited to attend.

> I asked him the reason for this, and he informed me that he had vowed during the epidemic that, if it was lightened and a day passed without having to pray for any dead, he would arrange a feast. He then said to me: "Yesterday, I did not pray for any dead, so I will give the promised feast." I found that those whom I had known among the shaykhs of Jerusalem had almost all ascended to God the Almighty.[97]

[94] *as-Sulūk*, part 2, vol. 3, p. 774, gives the first of Jumādā I, 749/July 1348, for the outbreak of plague in Aleppo. Ibn al-Wardī would obviously be the more reliable source, but both agree that it occurred after it struck Gaza and Damascus, as related by Ibn Baṭṭūṭah. See also *ibid.*, p. 779; *'Iqd al-jumān*, chap. 24, part 1, p. 85; *Durrat al-aslāk*, p. 358; *Tadhkirat an-nabīh*, fol. 145b; and *Kunūz adh-dhahab*, p. 10.

[95] *as-Sulūk*, part 2, vol. 3, pp. 775, 779; *Risālat an-naba'*, p. 185; *'Iqd al-jumān*, chap. 24, part 1, p. 85; *Durrat al-aslāk*, pp. 358-359; *Kunūz adh-dhahab*, p. 10; *al-Bidāyah*, vol. 14, pp. 225-230 (dates the epidemic from 7 Rabī‘ I, 749 to Muḥarram 750 A.H.); Ibn Baṭṭūṭah, *Voyages*, vol. 1, pp. 227-229; aṣ-Ṣafadī and Ibn Nubatah quoted in *as-Sulūk*, part 2, vol. 3, pp. 789, 790; *Badhl*, fols. 128a-128b taken from *Daf' an-niqmah*, fols. 75a-76a.

[96] This can be dated from the sources to Thursday, 26 Rabī‘ II, 749/24 July 1348. See *al-Bidāyah*, vol. 14, p. 226; Ibn Baṭṭūṭah, *Voyages*, vol. 1, pp. 227-228.

[97] *Voyages*, vol. 4, pp. 319-321.

The plague pandemic obviously moved throughout Palestine and Syria. The following towns are specifically mentioned in the chronicles for their plague ordeal: Gaza, 'Asqalān, Acre, Jerusalem, Sidon, Beirut, Damascus, al-Mizzah, Barzah, Ba'labakk, Qārā, al-Ghasūlah, al-Jubbah(?), az-Zabadānī, Ḥomṣ, Ḥamā, Sarmīn, 'Azāz, al-Bāb, Tall Bāshir, Aleppo, Sīs, Ṣafad, Nābalus, Karak, Lyddah, Ramlah, Tripoli, Baysān, 'Ayn Ṭāb, Manbij, Jinīn, and the bedouin encampments.[98]

In 749/1348-1349, the pandemic assailed Antioch, and the people fled to Rūm (Anatolia) and carried the disease to the regions of Qaramān and Caesarea (in Cappadocia).[99] Since the inhabitants of Antioch sought refuge from the epidemic by fleeing northward, it is unlikely that plague had already been brought across Anatolia to northern Syria. Yet it is difficult to determine exactly in what manner it reached Antioch; the report of plague in Antioch by al-Maqrīzī seems to indicate a separate focus of infection apart from that in southern Syria. Most likely, the pandemic was brought to Antioch by sea; Ibn Khātimah relates that Christian merchants, returning to Almería, reported plague along the Turkish coast.[100]

Plague was present in Mardin[101] and Diyār Bakr[102] in southeastern Anatolia, where the Kurds tried unsuccessfully to flee from the scourge.[103] As mentioned before, the earliest date for plague from the Armenian sources is September 10, 1348. Again, it is impossible from the available data to know the precise route of its dissemination in this region. It may have come northward from Syria, but more probably it came southward to Greater Armenia and Azarbayjan from the Caucasus region or the southern shore of the Black Sea. Con-

[98] Compiled primarily from *as-Sulūk*, part 2, vol. 3, pp. 774-775, 779, and *Risālat an-naba'*.

[99] *as-Sulūk*, part 2, vol. 3, p. 773.

[100] *Taḥṣīl*, fol. 53a.

[101] *as-Sulūk*, part 2, vol. 3, p. 774.

[102] Claude Cahen, "Contribution à l'histoire du Diyār Bakr au quatorzième siècle," *JA*, vol. 243 (1955), p. 82.

[103] *as-Sulūk*, part 2, vol. 3, p. 774; *an-Nujūm*, Cairo ed., vol. 10, p. 196.

cerning the latter, we know that plague attacked Trebizond in September, 1347—roughly the same time that it reached Egypt. The epidemic lasted for seven months in Trebizond and was quite severe.[104] It would be natural to suggest that the pandemic was transported to this important Byzantine seaport by ships coming from the Crimea.

In 749/1348-1349, plague also struck Mecca, and large numbers died there. The epidemic was probably brought to Mecca by the pilgrimage traffic, for al-'Aynī remarks that plague befell the pilgrims that year.[105] Ibn Abī Ḥajalah notes that many students and inhabitants of Mecca perished as well.[106] This was the subject of detailed discussion among the Muslim scholars because the Prophet was supposed to have promised that no disease would ever enter the holy cities of Mecca and Medina. It was considered a miracle that it did not spread to Medina. Some believed that the plague in Mecca was due to the violation of the city by the presence of unbelievers.[107]

Beyond the Middle East, the Black Death extended its grasp to North Africa, being brought principally by merchant ships, as it was to Egypt, Sicily, and Italy. An Andalusian source states that it reached the western Mediterranean islands of Sicily, Majorca,[108] and Ibiza and then sprang across to the neighboring coast of Africa and from there moved westward.[109] All of Ifrīqiyah (Tunisia, Algeria, and Morocco) was affected by plague epidemics.[110] The pandemic attacked Tunis at a time when the Marinid ruler of Fez, Abū l-Ḥasan, was

[104] William Miller, *Trebizond, The Last Greek Empire of the Byzantine Era* (Chicago, 1969), p. 53.

[105] *'Iqd al-jumān*, chap. 24, part 1, p. 86.

[106] *Daf' an-niqmah*, fol. 74b.

[107] *Ibid.*, fols. 59b, 74b-75a; Ibn Iyās, vol. 1, p. 191; *Badhl*, fols. 55a-57a, 123b, 128a; *Mā rawāhu l-wā'ūn*, p. 155, and *Ḥusn al-muḥāḍarah fī ta'rīkh Miṣr wal-Qāhirah* (Cairo, 1968), vol. 2, p. 303; Shams ad-Dīn al-Ḥijāzī, *Juz' fī ṭ-ṭā'ūn*, Dār al-Kutub al-Miṣrīyah MS no. 102 *majāmī' m*, fol. 148a; al-Qalqashandī, *Ṣubḥ al-a'shā*, vol. 13, p. 79.

[108] Ziegler, pp. 113-114.

[109] *Taḥṣīl*, fol. 58a.

[110] *as-Sulūk*, part 2, vol. 3, p. 777.

attempting to conquer Tunisia.[111] He was decisively defeated near Kairouwan (al-Qayrawān) by a coalition of nomadic Arab tribes and was forced to withdraw his army to Tunis.[112] Concerning this battle at the beginning of 749/April 1348, the famous Tunisian historian, Ibn Khaldūn, says that "violent plague occurred and it settled the affair."[113] When Abū l-Ḥasan returned to Tunis, he found the city in disarray, since plague had ravaged its inhabitants. It was claimed that the epidemic was so severe that 1,000 people died daily during the month of Rabīʿ I, 749/June 1348.[114] Many of the notables who had accompanied the Marinid sultan to Tunis died of plague as did a large number of the native élite.[115] Ibn Khaldūn quotes the Tunisian poet Abū l-Qāsim ar-Raḥawī:

> Constantly, I ask God for forgiveness.
> Gone is life and ease.
> In Tunis, both in the morning and in the evening—
> And the morning belongs to God as does the evening—
> There is fear and hunger and death,
> Stirred up by tumult and pestilence. . . .[116]

[111] See R. Le Tourneau, "North Africa to the Sixteenth Century," *The Cambridge History of Islam*, vol. 2, pp. 229-232, for a general history of the region.

[112] Ibn Khaldūn, *The Muqaddimah*, vol. 1, pp. xxxix-xl, vol. 3, pp. 264, 471-475, and *Histoire des Berbères et des dynasties musulmanes de l'Afrique Septentrionale*, trans. by Baron de Slane and Paul Casanova (2nd ed., Paris, 1925-1956), vol. 3, pp. 26-37, vol. 4, pp. 246-268.

[113] *at-Taʿrīf* (Cairo, 1951), p. 27. Unaccountably, R. Brunschvig gives the year A.D. 1349 for plague in Africa (*La Berbérie Orientale sous les Hafsides* (Paris, 1940), vol. 1, p. 171).

[114] Ibn Abī Dīnār, *al-Muʾnis fī akhbār Ifrīqiyah wa Tūnis* (Tunis, 1967), p. 147; Pellissier, trans., *Histoire de l'Afrique* (Paris, 1845), p. 247; Guyon, *Histoire chronologique des épidémies du Nord de l'Afrique*, p. 175; Bloch, *La Peste en Tunisie*, p. 3.

[115] Ibn Khaldūn, *Histoire des Berbères*, vol. 4, p. 203, and *at-Taʿrīf*, pp. 44-45, *e.g.*, ʿAbd an-Nūr, the *qāḍī* of the Marinid army died of plague in Tunis (p. 46); Shaykh Muḥammad ibn an-Najjar (p. 47); and the king's physician, Abū l-ʿAbbās Aḥmad ibn Shuʿayb (p. 48). A friend of Ibn Khaldūn's family, ʿAbd al-Muhayman (secretary of Abū l-Ḥasan), died of plague and was buried in Ibn Khaldūn's family ceme-

Plague was not confined to the northern part of Tunisia, for we know that it struck the island of Jirbah in the same year.[117]

Beyond Tunisia, the Black Death reached along the coast of North Africa. Part of the Marinid army may have carried plague back to Tlemcen, which Abū l-Ḥasan had previously captured, on its return to Morocco. We are told that Abū l-Ḥasan released Abū Mūsā, one of his advisers, from the campaign in Tunisia and that, when Abū Mūsā came to Tlemcen, he died of plague in 749/1348.[118] While discussing the number of deaths in his native town of Almería, Ibn Khātimah remarks that it was relatively light compared to other cities, both Muslim and Christian. He had received credible reports about North African cities for his comparison.[119] Plague overtook Tāzah in Morocco, for Ibn Baṭṭūṭah learned in 750/1349 that his mother had died there of it.[120] And Ibn al-Khaṭīb gives an example of a man of Salé, on the Atlantic coast, who secluded himself from the disease and remained healthy. This author, who is famous for his theory of contagion, argues that the best evidence for it was that the tent-dwelling and nomadic Arabs of North Africa remained healthy during the pandemic.[121]

The Black Death was brought to the eastern shore of the Iberian peninsula from the Mediterranean islands, as already mentioned. In May, 1348, it appeared in Barcelona and Valen-

---

tery in Tunis (pp. 27, 38-41). See also Brunschvig, *La Berbérie Orientale*, vol. 2, pp. 293, 295; Ibn Baṭṭūṭah, *Voyages*, vol. 4, p. 330.

116 *The Muqaddimah*, vol. 3, p. 264.

117 Ibn Khaldūn, *Histoire des Berbères*, vol. 3, p. 163, vol. 4, p. 284.

118 Ibn Khaldūn, *at-Ta'rīf*, p. 31. In a discussion of the siege of Tlemcen in A.H. 765 by the Marinids and their allies, Ibn Khaldūn mentions that plague "which had reappeared in Africa after having carried off there many of the people in the year 747 [1346-1347]" (*Histoire des Berbères*, vol. 3, p. 447). This date for the pandemic may be an error since it would be very early for a plague incidence in the western part of North Africa—earlier than Egypt—and does not accord with Ibn Khaldūn's dates in the *Ta'rīf*.

119 *Taḥṣīl*, fol. 57b.

120 *Voyages*, vol. 4, p. 332.

121 *Muqni'at*, fol. 42b.

cia, after it had occurred in Majorca.[122] Ibn Khātimah relates that plague reached Almería at the beginning of Rabīʿ I, 749/ June 1348, and lasted through the summer and winter. The first case reportedly arose in a house in the poor quarter of Almeria belonging to a family called Beni Dhannah.[123] We know that plague overtook Granada in 749/1348, since Ibn al-Khaṭīb was appointed the chief secretary of Sultan Abū l-Hajjāj Yūsuf I when his predecessor was carried off by plague.[124] The pandemic then swept inland through Andalusia.[125] By the time Ibn Khātimah wrote his treatise on plague, it had reached the greater part of Castile and the city of Seville.[126]

Plague afflicted the Muslim armies confronting the forces of King Alfonso XI, who was besieging Gibraltar in 1349.[127] It was said that the Muslims were so deeply disturbed by their suffering while the Christian army was unaffected that many of them seriously thought of adopting Christianity. Fortunately for their faith, however, the Black Death was soon raging quite as disastrously among the troops of Castile. In March, 1350, plague attacked the troops of King Alfonso, who would not leave his men; he duly caught the disease and died on Good Friday, March 26, 1350.[128]

122 Charles Verlinden, "La Grande peste de 1348 en Espagne," *Revue Belge de philologie et d'histoire*, vol. 17 (1938), p. 116; see also Ziegler, pp. 113-116 for Christian Spain.

123 *Taḥṣīl*, fol. 57a.

124 Ibn Khaldūn, *Histoire des Berbères*, vol. 4, p. 391; *as-Sulūk*, part 2, vol. 3, p. 777, is wrong in the statement that plague did not attack Granada.

125 *Taḥṣīl*, fol. 58a; *as-Sulūk*, part 2, vol. 3, p. 777.

126 Verlinden, "La Grande peste de 1348 en Espagne," p. 118.

127 Ibn Khaldūn, *Histoire des Berbères*, vol. 4, p. 476. Campbell, p. 129 quotes Casiri, *Bibliotheca Arabico-Hispana Escurialensis* (Madrid, 1760-1770), vol. 2, p. 89, that a Muslim, Muḥammad ibn Ahmad al-Anṣārī, fled before the Christian army, and that he came to Ceuta and wrote a book advocating a war against the Christians. al-Ansārī was, however, stricken by plague in Ceuta and died. This may be Muḥammad ibn Aḥmad ibn ʿAlī al-Anṣārī al-Ishbīlī, who is only mentioned in *GAL, Supplement*, vol. 1, p. 768 for his commentary on a work by as-Salālijī.

128 Ibn Khaldūn, *Histoire des Berbères*, vol. 4, pp. 378-379; Ziegler, p. 114.

Ibn Khaldūn gives the most succinct and perceptive contemporary summary of the far-reaching significance of the Black Death in Muslim lands. The great historian himself had lost his mother and father and a number of his teachers during the Black Death in Tunis.[129] He wrote in the introduction to his universal history:

> Civilization both in the East and the West was visited by a destructive plague which devastated nations and caused populations to vanish. It swallowed up many of the good things of civilization and wiped them out. It overtook the dynasties at the time of their senility, when they had reached the limit of their duration. It lessened their power and curtained their influence. It weakened their authority. Their situation approached the point of annihilation and dissolution. Civilization decreased with the decrease of mankind. Cities and buildings were laid waste, roads and way signs were obliterated, settlements and mansions became empty, dynasties and tribes grew weak. The entire inhabited world changed. The East, it seems, was similarly visited, though in accordance with and in proportion to [the East's more affluent] civilization. It was as if the voice of existence in the world had called out for oblivion and restriction, and the world responded to its call. God inherits the earth and whomever is upon it.[130]

129 *at-Ta'rīf*, pp. 19, 55.

130 *The Muqaddimah*, vol. 1, p. 64. A central concept of Ibn Khaldūn's historical thinking is *'umrān*, which may be translated as "social organization" or "civilization"; Rosenthal asserts that "progress in civilization is in direct proportion to the number of people co-operating for their common good. Thus, *'umrān* acquired the further meaning of 'population' and Ibn Khaldūn frequently uses the word in this sense. Wherever people are co-operating with each other, no matter on how limited a scale, there is *'umrān*. When the number of these people increases, a larger and better *'umrān* results. This growth in numbers, with a corresponding progress in civilization, finally culminates in the highest form of sedentary culture man is able to achieve; it declines from this peak when the number of cooperating people decreases" (vol. 1, pp. lxxvi-lxxvii). See also vol. 1, pp. 135-137, vol. 2, pp. 236, 270-283, 290-291, 314-315, and Brunschvig, *La Berbérie Orientale*, vol. 2, p. 374.

III

THE NATURE OF PLAGUE

A. MODERN MEDICAL PATHOLOGY[1]

We have an enormous advantage over our predecessors, particularly Ibn Khaldūn and his contemporaries, in knowing the true nature of the Black Death. Not only can we now control plague infection, but we can also see the seemingly incoherent pattern of plague epidemics in the past. Until the late nineteenth century, plague remained incomprehensible—a morbid riddle which could be neither solved nor avoided. Medieval man was without any form of effective medical defense against violent plague epidemics. In stark contrast, we are able today to conduct a post-mortem on the victims of the Black Death. It seems appropriate, therefore, at this point to review briefly the relevant aspects of our current knowledge of the pathology of plague, in order to interpret the descriptions of the disease during the Black Death and later plague epidemics in the Middle East.

The third pandemic of plague, which reached Canton and Hong Kong in 1894 and then spread throughout the world, afforded the opportunity for epidemiologists to gain an extensive knowledge of plague. Bacteriological techniques previously developed by Koch and Pasteur were applied to the ancient problems of the etiology of plague. In 1894, these techniques were employed in Hong Kong by Professor Kitasato and Dr. Yersin, sent by the Japanese and French governments respectively, to investigate the plague epidemic. Almost simultaneously but independently, they discovered the plague bacillus in the blood and tissues of plague victims and in the organs

[1] The most complete survey of the pathology of plague may be found in Pollitzer, *Plague*.

of dead rats found in plague regions. *Pasteurella pestis* was fully established as the infective micro-organism of plague. Yersin was the first to suggest that the rat was the principal vehicle of contagion and that an effective vaccine could be developed from the bacillus.

Subsequent work on plague was devoted to the complex nature of the interrelationships among the bacillus, rats, and men. Various theories of plague transmission were proposed, including alimentary transmission, simple infection as in cholera, and the ancient theory of miasma.[2] Finally, the flea was proved to be the vital mechanism of plague transmission from rats to human beings.

The discovery of the flea as the missing link in the chain of plague contagion was made by Paul Louis Simond and formulated in his classic paper in the *Annals of the Pasteur Institute* (Paris, October, 1898). We now know that the flea alighting on an afflicted rodent ingests the plague bacilli from its host. Because of a blockage of bacilli in the esophagus of some types of fleas, the flea becomes increasingly hungry, seeks a host, and attempts to feed but instead regurgitates the bacilli into its host or an alternative victim. The latter is sought particularly after the host dies and grows cold. The infected flea may attack any available man or animal while itself remaining immune to the disease. The infected flea may also cause infection through the entry of its faeces into its bite. The most efficient vector for bubonic plague is *Xenopsylla cheopis*, which probably had a Nilotic origin and is still the most common flea in present-day Egypt.[3] Fleas usually hibernate in

[2] See Hirst, chap. v.

[3] The significance of the *Xenopsylla cheopis* is due to the "blockage phenomenon" which invariably occurs in this type of flea. For an explanation of this phenomenon, see Hirst, pp. 183-187. For the current study of the flea in modern Egypt, see R. E. Lewis, "The Fleas (Siphonaptera) of Egypt," *The Journal of Parasitology*, vol. 53, no. 4 (1937), pp. 863-885, particularly p. 867; H. Hoogstraal and R. Traub, "The Fleas (Siphonaptera) of Egypt," *The Journal of the Egyptian Public Health Association*, vol. 40, no. 5 (1965), pp. 343-379: "The most numerous rodent of Egyptian cultivated areas, the Grass Rat, *Arvican-*

winter, and therefore, in temperate climates, the height of the bubonic plague season is the summer.

As a result of the study of the British Commission for the Investigation of Plague in India between 1905 and 1910, the entire epidemiology of plague was elucidated. Specifically, it was shown positively that rat plague is flea-borne, and bubonic plague cannot be transmitted continuously as an epizootic in the absence of rat fleas. Further research has concentrated on the ecological problem of immense complexity concerning the factors governing the fourfold relationship between man, microbe, rat, and flea and the emergence of the disease in epidemic proportions. The progress of plague is affected by the habits of man and the nature of his commerce and communications, and by the density of population and behavior of a vast variety of species of rodents and their parasites; they in turn are influenced by climate, harvest, and natural ecological changes. Perhaps it is sufficient for our purposes to say that plague is primarily a disease of rodents, and man enters only accidentally into the enzootic cycle.

With regard to the Black Death's origin in Central Asia, it should be emphasized that plague has been endemic for a very long time in the wild rodents of Transbaikalia, Mongolia, Manchuria, and Russian Turkestan, especially among the tarabagan (Siberian marmot). The inhabitants of these regions have been aware for generations of the periodic occurrence of a

---

this n. niloticus, is universally parasitized by *Xenopsylla cheopis*. . . . These animals and their numerous fleas live in close proximity to the dense human and domestic animal population of rural Egypt, and opportunities for transfer of fleas to and from people and domestic animals appear to be especially favorable. . . . *Rattus Rattus* and *R. Norvegius* harbor chiefly *X. cheopis* and smaller numbers of several other species, among them *Leptopsylla Segnis*" (pp. 376-377). See also vol. 23, nos. 2-3 of the *Bulletin of the World Health Organization* (Geneva, 1960), which is devoted to plague; particularly M. Baltazard, "Recherches sur la peste en Iran," pp. 141-156; M. Baltazard and B. Seydian, "Equête sur les conditions de la peste au Moyen-Orient," pp. 157-168; and R. Pollitzer, "A Review of Recent Literature on Plague," pp. 313-400.

fatal contagious disease in the tarabagan, which was apt to be transmitted to man. The natives of Transbaikalia and Outer Mongolia possessed a working knowledge of the disease and adopted elaborate precautionary measures. The mysterious illness among the tarabagan was also the subject of numerous legends of the Buriats and Mongols. The disease among these animals and men is mentioned in the old Tibetan sacred books.[4] Marco Polo described the peoples of the steppe and the tarabagan in his *Travels*: "The Tartars subsist entirely upon flesh and milk, and a certain small animal, not unlike a rabbit, called by our people Pharaoh's mice, which during the summer season are found in great abundance in the plains."[5]

Thus, the wild rodent population of the Asiatic steppe is one of the oldest plague foci in the world. A permanent reservoir of plague among wild rodents extends today into southeastern Russia, where susliks are of prime importance, and Iranian Kurdistan and Transcaspia, where gerbils are the reservoir hosts.[6] An epizootic may become entrenched among rats by the interchange of their fleas. The long-distance transmission of plague is usually not the result of the active migrations of rats, but the result of the passive transportation of rats or their fleas by humans. Modern research has shown that infected fleas can survive for a prolonged period in grain, clothing, and merchandise. A blocked flea, in favorable conditions, can remain alive and infectious for up to fifty days, even without food.[7] These facts, established largely by investi-

[4] Pollitzer, *Plague*, p. 252; Wu Lien-Teh, "The Original Home of Plague," p. 294.

[5] Wu Lien-Teh, "Plague in Wild Rodents, Including the Latest Investigations into the Role Played by the Tarabagan," *Far Eastern Association of Tropical Medicine: Transactions of the Fifth Biennial Congress* (Singapore, 1923), p. 320.

[6] Pollitzer, *Plague*, p. 256, and *Plague and Plague Control in the Soviet Union*, pp. 1-57, especially p. xiv: "Sketch map of the natural plague foci in the Soviet Union and the adjacent countries."

[7] Pollitzer, *Plague*, pp. 300-301; Wu Lien-Teh, J.W.H. Chun, R. Pollitzer, and C. Y. Wu, *Plague, A Manual for Medical and Public Health Workers* (Shanghai, 1936), p. 269.

gations of plague in modern Russia, do not take into account, however, the possible large-scale migration of wild or domestic rodents resulting from violent changes in the environment, as may have been the case before the Black Death.

Plague itself may take three clinical forms in animals and men: bubonic, pneumonic, and septicaemic. Misleading use of the word "bubonic" has given rise to the erroneous idea that true plague is necessarily bubonic and that non-bubonic forms are a different disease. Bubonic plague is contagious, depending almost entirely on flea-bite, and affects the lymphatic system of the body. The observable pathognomonic sign is the appearance of buboes, or inflamed nodes, which appear early in the illness, usually during the second or third day. They are located in or near the groin (Greek *boubōn*: hence "bubonic") in about two-thirds of the cases; the buboes are also commonly found in the armpits and the neck (behind the ear). The glands in other areas are rarely affected. Buboes may be multiple, but usually there is only one, though there may be secondary enlargements on the same chain of lymphatic glands. The size of the bubo varies from that of an almond to an orange and, until it begins to discharge, the bubo may be extremely painful. Most buboes break down and suppurate, but sometimes the inflamed swelling resolves itself. The typical case may be accompanied, at first, by shivering followed by a rise of temperature with vomiting, headache, giddiness, and intolerance to light; pain in the abdomen, back, and limbs; and sleeplessness, apathy, and delirium. The severity of the bubonic form varies greatly in different epidemics and at different stages of the same epidemic. Being insect-borne, bubonic plague depends directly on flea population density and the persistence of the infection in rodents.

Unlike bubonic plague, primary pneumonic or pulmonary plague is infectious. For reasons that are not yet known, bubonic plague may produce a secondary pneumonia, and consequently an epidemic of pneumonic plague may arise. In some conditions, plague may take a primary pneumonic form from the outset. The onset of the infection is marked by shivering, with difficult and hurried breathing, coughing, and expectoration. The expectoration shows an admixture of blood containing plague bacilli, indicating a massive infection of the lungs. The bacilli are sprayed into the air each time the victim coughs and are transmitted aerially to others. The physical signs are those characteristic of bronchopneumonia. In contrast to the bubonic type of plague, therefore, pneumonic plague is independent of rodent and flea infection. Prostration is great, and the course of the illness is rapid; death usually occurs within three days. The mortality rate is almost 100 percent; the demographic importance of this form of plague cannot be overemphasized.

Septicaemic plague results from the introduction of the bacillus into the bloodstream and is invariably fatal. This form of plague may be caused by the injection of bacilli from the flea directly into the bloodstream of the victim or by the failure of the bacilli to be localized in the lymphatic regions of the body. In septicaemic cases, the human flea (*Pulex irritans*), normally a poor vector of plague, may become an effective means of transmission. The course of this form of the disease is very acute, and the victim may die suddenly without visible symptoms within a few hours, with the possible exception of a few petechial haemorrhages in the serous and mucous membranes. Prostration and cerebral symptoms are particularly marked; the temperature rises rapidly and becomes very high. This type of plague is often found in the bloodstream of those with advanced cases of bubonic and pneumonic plague.[8]

[8] "There are also rarer clinical types of plague such as the cellulocutaneous or carbuncular, the tonsillar, and the vesicular. In some modern epidemics inflammatory lesions of the skin, often followed by extensive sloughing, were not uncommon and may amount to 6% of all cases. In former times extensive skin lesions were commonly reported. The prognosis is relatively favorable. The vesicular variety of plague may simulate smallpox, but the pustules contain plague bacilli. The tonsillar or anginal type is suggestive of diphtheria; these last two types are deadly" (Hirst, p. 30). For possible tonsillar incidences, see the discussions in *Badhl*, fols. 13a-13b, and *Taḥṣīl*, fol. 73b. The vesicular form of plague may have played a significant role in the plague epidemics in early Islamic history.

As a rule, if the disease is bubonic or septicaemic, plague does not spread directly from one human being to another. Rarely are there enough bacilli in men to infect the fleas that ingest their blood. However, when the bacilli become localized in the lungs (pneumonic plague) and are eliminated in large numbers in respiratory discharges, and when environmental and climatic conditions favor aerogenic droplet transmission, the disease becomes infectious among men. The pulmonary plagues in Manchuria in 1910-1911 and 1920-1921 and later in eastern India amply attest to the importance of cool weather and crowding in badly ventilated dwellings as contributory factors in creating pneumonic epidemics.[9] Accordingly, the pneumonic form of plague is most commonly found in the winter months in the Middle East.

B. MEDIEVAL OBSERVATIONS OF PLAGUE

Historically, the symptomatology of plague is vitally important for the recognition of the various forms of the disease.[1] The

[9] In my discussion of the Muslim prohibition of the idea of infection, I have interpreted "infection" (*'adwā*) in the Arabic texts in a broad sense to mean both contagion and infection. In modern medical terminology, as in the description above, this is unacceptable. "Contagion" means the transmission of the disease by an agent while "infection" implies the lack of such an agent and the communication of the bacilli directly. With regard to plague, the distinction is an important one; bubonic plague is contagious, whereas pneumonic plague is infectious. While this distinction is helpful in understanding the historical phenomenon of the Black Death, no such distinction was made in the medieval treatises on plague. Moreover, the statement that there is no infection should be understood to mean that the disease came directly from God. In this sense, infection should not be interpreted as distinct from contagion. Therefore, I have felt free to use the two terms "contagion" and "infection" interchangeably, particularly in the discussion of Ibn al-Khaṭīb's theory of inter-human plague transmission.

[1] See the modern symptomatology of plague in Pollitzer, *Plague*, pp. 411-446. In some instances the identification of symptoms described by Muslim witnesses of the Black Death is uncertain. For example, al-Maqrīzī describes plague in Baghdad and states that a man would find abscesses (*tulū'*) on his face; the man would put his hand to them and

plague bubo was the most conspicuous sign of a plague epidemic, but proof of pneumonic plague is also abundant. For example, al-Maqrīzī attests to these two forms of plague in his description of the Black Death in Damascus:

> The malady manifested itself in the following manner: a small swelling grew behind the ear which rapidly suppurated. There was a bubo under the arm and death followed very quickly. One noticed also the presence of a tumor[2] which caused a serious mortality. They were occupied with this for a time; then they spat blood, and the population was terrified by the multitude of the dead. The maximum of survival after the spitting of blood was fifty hours.[3]

The buboes in the lymphatic regions of the body clearly refer to bubonic plague; the spitting of blood which ensued, together with a high mortality, is characteristic of secondary pneumonic plague. The buboes were variously described; the term *khiyārah* ("cucumber") is frequently used by the Arabic writers to indicate the large inguinal bubo that is most common in bubonic epidemics. Aṣ-Ṣafadī refers precisely to "a *khiyārah* in the groin" during the Damascus plague.[4] Ibn Ḥabīb describes the distinctive bubonic symptoms as "the pustule, the almond, and the cucumber."[5]

The later writers on plague drew on their predecessors' descriptions; yet there is evidence of genuine observations of

---

would die suddenly (*as-Sulūk*, part 2, vol. 3, p. 774). This may refer to cervical buboes or subcutaneous haemorrhaging, but the report is too vague to be certain. Another imprecise report is the strange appearance of a "bubo" on the tip of the nose given by Ibn Abī Ḥajalah (*Kitāb at-ṭibb*, fol. 145a) and repeated because of its uniqueness by Ibn Ḥajar (*Badhl*, fol. 45a). This may refer to the plague pustules and not to the more familiar buboes.

[2] *khiyārah*.

[3] *as-Sulūk*, part 2, vol. 3, p. 775. The references to the buboes in the Arabic sources are too numerous to cite; see, however, the various Arabic terms used for the bubo in Appendix 2.

[4] Dār al-Kutub al-Misrīyah MS no. 102 *majāmī' m*, fol. 199b.

[5] *Durrat al-aslāk*, p. 358.

the disease.[6] During the plague epidemic of 833/1429-1430 in Cairo—which undoubtedly included pneumonic plague—Ibn Ḥajar states in his plague treatise that plague "occurred after eighty-eight years[7] and was similar to it in every way."[8] A sixteenth-century treatise correctly observes a number of accompanying symptoms of plague not usually found in the earlier works: high fever and severe dizziness, often occurring with vomiting, rapid heartbeat, and fainting.[9] The greatest lack of originality in the treatises is the slavish repetition of the accepted etiology of plague drawn primarily from Ibn Sīnā, which will be dealt with in the next chapter.[10]

From the medical treatises in southern Spain, we have the most detailed descriptions of the plague symptoms, while most of the Middle Eastern tracts are mainly religio-legal discussions of plague and deal only peripherally with the clinical aspects of plague. The works of the three Andalusian authors, Ibn Khātimah, ash-Shaqūrī, and Ibn al-Khaṭīb, are the only Arabic medical tracts contemporary with the Black Death that have survived. Their treatises, therefore, are valuable for the careful medical observations of the Black Death, and there seems to be no reason not to consider their accounts representative. Without the advantage of comparable Middle Eastern medical treatises, their observations appear more empirical than the traditional explanations found in the standard medical manuals, although entirely consistent with them.[11]

In general, most of the Muslim writers emphasized the pre-

[6] Ibn Abī Sharīf, *Kitāb fī aḥkām aṭ-ṭā'ūn*, Dār al-Kutub al-Miṣrīyah MS no. 102 *majāmī' m*, fol. 157a; *Badhl*, fols. 12a-14a, 45a; *Daf' an-niqmah*, fols. 40b-41b; *Kitāb aṭ-ṭibb*, fol. 145a; and al-Ḥijāzī, *Juz' fī ṭ-ṭā'ūn*, fols. 148a-149a.

[7] The Black Death in A.H. 748.

[8] *Badhl*, fol. 110a.

[9] Ṭāshköprüzāde, fol. 33b. Ibn Khātimah does note a number of symptoms besides the buboes and pulmonary infection; they include severe pains, sore throat, acute ulcers, headache, diarrhea, vomiting, and extreme thirst.

[10] See the discussion of etiology below, chap. IV.

[11] Donald Campbell, *Arabian Medicine and Its Influence on the Middle Ages* (London, 1926), vol. I, p. 85.

disposition of a man's body to disease, following classical medical tradition; the difference in men's states of health was used to account for the irregularity of the pestilential miasma in striking some men and not others. Ibn al-Khaṭīb's lengthy discussion of predisposition concludes with a comparison of men's receptivity to disease with a wick that is brought near a flame. A man's temperament is like the wick that can be easily ignited after it has been recently put out; a dry wick takes longer, and a damp wick—a man whose temperament is antithetical to disease—takes a long time to ignite, if it will do so at all.[12] Ibn al-Khaṭīb is in complete accord with the view of Galen[13] that susceptibility to disease depends on the condition of the individual human body. This was governed by the dominant humor and the effects of acquired habits and mode of life. Ibn Khātimah maintained that persons of hot, moist temperament should be very careful during a plague epidemic. Especially susceptible were young women of strong sensuality and passionate nature, and the young and corpulent of either sex.

The two Andalusian writers, Ibn Khātimah and Ibn al-Khaṭīb, identified the buboes (*ṭawā'īn*) behind the ears, under the arms and in the groin.[14] As explained by Ibn Khātimah, these tumors were a result of the expulsion by the vital organs —the brain, heart, and liver—of the destructive substances through agitated blood to the cervical, axillary, and inguinal cavities respectively.[15] It was believed that in a healthy body the corrupt substance would be localized and the patient would recover. Otherwise, the poisonous matter would be diffused in the body, affecting the major organs, especially the lungs, and the individual would die.[16] This theory of emunctories

12 *Muqni'at*, fols. 41a-42a.

13 *Medicorum Graecorum Opera Quae Exstant*, ed. by C. G. Kühn (Leipzig, 1821-1833), vol. 7, pp. 291-292.

14 *Taḥṣīl*, fols. 73b-74a; *Muqni'at*, fol. 39b.

15 *Tahsīl*, fols. 51b, 72b, 73b-74a. See also *Muqni'at*, fol. 40b; *Badhl*, fols. 12b-13b, and Ṭāshköprüzāde, fol. 34a.

16 *Tahsīl*, fols. 73b-74a.

was taken from Arabic medicine and had a long life in European medicine; it may be found from the early treatise on plague by John of Burgundy (1365) to the investigation of plague by Sydenham in the seventeenth century.[17]

Only these two Andalusians clearly distinguished between the buboes and the cutaneous pustules or petechial spots.[18] Primary plague lesions, or carbuncles, usually form at the site of infection, but secondary carbuncles or necrotic ulcers of haematogenous origin may develop on all parts of the body;[19] these are described by the Arabic authors. Ibn Khātimah describes the pustules as black sores resembling blistering (*tafqī'*) accompanied by inflammation. These black spots are also depicted as grains (*ḥubūb*) and contain watery fluid when they are broken—possibly a reference to vesicular plague.[20] The author interprets these pustules according to the emunctory theory: finding the vital organs of the body weak, the corruption pushes out onto the surface of the body as black, visible sores (*qurūḥ*) on the back, neck, and extremities.[21] Ibn al-Khaṭīb refers to the green, blue, or black-colored pustules.[22]

Aṣ-Ṣafadī wrote that the plague-stricken Damascenes during the Black Death "looked like roses," which may reasonably refer to these conspicuous skin blemishes.[23] This symptom recalls, in a morbid manner, our common children's song, "Ring Around the Rosy," which originally applied to these inflamed pustules during European plague epidemics. At the time of

[17] Hirst, pp. 42-43. For the widespread knowledge of emunctories in Portugal in the fifteenth century, see Ricardo Jorge, "Les anciennes épidemies de peste en Europe, comparées aux épidemies modernes," *Comptes-Rendus*, Ninth International Congress of the History of Medicine (Bucharest, September, 1932), p. 365.

[18] See Appendix 2; cf. Procopius' description of the pustules (*History of the Wars*, vol. 1, pp. 462-463).

[19] Pollitzer, *Plague*, pp. 424-427 and fig. 32, p. 743.

[20] *Tahsīl*, fols. 82a-83b. *Badhl*, fols. 12b-13b completely confuses the two symptoms; other writers simply describe the two more conspicuous forms.

[21] *Taḥṣīl*, fols. 73a, 74a.

[22] *Muqni'at*, fol. 40a.

[23] Dār al-Kutub al-Miṣrīyah MS no. 102 *majāmī' m*, fol. 199b.

the plague epidemic of 790/1388 in Egypt, Ibn al-Furāt, who had witnessed the Black Death in Cairo, also distinguished between these blisters (*naffāṭah*), appearing mostly on the back, and the bubo (*ḳubbah*).[24]

The historical evidence for pneumonic plague (either primary or secondary) is clearly evident in the Arabic sources for the Black Death, as already indicated, and for plague recurrences over the following century and a half. Pneumonic plague was common during the Black Death in Europe and the Middle East as a complication of severe bubonic plague.[25] Primary pneumonic plague, because of its relation to pneumonia, is usually found in the winter months. Al-Maqrīzī reports that the Black Death was most severe in Egypt during the months of Sha'bān, Ramaḍān, and Shawwāl 749/November 1348 through January 1349,[26] indicating the presence of pneumonic plague infection. Later, during the plague of 833/1429-1430 in Egypt, which included pneumonic plague, the same author was a direct observer of the event and wrote:

> This was reckoned among the strange things, that the plague was during the winter and not at a time in which we are accustomed. The plague usually struck in the spring [bubonic plague], and the doctors ascribed this to the flowing of the mixtures in the spring and the hardening of them in the winter, but God makes what appears.[27]

In the same plague epidemic, al-Maqrīzī compares the lengthened period of illness, after spring had come, with the speedy death before. He was almost certainly observing one of the differences between bubonic and pneumonic plague.[28]

The conspicuous symptoms of pneumonic plague are spitting

[24] *Ta'rīḳh*, vol. 9, p. 26.

[25] Wu Lien-Teh, *A Treatise on Pneumonic Plague* (Geneva, 1926), pp. 3-4.

[26] *as-Sulūḳ*, part 2, vol. 3, p. 772.

[27] *Ibid.*, part 4, vol. 2, p. 821 (Bodleian MS Marsh no. 121, fol. 17b).

[28] *Ibid.*, part 4, vol. 2, p. 829. Similarly, Ibn Taghrī Birdī writing on the same plague in Cairo (833/1429-1430) observed: "Then sickness also began to be protracted and physicians and surgeons went to the sick." (*an-Nujūm*, Popper trans., vol. 18, p. 73.)

blood and rapid death. Because of its infectious nature, there is a much higher mortality rate than during a bubonic plague epidemic.[29] On the basis of observations of the spitting of blood, we can be certain of its presence during the Black Death. Al-Maqrīzī has been quoted for the occurrence of pneumonic plague in Damascus. In another instance, the famous scholars as-Subkī and aṣ-Ṣafadī wrote for one another poetic accounts of the plague in 749/1348-1349.[30] (Both men ultimately died of plague, in 771/1370 and 764/1363 respectively.) Aṣ-Ṣafadī wrote about Damascus:

> Then came the worst calamity that brought tears to every eye. People spat bits of blood, and one was covered with blotches and died. . . . Every person in the morning or evening breathed out blood from his throat as if he had been slain without a knife.[31]

Ibn Abī Ḥajalah, who was also an eyewitness to the Black Death in Damascus, incorporated his observations of blood-spitting, as well as the buboes, into his treatise written after the plague epidemic of 764/1362-1363.[32]

Al-Maqrīzī refers to the existence of pneumonic plague in Cairo during Shawwāl 749/January 1349, when "new symptoms appeared consisting of spitting blood. The sick would feel an internal fever followed by nausea and spitting blood, and then die."[33] Again, he tells us that in Cairo and Fusṭāṭ (Old Cairo) "an individual who was struck by the plague

[29] See chap. v for the determination of later recurrences of pneumonic plague in Egypt and Syria.

[30] The works are found in Dār al-Kutub al-Miṣrīyah MS no. 102 *majāmī' m*, fols. 197a-200a. The account of as-Subkī is quoted in *Badhl*, fols. 129b-130a, which Ibn Ḥajar attributes to the plague epidemic of A.H. 764; Ibn Hajar only refers to a *risālah* of aṣ-Safadī (fols. 45b, 129a), which may be identified with this poetic description by as-Safadī in MS no. 102.

[31] Dār al-Kutub al-Miṣrīyah MS no. 102 *majāmī' m*, fol. 200a. This morbid metaphor was very popular with other writers: *as-Sulūk*, part 2, vol. 3, p. 789; *Badhl*, fols. 129a-129b.

[32] *Daf' an-niqmah*, fol. 75a.

[33] *as-Sulūk*, part 2, vol. 3, p. 781.

spat blood, uttered cries, and died."[34] In the same year, Ibn Ḥabīb (d. 779/1377) described a Cairene who spat blood as "a messenger drawing others to death."[35] Another historian, al-'Aynī, states simply that during the Black Death "their death was from spitting blood. A man would eat, walk, converse with his friends, and then spit. When he proceeded on a little further, he might suddenly be dead."[36]

Besides the numerous references to the plague buboes, Ibn al-Wardī observed the spitting of blood in Aleppo during the pandemic and its extreme infectiousness: if one member of a household spat blood, all were sure to perish. "Whoever tasted his own blood was certain of death."[37] Even in the *Decameron*, Boccaccio alludes vaguely to the "eastern countries" (the Orient), where "bleeding at the nose"—a sign of pulmonary infection—was a manifest warning of inevitable death during the Black Death.[38]

We are equally certain of the pneumonic form of plague in Andalusia. Ibn Khātimah, who experienced the pandemic in Almería in 749-750/1348-1349, observed the infectiousness of pneumonic plague and the high mortality rate.[39] He recognized that the disease attacked the lungs, producing the symptom of expectoration of blood, and that this pulmonary type of plague coincided with the winter months.[40] He knew of only one man who had recovered from the malady. Despite all the remedies that the writer offered for the buboes and

[34] *Ibid.*, p. 773.

[35] *Durrat al-aslāk*, p. 358.

[36] *'Iqd al-jumān*, p. 85; copied by al-Mu'minī, *Kitāb futūḥ an-naṣr*, vol. 2, p. 295.

[37] See my "Ibn al-Wardī's *Risālat an-naba' 'an al-waba'*," *Near Eastern Numismatics, Iconography, Epigraphy and History*, ed. by Dickran K. Kouymjian (Beirut, 1974), p. 451. Another example of this description is found in a poetic account of the pandemic attributed to Ibn al-Wardī (Dār al-Kutub al-Miṣrīyah no. 102 *majāmī' m*, fol. 197b). Also, for Aleppo in A.H. 749, see *Kunūz adh-dhahab*, vol. 2, p. 10 (p. 156 of the Arabic text).

[38] See Wu Lien-Teh, *A Treatise on Pneumonic Plague*, p. 4.

[39] *Tahṣīl*, fols. 64b, 73a.

[40] *Ibid.*, fol. 57a.

pustules, he could offer no treatment for the pneumonic form of plague.[41]

Slightly later, Ibn al-Khaṭīb described the plague in Granada and stressed the spitting of blood among the other signs of plague; in an unhealthy body the disease killed by attacking the lungs.[42] The spitting of blood was considered the easiest way of spreading the epidemic, as well as being incurable.[43] Because of the widespread prevalence of pneumonic plague during the pandemic, it was natural that Ibn al-Khaṭīb would have argued so strongly for the infectious nature of plague. Other Arabic writers, both before and after him, disagreed with the traditional Islamic doctrine that denied contagion-infection but shrank from open confrontation with the religious scholars.[44] Because of his forthright statement in favor of the infection theory during the Black Death, Ibn al-Khaṭīb has gained considerable notoriety in the West.[45]

Finally, the septicaemic form of plague has no distinctive symptoms except severe prostration and a very rapid death. In a number of historical descriptions of plague victims, it is very probable that this form of plague was being observed. For example, during the Black Death as-Subkī noted the rapid death of plague victims without any visible bodily signs.[46] Ibn al-Khaṭīb emphasized the fainting and prostration of the plague-stricken in Granada.[47] In the plague epidemic of 833/1429-1430, one observer tells us of a slave girl in his household who was ill in the morning and died before sunset.[48] In general, fatal cases of bubonic plague usually resulted from the infection of the bloodstream.

[41] *Ibid.*, fols. 81a-82a.

[42] *Muqniʿat,* fols. 39b-41a. [43] *Ibid.*, fol. 45a.

[44] See Ullmann: "Das Problem der Infektion" (pp. 242-250), and Seidel, "Die Lehre von der Kontagion bei den Arabern," pp. 82-83.

[45] T. W. Arnold and A. Guillaume, eds., *The Legacy of Islam* (Oxford, 1931), pp. 340-341. See the discussion of this topic below, chap. IV.

[46] Dār al-Kutub al-Miṣrīyah MS no. 102 *majāmīʿ m,* fol. 198a.

[47] *Muqniʿat,* fol. 40a.

[48] *an-Nujūm,* Popper trans., vol. 18, p. 72.

On the basis of the foregoing summary of the modern medical pathology of plague and the symptoms of the Black Death, there can be no question that it was a plague pandemic. Furthermore, the three major forms of plague were clearly prevalent in the Middle East during the Black Death and recurrent plague epidemics. Ignorant of the actual nature of plague, Muslim communities were completely vulnerable to the disease; men explained the terrible pestilence and healed the sick as best they could. The medical ignorance in which they floundered may convey to us an exaggerated sense of confusion and desperation that may only partly describe the medieval response. For a medical explanation *was* produced largely within the framework of religious belief; within this framework, men also resorted to related magical beliefs to allay their justifiable fears. Their understanding of plague offers us an explanation for their social responses and, more generally, a glimpse into the medieval Muslim mind.

IV

MEDIEVAL MUSLIM INTERPRETATIONS OF PLAGUE

A. MEDICAL INTERPRETATIONS

1. Etiology

When confronted by the Black Death, Muslims generally ascribed its ultimate cause to the will of God. The manner by which God caused it to occur among men, however, was the subject of innumerable and often contradictory explanations.[1] The majority of the Muslim legal scholars who wrote plague treatises were more interested in the theological explanation of the disease than in the physical causation; the latter was of greater concern to the physicians, although the physicians were not free from definite religious strictures in their medical interpretations. Apart from the medical tracts of the physicians, various naturalistic interpretations are usually found randomly lumped together with religious explanations, differing only in degrees of emphasis according to an individual author's point of view. What has been said about the fourteenth-century European plague treatises is true for the Middle Eastern treatises:

[1] There is no satisfactory modern study of Arabic medical history during the medieval period. For a general introduction and bibliography, see F. M. Pareja, *Islamologie* (Beirut, 1964), pp. 993-1002, 1014-1016; for Persia, see Elgood, *A Medical History of Persia*. Ullmann's recent work, *Die Medizin im Islam*, is largely a bibliographical study of Arabic translations of Greek works and Arabic medical compendia. See also the older bibliographical study of Arabic medical works for the fourteenth and fifteenth centuries in L. Leclerc, *Histoire de medécine Arabe* (Paris, 1876), vol. 2, pp. 261-301, and the survey of the subject that is still very useful: E. G. Browne, *Arabian Medicine* (Cambridge, 1921).

> Men's minds seem to have been unusually open to entertain any and every hypothesis concerning the origin of the great calamity, and often in the plague treatises of the period a variety of causes were accepted as being simultaneously and successively in operation.[2]

Out of this confusion arising from ignorance, the predominant etiological view of the Middle Ages that emerges, in both the Orient and the Occident, was that the disease was produced and spread by corruption of the air, or miasma.[3] This miasma was believed to damage men and animals, waters and plants. The miasmatic hypothesis was paramount in Europe and the Middle East because it could readily be integrated and supported by accepted theological beliefs and classical medical texts.

The Arabic writers at the time of the Black Death adopted this miasmatic theory of epidemics primarily from Hippocrates and Galen, either directly or indirectly through the commentaries of Muslim doctors, especially Ibn Sīnā (Avicenna: 370-428/980-1037).[4] The study of Hippocrates and Galen was the mainstay of medical education in the medieval period.[5] For example, the works of these classical authors are known to have been conspicuous in the libraries of Jewish physicians in Fusṭāṭ during the twelfth and thirteenth centuries. "Studying medicine meant in the first place memorizing selected writings of Hippocrates and even more of Galen."[6]

The miasmatic theory is found in Hippocrates' *Epidemics I and III*[7] and in Galen's commentary on the *Epidemics* in his

[2] Hirst, p. 25.

[3] Campbell, pp. 36-37, 48-56. The earliest Arab medical statement of this theory derived from Hippocrates may be found in 'Alī ibn Rabban aṭ-Ṭabarī, *Firdausu l-Ḥikmat*, p. 330.

[4] *EI*[2]: "Ibn Sīnā" (A.-M. Goichon); see also Tholozon, *Histoire de la peste bubonique en Perse*, p. 5.

[5] *GAS*, vol. 3, pp. 23-47, 88-140; see also F. Rosenthal, *Four Essays on Art and Literature in Islam* (Leiden, 1971), p. 3.

[6] Goitein, *A Mediterranean Society*, vol. 2, p. 249.

[7] *Hippocrates*, trans. by W.H.S. Jones (New York, 1923), vol. 1, pp. 139-211. The Arab adoption of the Hippocratic theory of epidemics

De differentiis febrium (Book I, Chapter VI).[8] In his commentary, Galen develops Hippocrates' idea of miasmatic corruption of the air and incorporates the idea of an energizing spirit or *pneuma*, which is absorbed by the body from the atmosphere and is radiated to all the vital organs. This was part of Galen's theory of humors that dominated medieval medicine and formed the framework for most of the medical accounts of the Black Death.[9]

The humoral theory not only was wrong but subverted clinical observation. The theory presupposes that the world is composed of four elements: fire, air, water, and earth. Each of the elements is linked with one of the four principal body fluids, and each of the fluids thereby assumes certain qualities of the elements. Thus, since fire is hot and dry, and since fire is linked with yellow bile (choler), yellow bile is hot and dry. Air is associated with blood, and blood is therefore hot and moist; water is the element of phlegm, the humor which is moist and cold; and earth is the element of the melancholic humor, black bile, which is cold and dry. Moreover, each humor is associated with a color, a taste, an age, a season of the year, and a temperament.

---

is interestingly demonstrated by the important (lost) Berlin MS no. 6380 (Ahlwardt), which contained eleven Arabic treatises on plague. The last ten treatises may be dated from the time of the Black Death; the first was an Arabic translation of Hippocrates' *Epidemics*: "al-Abīdhīmīan [ἐπιδήμιον] al-amrāḍ al-wāfidah" (see Appendix 3).

[8] *Medicorum*, vol. 7, pp. 287-294; see also vol. 19, p. 391. It should be borne in mind that almost the entire Galenic corpus was translated into Arabic and reached the West through Latin and Hebrew translations from Arabic. For plague specifically, see the selection from Galen's work on plague and its symptoms: *Jawāmiʿ kitāb Jālīnūs fī l-dubūl wa dalāʾilhu*, MS no. A84, no. 3, The National Library of Medicine (D. M. Schullian and F. E. Sommer, *A Catalogue of Incunabula and Manuscripts in the Army Medical Library*, New York, 1950, p. 325; *GAL*, vol. I, p. 217).

[9] For a thorough modern exposition of Galen's humoral theory, see R. E. Siegel, *Galen's System of Physiology and Medicine* (Basel, 1968), pp. 196-359.

The corruption of the air is a disturbance of the healthy balance of the four elements that, in turn, upsets the proper balance of the four corresponding bodily humors. For example, Ibn Ḥajar describes an epidemic as the corruption of the essence of the air, which is a substance and nutrient of the soul.[10] Ibn al-Khaṭīb explains that the putrid air changes men's humors so that fever and blood-spitting ensue.[11] The prophylaxes against plague recommended by Ibn Sīnā and others were directed precisely to righting these imbalances in one's surroundings and in one's body, and many remedies naturally go back to Galen.

The influence of Galen's *De differentiis febrium* on Islamic medicine can be traced directly to the work's early translation into Arabic by Qusṭā ibn Lūqā al-Ba'labakkī (d. ca. 300/912),[12] who was also the author of two early works on infection and epidemics.[13] Ibn Sīnā's explanation of epidemics in his important medical manual, the *Qānūn fī ṭ-ṭibb*, is based primarily on Galen's work. In addition, the description by Ibn Sīnā of plague in various parts of the *Qānūn*[14] seems to show that he was familiar with the disease or had access to well-informed medical sources.[15] For he was able accurately to relate the plague symptoms in Arabic to their Greek terminology and to give the relevant medical treatment and remedies. From all indications, the influence of Ibn Sīnā's interpretation of plague was enormous in the Middle East, as well as in Europe. The *Qānūn* governed European medicine for several

[10] *Badhl*, fol. 13a; the author quotes Ibn Kathīr's *al-Bidāyah* that the epidemic corrupts the air consequently the humors (*Badhl*, fols. 11a-12a). He also cites al-Ghazzālī's *al-Iḥyā'* that the corrupt air does no harm when it meets the outside of the body, but the illness depends on the duration of its inhalation (*Badhl*, fol. 98a).

[11] *Muqni'at*, fol. 39b.

[12] *GAL, Supplement*, vol. 1, p. 366; see also Seidel, "Die Lehre von der Kontagion bei den Arabern," p. 85.

[13] *Kitāb fī l-i'dā'* ("On Infection") and *Kitāb fī l-wabā' wa asbābihi* ("On the Epidemic and Its Causes").

[14] *al-Qānūn fī ṭ-ṭibb* (Cairo, 1877), vol. 3, pp. 64-66, 121-122. Cf. Campbell, p. 77, n. 43 is clearly erroneous concerning Ibn Sīnā.

[15] Sticker, *Abhandlungen*, vol. 2, p. 37.

centuries after its translation by Gerard of Sabloneta in the thirteenth century. It has been recently stated, in a rather curious manner, that in the *Qānūn* of Ibn Sīnā "are to be found most of the germs of European medieval thought in regard to epidemiology."[16]

Ibn Khātimah, in his lengthy discussion of the corruption of the air, conveniently distinguishes for us the three remote causes of plague miasma frequently encountered in the medieval accounts: (1) the irregularity of the seasons, either in temperature, rains, or winds; (2) the putrid fumes arising from decaying matter on the earth; and (3) astrological events. The first explanation is considered by the author to be the most probable one for the pandemic. Ibn Khātimah drew this theory of natural causation of the disturbance of the four natural elements from Hippocrates.[17]

Evidence of these three beliefs, as well as an illustration of Ibn Sīnā's preponderant influence on later Arabic medicine, is apparent in the following quotation from Ibn Ḥajar's plague treatise. The Egyptian physician Ibn an-Nafīs, who wrote an important commentary (*Mūjaz al-qānūn*) on Ibn Sīnā's *al-Qānūn*,[18] is cited for his discussion of the causes of the plague miasma:

> The pestilence resulted from a corruption occurring in the substance of the air due to heavenly and terrestrial causes. In the earth the causes are brackish water and the many cadavers found in places of battle when the dead are not buried, and land which is water-logged and stagnant from

[16] C.E.A. Winslow, *The Conquest of Epidemic Diseases* (Princeton, 1943), p. 95. For example, the important plague treatise of Gentile of Foligno (*Consilia contra pestilentiam*, A.D. 1348) draws explicitly upon Arabic sources. Besides those of Ibn Sīnā, he utilized the works of 'Alī ibn 'Abbās al-Majūsī (Haly Abbas) and Abū Marwān Zuhr (Avenzoar). See Campbell, p. 60.

[17] *Tahsīl*, fols. 52a-56b. Ibn al-Khaṭīb denied the essential change in the nature of the air but was correct in interpreting the air as the vehicle for plague infection (*Muqni'at*, fol. 39b).

[18] *al-Qānūn*, vol. 3, pp. 64-65 (translated in Seidel, "Die Lehre von der Kontagion bei den Arabern," pp. 87-88): "Faṣl fī ḥummayāt al-wabā' wamā yujānisuhā wa-hiya ḥummā l-judarī wal-haṣbah."

rottenness, vermin, and frogs. As regards the heavenly air, the causes are the many shooting stars and meteorites at the end of the summer and in the autumn, the strong south and east winds in December and January, and when the signs of rain increase in the winter but it does not rain.[19]

Turning to Ibn Sīnā's original discussion of plague in the *Qānūn*, from which Ibn an-Nafīs and Ibn Khātimah drew their information, we find that Ibn Sīnā mentions as a sure sign of an approaching plague epidemic that rats and subterranean animals flee to the surface of the earth, behave as if they were intoxicated, and die.[20] Although this is an exact description of the effects of a plague epizootic, it was believed at that time that animals perceived the evil miasma before men; as *only* a forewarning of disease, creatures such as rats were observed to flee from the contaminated soil. In no case, either in the East or in the West, was the causal relationship between rats and plague recognized during the medieval period.[21]

[19] *Badhl*, fols. 13b-14a. The passage is frequently quoted by the Muslim authors in their treatises: *Kitāb ṭ-ṭibb*, fol. 144b; Ibn Abī Sharīf al-Kāmilī, *Kitāb fī aḥkām aṭ-ṭā'ūn*, Dār al-Kutub al-Miṣrīyah no. 102 *majāmī' m*, fols. 157a-157b.

[20] *al-Qānūn*, vol. 3, pp. 66 (quoted in *Badhl*, fol. 14a *et passim*). While Ibn Sīnā derived a large portion of his etiology of epidemics from Galen, as mentioned above, there is no observation by Galen of the behavior of rats, which are the essential vehicles of flea transmission. The question naturally arises: What was the source of this important observation? To repeat, there is no evidence that this phenomenon was derived by Ibn Sīnā from Galen (see Heinrich G. Schmitt, *Die Pest des Galenos*, diss., Medical Faculty, Würzburg, 1936). Therefore, the observation of the rats' behavior may have been taken from earlier Arabic medical commentaries on Galen, from non-medical writers, such as al-Jāḥiẓ, or was a genuine personal observation of Ibn Sīnā himself. From a different point of view, Major Greenwood maintains that Ibn Sīnā was merely applying the miasmatic theory to rodents since the miasma was believed to arise from the earth, and that he was, consequently, not recording an empirical fact (*Epidemics and Crowd-Diseases*, p. 295).

[21] See Otto Neustatter, "Mice in Plague Pictures," *The Journal of the Walters Art Gallery*, vol. 4 (1941), pp. 105-114.

On the basis of the idea of the terrestrial corruption of the air as expressed by these Arabic medical works, Ibn Khaldūn asserts that pestilences resulted from famines and the corruption of the air produced by over-population, according to his original theory of the dissolution of human society. Ibn Khaldūn writes:

> In the later [years] of dynasties, famines and pestilences become numerous. . . . The large number of pestilences has its reason in the large number of famines just mentioned. Or, it has its reason in the many disturbances that result from the disintegration of the dynasty. There is much unrest and bloodshed, and plagues occur. The principal reason for the latter is the corruption of the air [climate] through [too] large a civilization [population]. It results from the putrefaction and the many evil moistures with which [the air] has contact [in a dense civilization]. Now, air nourishes the animal spirit and is constantly with it. When it is corrupted, corruption affects the temper of [the spirit]. If the corruption is strong, the lung is afflicted with disease. This results in epidemics, which affect the lungs in particular.[22]

Because of Ibn Khaldūn's exposure to the Black Death in Tunis, it is very likely that he is referring specifically in the last two sentences to pneumonic plague. In any case, he observes the significant role of famines that have frequently preceded plague epidemics in the Middle East and North Africa. As for the underlying conception of the air and its corruption, certain classical ideas of epidemics, which we have already discussed, are clearly recognizable.

The cause of the poisonous miasma was also sought in unusual heavenly phenomena that preceded an epidemic. A remote cause of the great pestilences was considered to be the unfavorable conjunction of the major planets. The Arabs had previously developed the theory that the celestial bodies have an important effect on human activity, and their beliefs greatly

[22] *The Muqaddimah*, vol. 2, pp. 136-137.

influenced Western astrology.[23] The Middle Eastern astrologers attached particular importance to the conjunction of the planets in explaining pestilence and plague.[24] However, planetary ideas are present but not prominent in the plague treatises and accounts of the Black Death in the Middle East. This was due to the fact that the learned Muslim scholars and physicians of this period were generally opposed to such occult sciences as astrology. Ibn Khaldūn's attitude that astrology was incompatible with Islam may be representative of the opinion of the educated class.[25] Ibn Sīnā, particularly, gives only slight and obscure references to the remote influence of celestial conditions in his description of plague miasma because of his personal hostility toward astrology.[26] Discussion of astrology is found in the later plague treatises primarily in connection with magical beliefs and practices, which leads us to the suspicion that astrological explanations were popular

[23] Sarton, *Introduction*, vol. 2, part 1, pp. 91-93, 112. The foretelling of plague by atmospheric changes is discussed in detail by Ṭāshköprüzāde in his sixteenth-century treatise, *Majmūʿat ash-shifāʾ*, fol. 33a. Parenthetically, there is a modern medical interest in the effects of unusual celestial and terrestrial changes that precede epidemics, as before the Black Death. The science of epidemiology has yet to explain the difficult question of why an epidemic suddenly begins; earthquakes, floods, sun-spots, etc. may have an effect on the nature of plague bacilli. This belief had a strong influence on nineteenth-century historical studies; see, for example, V. Seibel, *Die Grosse Pest zur Zeit Justinians*, and *Die Epidemienperiode des fünften Jahrhundert vor Christus und die gleichzeitigen ungewöhnlichen Naturereignisse* (Dillingen, 1857).

[24] See Māshāʾallāh's "On Conjunctions, Religions, and Peoples," which influenced medieval European astrology; specifically, Māshāʾallāh ascribed the plagues in the ʿAbbāsid Period to the conjunction of Mercury with the other major planets (Saturn, Jupiter, and Mars): E. S. Kennedy and David Pingree, *The Astrological History of Māshāʾallāh* (Cambridge, Mass., 1971), text: fol. 217r; trans.: pp. 54-55. See also Ibn Khaldūn, *The Muqaddimah*, vol. 2, p. 213.

[25] *The Muqaddimah*, vol. 1, pp. lxxii-lxxiii; vol. 3, pp. 169, 246, 258-267.

[26] *al-Qānūn*, vol. 3, p. 65. Ibn Sīnā wrote a work expressly against the theory of astrological causation; see Ullmann, p. 254.

among the lower classes, although not with the treatise writers and physicians.

The Andalusian physicians mention astral influences perfunctorily as only a possible prior cause of plague. As Ibn al-Khaṭīb asserted, the ultimate cause of plague was a subject beyond the competence of most men to determine.[27] In marked contrast, the European writers attributed to the stars a primary role in the causation of the Black Death and subsequent epidemics.[28]

Alongside these terrestrial and celestial explanations for the causation of the pestilential miasma, an immediate cause was believed to be contagion, which was recognized by many Muslims, such as Ibn al-Khaṭīb, during the Black Death.[29] Although Ibn Khātimah denied the theory of contagion on religious grounds,[30] no other treatise contains clearer clinical evidence of the contagious nature of the pandemic. Contamination of the air, according to Ibn Khātimah, may arise from the sick and their clothing, bedding, and utensils. In an interesting illustration of contagion, Ibn Khātimah observed that among the inhabitants of the Sūq al-Khalq in Almería, where the flea-laden clothes and bedding of the sick were sold, almost everyone perished.[31] Similarly, Ibn al-Khaṭīb attributed the

[27] *Muqni'at*, fol. 39b.

[28] For the unfavorable conjunction of the planets, occurring in 1345, which was related by the European astrologers to the Black Death, see Campbell, pp. 16, 18, 22, 30-33, 37-44, 63, 65-68, 70, 74-76, and Lynn Thorndike, *History of Magic and Experimental Science* (New York, 1923-1958), vol. 3, pp. 224-232 *et passim*. Particularly influential on the European plague treatise writers was the *Compendium de Epidimia* issued by the medical faculty of the University of Paris in October, 1348, at the request of Philip VI of France (text: *AGM*, vol. 17, pp. 65-76). The European treatises commonly attribute to earthquakes as well the production of pestilences (Campbell, pp. 44-46, 55), but this cause is entirely lacking in the Arabic sources except for the plague treatise of al-Isbānī (see Appendix 3).

[29] For the European view of contagion, see Campbell, pp. 56-63.

[30] It has been suggested that Ibn al-Khatīb's treatise in defense of the theory of contagion was in reply to Ibn Khātimah's denial of contagion on religious grounds (*ibid.*, p. 28).

[31] *Tahsīl*, fol. 64b.

spread of the epidemic to men's coming into contact with the ill, their clothing and furnishings, and attending their funerals.[32]

Unlike all other Muslim commentators on plague, and possibly as a rebuttal to Ibn Khātimah's maintenance of orthodoxy specifically, Ibn al-Khaṭīb denied the *fatāwā* or legal decisions of the jurists against the theory of contagion and stated: "The existence of contagion is well-established through experience, research, sense perception, autopsy, and authenticated information, and this material is the proof."[33] He recognized that the plague outbreaks coincided with the arrival of contaminated men from lands where plague was raging. Some isolated communities, on the other hand, remained healthy, such as that of the Muslim prisoners in Seville, who were protected in prison while the city close-by was destroyed. More convincing proof to Ibn al-Khaṭīb were the reports of the nomadic Arabs in North Africa who remained uncontaminated.

Fighting *ḥadīth* with *ḥadīth*, Ibn al-Khaṭīb quoted the tradition about the owner of a flock of healthy animals who should not bring his herd near an owner of sick animals. He also cited the advice of the Caliph 'Umar, who was reported to have said during the plague of 'Amwās that one is justified in fleeing from a plague-stricken region to safety.[34] Although Ibn al-Khaṭīb did not develop a theory of contagion, as Jerome Francastor did in his famous *De Contagione* (1546), he did observe contagion-infection empirically. It should be borne in mind as well that Ibn al-Khaṭīb's treatise was conceived within

[32] *Muqni'at*, fol. 45b. Volney noted in the late eighteenth century the similar practice of selling the property of the plague dead in Istanbul. It was bought by merchants, who then took it to the bazaars of Alexandria; the merchandise, he believed, perhaps correctly, effectively spread plague to Egypt (*Voyage*, p. 242). See also Niemeyer, *Ägypten zur Zeit der Mamluken*, p. 109, for this practice among the Jewish merchants in Egypt.

[33] *Muqni'at*, fol. 42a.

[34] *Ibid.*, fols. 42b-43a; for the *hadīths*, see al-Bukhārī, *Le Recueil des traditions mahométanes*, ed. by M. L. Krehl and T. W. Juynboll (Leiden, 1862-1908), vol. 4, pp. 59-60.

the framework of the miasmic theory, which differs radically from modern germ theory of disease. In any case, the human transmission of plague as interpreted by Ibn al-Khaṭīb was unacceptable to the orthodox Muslim view of a divine act. The treatise is a clear example of innovation, at a time of crisis, within a traditional and authoritative body of thought. In general, Professor Hirst considers Ibn al-Khaṭīb's work as perhaps "the most instructive of all those treatises written about the Great Mortality."[35] But as a personal consequence, Ibn al-Khaṭīb's defense of the contagion theory is probably one of the portions of his writings which gave support to his enemies in their later persecution of him as a heretic.

The reason for this unorthodox belief in contagion-infection during the Black Death was undoubtedly the presence of highly infectious pneumonic plague. Whenever pneumonic plague has been predominant in a plague epidemic, it has naturally lent weight to a theory of contagion-infection over the purely miasmatic theory. The observable effect of pneumonic plague would be to increase the belief in the interhuman transmission of the disease as opposed to miasma. Contagion-infection could account for the spatial irregularity of plague incidence, which was always the major difficulty with the miasmatic theory. Because pneumonic plague recurred in the Middle East after the Black Death, the controversy over infection versus miasma was kept alive.

The debate lasted until the late nineteenth century in the Middle East.[36] The difference between the two views had considerable practical effect on the nature of preventive mea-

[35] Hirst, p. 51.

[36] *Ibid.*, pp. 283-296. A lively summary of the debate on plague in the nineteenth century may be found in E. H. Ackerknecht, "Anticontagionism Between 1821 and 1867," *Bulletin of the History of Medicine*, vol. 22 (1948), pp. 562-593. I was very fortunate during my research in Cairo (1969-1970) to benefit from the work of Dr. Laverne Kunke, who was preparing her dissertation on "The Introduction of Preventive Medicine in Egypt in the Nineteenth Century" for the University of Chicago. Her discussion of plague is in many ways a natural sequel to the present study.

sures. It can only be remarked here that the last serious medical dispute regarding the nature of plague and its prevention arose at the time of the Egyptian plague epidemic of 1834-1835. The leading exponent of the miasmatic theory was Clot-Bey, the pioneer of western medicine in Egypt under Muḥammad 'Alī; a large part of the European community in Egypt upheld the contagion theory and, hence, believed firmly in the value of traditional methods of quarantine.[37] Because of the irregularities of plague incidence and its restriction to certain geographical areas, such as the Middle East, from the time of the Black Death to the nineteenth century, the miasmatic theory was refined over time according to a number of "localist" theories: the belief that the miasmatic poison arose from particularly unhealthy regions. In this manner, Clot-Bey was a true disciple of Galen, Ibn Sīnā, and Sydenham. Consistent with the medieval Muslim plague treatises, the only prevention against the pestilential effluvium was to change the air by some type of fumigation or possibly by flight to an uncontaminated area.[38]

These two rather crude conceptions of the nature of plague were constantly reiterated and refined in the Arabic plague treatises especially because flight from plague and the belief in contagion were proscribed by Muslim religious law. There were naturally a number of compromise explanations presented. Some contagionists held that the sick could radiate contagion through the air in their immediate vicinity and thus set up a kind of local miasma. This seems to be the case with Ibn al-Khaṭīb's interpretation. The miasmatists were willing to admit a limited degree of contagion at the acme of a severe epidemic, which usually included infectious pneumonic plague.

Whether plague was considered contagious or not, the Arabic historical and literary accounts of the Black Death clearly attest to the belief that plague resulted from an atmospheric miasma. Writing about the origin of the Black Death,

[37] Hirst, pp. 65-72.
[38] Ibn Sīnā, *al-Qānūn*, vol. 1, p. 182.

al-Maqrīzī echoes Ibn Sīnā when he states: "The wind transmitted the stench of these cadavers [Khiṭai and Mongols] across the world. When this empoisoned blast dwelt on a city, an encampment, or some region, it struck with death both men and beasts at the same instant."[39] Referring to the inhabitants of the Mediterranean islands, the same chronicler attributes the death to a wind coming from the open sea; anyone who breathed this wind fell down, stricken by plague, and struck his head against the earth until death ensued.[40] Such a terrible wind was also considered to have stopped a group of Arabs from North Africa in their attack on Christian Spain after plague had greatly weakened the Christian army.[41]

A well-known incident occurred in Damascus during the height of the Black Death. According to Ibn Abī Ḥajalah, who witnessed the plague in the Syrian capital, the plague "blew with the blowing of the wind" in Egypt and Syria.[42] On Tuesday, 12 Rajab 749/6 October 1348,[43] following the afternoon call to prayer,

> there appeared a mighty wind which provoked a great yellow dust cloud, then red, then black until the earth was darkened by it entirely and the people remained in it for nearly three hours. They turned to God Almighty and begged His forgiveness. And the people hoped that this cataclysm marked the end of their distress. But the number of deaths did not decrease; it did not prevent a terrible mortality.[44]

[39] *as-Sulūk*, part 2, vol. 3, p. 773. Ibn al-Khaṭīb also places the origin of plague in the Far East, where it resulted from decaying corpses on the battlefields that corrupted the air (*Muqni'at*, fol. 43b). See also the late fifteenth-century *Risālah fī taḍ'īf al-madhbah* by Luṭfallāh at-Tūqātī, Istanbul MS no. 3596, fol. 4b or Leiden MS no. 1229, fol. 15b.

[40] *as-Sulūk*, part 2, vol. 3, p. 776.

[41] *Ibid.*

[42] *Daf' an-niqmah*, fols. 74b, 75a, 85b.

[43] *al-Bidāyah*, vol. 14, p. 228, where the date is given as Rajab 11.

[44] *Daf' an-niqmah*, fol. 75b. The account with modifications is also found in *al-Bidāyah*, vol. 14, p. 228; *as-Sulūk*, part 2, vol. 3, p. 779; and *Badhl*, fol. 128b.

Another witness of the Black Death in Damascus in 749/1348-1349, aṣ-Ṣafadī, used a mélange of metaphors to describe plague. In one instance, he addressed the plague: "Oh, how many times have we seen your wind blowing through us—the wind which drives the mills of plague!"[45] Ibn Ḥabīb quotes the poetry of aṣ-Ṣafadī that plague encircled Damascus and would kill with its smell.[46]

Similarly, it was reported that during a plague epidemic in Cairo in Rabīʿ I, 790/March-April 1388, a great wind with dust blew so that it nearly blinded the people in the roads, and plague increased during this month.[47] The plague epidemic of 806/1403-1404 in Cairo was also observed to follow immediately after the blowing of a southern wind that was very cold and wet.[48]

A noteworthy example of this belief in miasma is a statement by Ibn Abī Ḥajalah about the plague epidemic of 764/1362-1363. He tells us that he had seen Arabic books in Egypt which related that near the well-known mosque of at-Tannūr on the Muqaṭṭam Hills, overlooking Cairo from the east, fires were lit at times of plague. Usually, when the people of Cairo saw these fires, they knew that the sultan was planning to leave the Citadel on an expedition, and they would prepare for him. But the sultan also would have fires kindled with tamarisk and *bān* or *ṣadrūs* to take away the pestilential air from the city.[49] During the Black Death in Europe, Gentile of Foligno recommended to his fellow Perugians various remedies, including building fires in the streets.[50] Likewise, bonfires were set in London at the end of the Great Plague of 1665, and

[45] Dār al-Kutub al-Miṣrīyah MS no. 102 *majāmīʿ m*, fol. 198b.

[46] *Durrat al-aslāk*, p. 359.

[47] Ibn Hajar, *Inbāʾ al-ghumr bi-anbāʾ al-ʿumr* (Cairo, 1969-1972), vol. 1, pp. 350, 353-354.

[48] *Ibid.*, vol. 2, p. 260; see also *an-Nujūm*, Popper trans., vol. 14, p. 80.

[49] *Jiwār al-akhyār*, fol. 86a, and *Kitāb aṭ-ṭibb*, fol. 143a.

[50] Campbell, p. 68.

in the towns of Austria and Germany.[51] This practice is almost certainly derived from Galen, who attributed to Hippocrates the instructions to build fires throughout the city during the great Athenian pestilence to purify the polluted air.[52]

Finally, there was a common belief among Muslims that plague was caused by evil jinn or demons that attacked mankind directly. This view is found in the religio-legal treatises, especially in the tract of Ibn Ḥajar, and is most vividly illustrated in the popular magical beliefs and practices.[53]

2. Prevention

The clearest evidence for the widespread belief in the miasmatic theory of plague at the time of the Black Death is the prophylaxes recommended by the contemporary authors. Since a good Muslim was ideally not supposed to flee if he found himself in a plague-stricken land, there may have been an additional emphasis in the non-medical as well as the strictly medical works on ways to improve his fate. In any case, the extensive advice for prevention and treatment suggests what was common medical practice in medieval Muslim society.

It must be mentioned at the outset in a discussion of plague prevention that a number of writers of plague treatises, particularly the Andalusian doctors, felt compelled to argue for the acceptability and benefit of medicine itself in understand-

[51] Hirst, p. 44; see also Campbell, p. 41, and Shrewsbury, *A History of Bubonic Plague*, pp. 190, 461.

[52] *Medicorum*, vol. 14, p. 281, which attributes to Hippocrates the advice to build fires throughout the city during the Athenian pestilence and to cast on the fires flowers and wreaths. Ibn Sīnā apparently does not mention the use of such fires.

[53] A comparable interpretation of demons as the vehicle of pestilence in medieval Europe is presented by Marsilio Ficino (d. 1499); see Thorndike, *History of Magic*, vol. 4, p. 564. In attempting to account for Chaucer's relative silence about plague, Shrewsbury states "that in adult life he believed in the superstition of the personification of pestilential disease—which was a common aberration of the public mind up to the eighteenth century—in which case the less he said about plague the better it would be for his personal safety." (*A History of Bubonic Plague*, pp. 41-42.)

ing and treating plague. This was opposed to the fatalistic view that plague was sent by God and should be simply endured. Because of this pervasive attitude, most of the Muslim authors recommended penance, supplication, and prayer along with their medical instructions.

Because they have a common source, the Middle Eastern and Andalusian remedies for plague are very similar in nature. This common source of information for prevention and treatment, often poorly distinguished in the plague treatises, was of course the classical texts or the derivative advice of Arabic doctors, primarily Ibn Sīnā's *al-Qānūn*[54] or one of the numerous commentaries on his work.[55] In addition to relying on the counsel of Ibn Sīnā, one treatise explicitly draws its preventive measures from the early 'Abbāsid physician, Yūḥannā ibn Māsawayh (d. 243/857), who suggested the sucking of an acrid pomegranate or plum at the time of an epidemic and the eating of lentils, Indian peas, and pumpkin seeds to guard oneself from plague. Further, one should drink sour fluids such as juices from lemons and pomegranates, grapes and onions. The treatise writer comments that eating a pickled onion every day before breakfast would certainly prevent a person's being struck by plague.[56] Such unappetizing remedies are fairly typical of methods of plague prevention found in the treatises.

Ibn Khātimah gives a more detailed discussion of preventive medicine; he lists six ways that would both improve the air and make men's bodies more resistant to the disease.[57] Con-

[54] *al-Qānūn*, vol. 1, p. 182.

[55] Ibn Abī Ḥajalah explicitly takes his remedies from Ibn Sīnā, Ibn an-Nafīs, and Ibn al-Akfānī (*Kitāb aṭ-ṭibb*, fols. 142b-143b). Cf. *Badhl*, fol. 113b; al-Hijāzī, *Juz' fī ṭ-ṭā'ūn*, fol. 154b; Tāshköprüzāde, fols. 35a, 36b; and Ibn Abī Sharīf al-Kāmilī, *Kitāb fī aḥkām aṭ-ṭā'ūn*, fol. 157b. See also Ata, "Évolution de la médicine en turquie," p. 100.

[56] Ṭāshköprüzāde, fol. 35a.

[57] *Taḥṣīl*, fols. 65a-69b. The third Andalusian physician, ash-Shaqūrī, discusses prophylaxes and treatment in his treatise, *Taḥqīq an-naba' 'an amr al-waba'* (see Appendix 3). While very similar to Ibn Khātimah's medical advice, it is entirely a layman's guide to plague prevention and treatment. This unpublished work was probably written during or

cerning the air, one should seek fresh air, live in a house facing north, and surround oneself with cool fragrances of flowers such as myrtle and eastern aspen. A house and its occupants should be sprinkled with rosewater mixed with vinegar. One should rub his face and hands with other scents as citron, lemon, and cool flowers such as roses and violets. It is recommended that one burn sandalwood together with some aloes-wood and drink a mixture of aloes-wood with rosewater. Also, one should guard against the sun, warm winds, ovens, etc.[58]

One of the earliest Arabic medical compendia, written by 'Alī ibn Rabban aṭ-Ṭabarī (d. 240/855), relates from Hippocrates that sweet-smelling shrubs should be piled up around the cities and towns; thereby the scent would prevent the pestilential air from reaching the inhabitants.[59] According to a late fifteenth-century account of plague, the open places were believed to be deadly during an epidemic; to stay indoors was considered preferable. The places of smoke and dirt were supposed to be effective against the plague miasma, apparently because of their stronger stench. A popular proverb was that dirty areas were the most healthful places during an epidemic![60]

---

shortly after the Black Death while the author was in Granada. Because this opuscule has never been the subject of any investigation, it may be useful to outline its contents. The author begins by saying that it is permissible for Muslims to use medicine and that it does not violate God's order. Plague is caused by a corruption sent to the stable air, and it is detestable that most people are not usually conscious of the air and the need for it. After these remarks (fols. 106b-107b), the treatise is devoted to the improvement of the air (fols. 107b-108b) and the improvement of the human body by nutrition and medicine (fols. 108b-110b), with a digression on matters that do not necessitate consulting a doctor (fols. 110b-111a). The digression includes a number of magical practices.

[58] Cf. the similar preventive measures recommended by al-Majūsī, *Kitāb al-malakī*, vol. 2, pp. 62-65.

[59] Ullmann, p. 244. This was also advised by Ibn Khātimah.

[60] al-Manṣūrī, Dār al-Kutub al-Miṣrīyah MS no. 102 *majāmī' m*, fol. 201b.

Because of his belief in the theory of contagion, Ibn al-Khaṭīb naturally suggested avoiding congested areas, where one suspected a corruption of the air by the plague-stricken and their clothing and utensils.[61] As-Subkī stated that he saw the people prohibited from visiting the sick during the Black Death to the point that no one visited the afflicted, but Ibn Ḥajar denied this.[62] Ibn Abī Ḥajalah, who witnessed the Black Death in Damascus, directed the reader of his treatise not to sit too close to the ill because the corruption of the air by the sick was the reason for infection. He cites as support for this advice the interesting tradition of the Prophet that the Prophet found leprosy on a new wife and sent her away immediately.[63]

The second factor for the prevention of plague infection, according to Ibn Khātimah, is to keep oneself as quiet as possible and to be moderate in movement, so as to avoid accelerating one's breathing. In another plague treatise, the *'ulamā'* or Muslim scholars are said to have argued in favor of the traditional prohibition against fleeing because traveling would excite the humors and make one more vulnerable to the disease.[64]

Third, Ibn Khātimah suggests that one should take care with his diet, as in the choice of bread—coarse bread is better than fine and black better than coarse.[65] Certain meats are beneficial, especially when cooked with lemon, sour citron, and grape leaves, and served with vinegar. Fruits are recommended, such as pears and pomegranates, but particularly plums and white grapes. Corn bread and everything made from corn should be avoided as well as all heavy foods such as thick broths, oatmeal, gruel, biscuits, mushrooms, and cheese-like foods. All old slaughtered meat should be avoided, along

[61] *Taḥṣīl*, fol. 4a.

[62] *Badhl*, fol. 114b. It should be recalled that Ibn Ḥajar was not a witness to the Black Death but wrote his treatise in the first half of the fifteenth century.

[63] *Kitāb aṭ-ṭibb*, fol. 142b. [64] *Ibid.*

[65] See Campbell's brief comparison of Christian and Muslim treatises with regard to diet, pp. 74-76.

with eggplant, cabbage, and garlic. One should not sleep after eating and should not miss meals or eat at irregular hours. Fresh, sweet, clear-flowing water from a spring is highly desirable. Ibn Khātimah also urges a number of concoctions, such as a daily drachma of syrup of basil, which the author himself had tried. Barley water, vinegar mixed with water, and most fruit juices would aid in calming the flow of blood and cool the body's bile. Furthermore, drinking Armenian clay is recommended on the authority of Galen.[66]

This last preventive measure is another example of the considerable influence of Galen in medieval Islamic medicine,[67] as well as of human credulity. Armenian bole is an argillaceous earth brought primarily from Persia and Armenia; its deep red color is due to iron oxide in the clay. Galen had first advised the use of Armenian bole as an astringent for wounds and ulcers before he advocated it as a specific for pestilence.[68] He recommended it as an anti-pestilential specific in his *De simplicium medicamentorum temperamentis et facultatibus libri* (Book 11, Chapter 1): "All those who used it were promptly cured. Those who felt no effect from it died; no other remedy could replace it, . . . those with whom this remedy failed were incurable."[69]

[66] *Taḥṣīl*, fol. 66b.

[67] See Ibn Khaldūn, *The Muqaddimah*, vol. 3, p. 149.

[68] Hirst, p. 43; Crawfurd, *Plague and Pestilence*, p. 74; *Oxford English Dictionary*: "bole." The whole subject of earth-eating is exhaustively treated by Berthold Laufer in his monograph, "Geophagy," *Field Museum of Natural History*, Publication no. 280, Anthropological Ser., vol. 18, no. 2 (Chicago, 1930), pp. 101-198, especially pp. 150-155 for this phenomenon among the Persians and Arabs. On the various types of edible clays, particularly Armenian clay for plague, see Ibn al-Bayṭār (d. 646/1248), *Jāmi' fī ṭ-ṭibb* (*GAL*, vol. 1, p. 492; L. Leclerc, trans., *Traité des simples* [Paris, 1881], vol. 2, pp. 421-427; cf. Carra de Vaux, *Les Penseurs de l'Islam* [Paris, 1921], vol. 2, pp. 289-296). Ibn al-Bayṭār cites Isḥāq ibn Imrān (*GAL*, vol. 1, p. 232, *Supplement*, vol. 1, p. 417), a tenth-century physician, that Armenian earth was salutary in cases of plague, being taken both internally and externally.

[69] *Medicorum*, vol. 12.

Armenian clay was used for both prevention and treatment of plague victims. Ibn Sīnā suggests using clay on the buboes,[70] and al-Maqrīzī is possibly referring to Armenian clay when he says that "some people devoted themselves to coating their bodies with clay" during the Black Death in Cairo.[71] This use of clays is included by Ibn al-Wardī in his description of the remedies contrived by "the nobles of Aleppo studying their inscrutable books of medicine" during the Black Death. He tells us that these doctors, too, advised smearing the buboes with Armenian clay.[72]

As for the later plague treatises, Ibn Haydūr suggests the general employment of Armenian clay.[73] Ibn Abī Ḥajalah states in his plague tractate, written shortly after the Black Death, that healing clay is "useful to drink for the plague, such as Armenian [clay] and blue bdellium."[74] The desirability of drinking Armenian clay with water and vinegar, as advocated by Galen, along with other healing clays, is still to be found in a sixteenth-century plague treatise.[75] Leo Africanus also witnessed the use of Armenian clay in North Africa during plague epidemics in the early sixteenth century.[76]

The utilization of Armenian bole for plague was known in Europe as well. Guy de Chauliac, the physician of Pope Clement VI, recommended consoling the bodily humors with this clay during the Black Death in Avignon.[77] The Medical

[70] *al-Qānūn*, vol. 3, p. 222. For other references to Armenian clay in Arabic medicine, see Dorothee Thies, *Die Lehren der arabischen Mediziner Tabari und Ibn Hubal über Herz, Lunge, Gallenblase und Milz* (Bonn, 1968), p. 176; the work contains a helpful appendix of Muslim *materia medica* ("Alphabetisches Verzeichnis der auftretenden Medikamente"). See also al-Majūsī, *Kitāb al-malakī*, vol. 2, p. 62.

[71] *as-Sulūk*, part 2, vol. 3, p. 763. [72] *Risālat an-naba'*, p. 186.

[73] Ibn Haydūr at-Tādalī, *Risālah fī al-amrāḍ al-waba'īyah al-kā'inah 'an fasād al-aghdhiyah*, Dār al-Kutub al-Miṣrīyah MS no. 183 *majāmī' m*, fol. 105b.

[74] *Kitāb at-tibb*, fol. 143a; the author took the information from Ibn al-Akfānī.

[75] Tāshköprüzāde, fols. 34b, 35a, 36b-37a.

[76] Quoted in Marchika, *La Peste en Afrique Septentrionale*, p. 14.

[77] Crawfurd, *Plague and Pestilence*, p. 12.

Faculty of the University of Paris in its official pronouncement on the Black Death gives a number of recipes for "smelling apples," which were carried in the hand and frequently inhaled to strengthen the principal organs.[78] The simplest recipe for these nosegays was taken from the Arabic physician, Yūḥannā ibn Māsawayh (John Mesuë). He had prescribed:

> Equal parts of black pepper, and red and white sandal, two parts of roses, half a part of camphor, and four parts of bol armeniac. All but the camphor are to be ground very fine, sifted and shaken, pounded during a week with rosewater, then the camphor mixed with them, and the apples made with paste of gum arabic and rosewater.[79]

Aside from Armenian bole, Ibn Haydūr prescribed another typical preventive concoction to ward off plague. One should take two parts of aloes and one part each of myrrh and saffron and heat them together. Then take a small *dirhem*'s weight of the mixture with an ounce of sweet basil every day. The author tried it, and he knew of no one who had followed this prescription and died of plague.[80]

According to Ibn Khātimah, men should avoid the permitted wines[81] as well as the prohibited wines, all kinds of milk because of the fermentation, and bad water. Fourth, it is

[78] See John M. Riddle, "Pomum ambrae. Amber and Ambergris in Plague Remedies," *Sudhoffs Archiv*, vol. 48, part 2 (June, 1964), pp. 111-122.

[79] Campbell, p. 68. Derived from a Latin translation of the *Qānūn* or from Galen directly is a fourteenth-century recipe for a plague preventive sent to the friars of Tegernsee; it contained Armenian bole together with *terra sigillata* moistened with citrus juice ("Ueber die grossen Seuchen," p. 103). Armenian bole continued to be used in Europe after the Black Death as a plague treatment; see J.-N. Biraben, "La Peste dans l'Europe Occidentale et le Bassin Méditérranéen," *Concours Medical*, vol. 35 (Paris, 1963), p. 789.

[80] *Risālah fī al-amrāḍ*, fol. 106a. This antidote is ascribed to Galen in Ṭāshköprüzāde, fol. 35b, in addition to a large number of various other concoctions.

[81] *nabīdh*: a beverage made of dates or raisins; before it ferments, it is a lawful drink.

best to get a normal night's sleep with the room open to the north wind. Fifth, whoever is exposed to plague should avoid constipation by eating cooked plums, violets, tamarind, etc. Baths and cohabitation should be avoided, while bloodletting is strongly recommended.[82]

Last and very interesting is Ibn Khātimah's psychological advice in order to maintain morale. It is best for the spirit to experience joy, serenity, relaxation, and hope; one should seek pleasant and attractive company—the best companion being the Qur'ān. Otherwise, there were history books, humorous works, and love stories to occupy the mind. Men should avoid talking about anything that would evoke sadness, and should refrain from all excitement. These measures, warns the author, should not be neglected because one believed that everything depended on God.

3. Treatment

Ibn Sīnā recommended bloodletting of the plague victim to relieve his fever and the excess of blood in the body.[83] Bloodletting was apparently quite common during the Black Death. Ibn Khātimah advocated it for the plague-stricken because the bad air increased the burning of the heart and thus increased the mass of blood that the heart could not control. According to this author, by decreasing the quantity of blood, bloodletting frees the life-force in the arteries. Ibn Khātimah had seen people having as much as eight pounds of blood drawn during the Black Death, although the usual amount was about five pounds. He himself had, at first, hesitated to prescribe it, but he tried it and was satisfied with its effects.[84]

> After people learned this and saw its effects, they began to have bleeding done for themselves, without medical prescription, several times a month, without consideration or fear, without feeling harm or weakness, and without contracting sickness in consequence.[85]

[82] *Taḥṣīl*, fols. 67a-68b. [83] *al-Qānūn*, vol. 3, p. 122.
[84] *Taḥṣīl*, fols. 68b-69b; see also *Muqni'at*, fol. 40a.
[85] Quoted in Campbell, pp. 72-73.

Ibn Khātimah recommended venisection and cupping for the treatment of plague victims, as well as for its preventive qualities. The victim should immediately be given a mixture of two ounces of both vinegar syrup and rose syrup and then be bled where the pain was most severe, but if the illness recurred or the patient had been in contact with the sick, there was little chance of curing him.[86]

Ibn Haydūr, writing in the half-century after the Black Death, saw no objection in bloodletting to relieve the plague-stricken. Ibn Ḥajar also believed in the utility of bleeding. He informs us that all the doctors of his time (d. 852/1449) and before him had completely ignored this measure advised by Ibn Sīnā. According to Ibn Ḥajar, they did not treat the plague victims with bloodletting because, until it became common among the people, they thought it was prohibited by religion.[87] A sixteenth-century plague treatise[88] cites Ibn Sīnā as well in favor of bloodletting during an epidemic, together with the same advice from Abū Hāmid Najīb ad-Dīn as-Samarkandī (d. 619/1222).[89]

There is surprisingly little information concerning the excising of the plague buboes in the Arabic sources, but it seems to have been common practice. Ibn Sīnā had recommended their removal if possible.[90] Ṭāshköprüzāde (d. 968/1560) mentions that the Turks did not consider the plague boils different from any other boils and simply cut them away immediately, and nothing remained except the scars of the surgery. This had been tried on a friend of the author's, and it had been successful. The writer related that a Turkish student had cut out a plague boil on his body, and the writer had seen the green-colored gland that had been removed.[91]

A number of remedies to be placed on the plague boils were

[86] *Taḥṣīl*, fols. 74a-75a; see also Campbell, pp. 86-88.

[87] *Badhl*, fol. 113b. Cf. Thorndike, *History of Magic*, vol. 4, p. 219.

[88] Ṭāshköprüzāde, fol. 36b.

[89] *GAL*, vol. 1, p. 491.

[90] *al-Qānūn*, vol. 3, p. 122. Cf. Galen, *Medicorum*, vol. 19, p. 524.

[91] Ṭāshköprüzāde, fol. 37b.

suggested. Besides Armenian clay, which has been discussed, Ibn Sīnā advised bathing the bubo with a sponge soaked in water and vinegar or oil of roses, apples, mastic, or myrtle. When the bubo suppurated, it should be bathed with camomile water, dill, and other delicate ointments.[92] While some recommended a great deal of cold water to relieve the pain of the boils, others placed the yolk of an egg on the bubo. When the yolk dried, it was expected to heal the boil.[93]

Ibn Ḥajar and others believed that nothing was more beneficial than violets which, in various forms, should be rubbed on the body or drunk.[94] Al-Ghazzalī is reported to have taken the advice of ash-Shāfi'ī that nothing that the latter had seen was more advantageous during an epidemic than violets rubbed on a patient or drunk.[95] As-Suyūṭī (d. 911/1505) questioned ash-Shāfi'ī's recommendation of violets as being applicable not to plague, but to another epidemic disease. However, as-Suyūṭī admitted that the people during his own lifetime used the ointment of violets to stop the disease at its advent.[96] A plague treatise written in Egypt as late as 1125/1713-1714 still regarded violets as the best treatment for the plague victim.[97]

In general, Ibn Sīnā urged those things for the plague-stricken that would preserve and strengthen the heart—for example, cooling fruit juices, scents such as roses, camphor, and sandal, and foods such as lentils with vinegar and meats cooked in vinegar. The frequent recommendation of fruit juices as a cure was probably due to its efficacy as a thirst-quencher, for dehydration was an invariable and distressing concomitant of the hyperpyrexia of bubonic plague. In addition, the bed of the ill should be covered with leaves of the

92 *al-Qānūn*, vol. 3, p. 22.

93 Tāshköprüzāde, fol. 37b.

94 *Badhl*, fol. 44b; al-Ḥijāzī, *Juz' fī ṭ-ṭibb*, fol. 151b; Ibn Haydūr, *Risālah fī amrāḍ*, fol. 105a.

95 Ṭāshköprüzāde, fol. 35a.

96 *Mā rawāhu l-wā'ūn*, p. 154.

97 'Abd al-Mu'ṭī as-Saḥalāwī, *Risālah taṭhīr ahl al-Islām biṭ-ṭa'n waṭ-ṭā'ūn al-'āmm*, Ṭanṭā Library (Egypt), section *kha*, no. 275, fol. 4a.

khilāf tree, violets, roses, white-lilies, and other flowers. And cool, strong "coatings," presumably plasters, should be placed over the heart.[98]

Ibn Khātimah offered a large number of treatments for the plague fever, the buboes, and the pustules.[99] The general prognosis depended on the symptoms; both Ibn Khātimah and Ibn al-Khaṭīb despaired of any remedy when the victim began to spit blood, indicating pneumonic plague. Nevertheless, their fellow countryman, ash-Shaqūrī, strongly warned that a doctor like himself should be consulted in any case where a person had contracted the disease:

> The men of religion and reason, who were appointed to deal with the affairs of the Muslims, should prevent the people of ignorance and adventure from harming the people by giving them medicines and bleeding them without consulting the doctors. . . . What would harm the druggist or the bloodletter if they acted according to the doctor's opinion![100]

Furthermore, a doctor is the best judge of compound medicines and their proper use for serious illnesses such as plague. In another plague treatise, Yūḥannā Ibn Māsawayh is quoted for his advocacy of simple, rather than compound, drugs for plague.[101]

Looking back from our vantage-point of modern science, it is impossible not to feel a certain impatience—but also a certain sympathy—with the largely futile advocacy of useless and

[98] *al-Qānūn*, vol. 3, p. 122.

[99] *Tahsīl*, fols. 69b-83b. Galen's theory of "contraries" is conspicuous in the Muslim plague treatises. According to this belief, a hot fever during an epidemic should be alleviated by a cooling remedy. To cite Galen on general diseases: "Let us suppose, for instance, that we want to cure a hot disease without realizing that first, to cure it, we need to know that opposites cure opposites. For it has been clearly shown that this knowledge is the all-embracing general preliminary to everything that is known about types of therapy." (Malcolm Lyons, *Galen on the Parts of Medicine* [Berlin, 1969], pp. 46-47.)

[100] *Tahqīq*, fols. 110a-110b.

[101] Ṭāshköprüzāde, fol. 35b.

sometimes harmful remedies that were earnestly devised. The medical and legal treatises must reflect what was, to some degree, actual practice during the calamity. Yet a writer at the time of the plague epidemics in the late fifteenth century perfunctorily mentions a number of such remedies but concludes with the adage: "For every disease there is medicine to cure it except for madness, plague and old age."[102]

B. RELIGIOUS INTERPRETATION

Along with the naturalistic views of plague, a consensus of orthodox Muslim belief may be extracted from the plague treatises. It must be borne in mind that the religio-legal conceptualization of the disease imposed itself on the imagination of all those who dealt with the problem of plague epidemics. Thus, the religious interpretation should not be understood as distinct from the naturalistic point of view—no matter how incongruous—nor should the religious explanation be considered a wholly static one.

The religious attitudes toward plague changed and provoked continual controversy until modern times. The debated points of interpretation, which have already been discussed, were the following three major tenets:

1. A Muslim should not enter or flee from a plague-stricken land.
2. The plague is a martyrdom and a mercy from God for a Muslim and a punishment for an infidel.
3. There is no infection (contagion).

These principles were operative in Muslim society from an early time, as we have seen, when plague appeared in the newly established Muslim empire in the Middle East. This is particularly clear in the case of the plague of 'Amwās,[1] which itself affected later interpretations of plague.

[102] al-Manṣūrī. Dār al-Kutub al-Miṣrīyah MS no. 102 *majāmī' m*, fol. 201b.

[1] See chap. II.

Despite the difficulty of the first *ḥadīth* or tradition for later generations, who were naturally anxious to avoid plague, the prohibition against flight appears to be a pragmatic medical principle, rather than a strictly theological one. It may argue historically for the recognition of contagion-infection in the plague epidemics that afflicted the early Muslims and the desire to limit the spread of epidemics. Theologically, the principle is consistent with the belief that God sent his mercy and martyrdom in the form of plague, which was not considered to be infectious, to a specifically favored community.

The principle that there was no contagion-infection among men should be interpreted from a theological point of view: only God can cause plague or other diseases. This belief, however, impinged on the presentation of the physicians' clinical observations of plague that demonstrated its contagious nature. We have seen how Ibn Khātimah felt constrained to accept this tenet as established by the *Sharī'ah* or Muslim Law in opposition to his empirical perception of the Black Death,[2] while his colleague, Ibn al-Khaṭīb, stood foursquare against the religious establishment by arguing in favor of contagion. In all three tenets, there is a tension between what the traditions prescribed and what may have been actually observed and felt by a Muslim community subjected to a plague epidemic.

Perhaps the best manner of grasping the predominantly religio-legal interpretations of the Muslim plague treatises, which deal with these principles and their ramifications, is to describe fully one of them as a representative type.

Ibn Ḥajar al-'Asqalānī's plague treatise, *Badhl al-mā'ūn fī faḍl aṭ-ṭā'ūn*,[3] is a good example of this literature because it presents the fullest explanation of the relevant tenets of ortho-

[2] *Taḥṣīl*, fols. 83b-90b, 92a-105a. The author's discussion of this tenet as well as the others has been completely omitted from Dinānah's translation of the text.

[3] as-Sakhāwī, *al-Jawāhir wad-durar fī tarjamat Shaykh al-Islām Ibn Ḥajar*, Paris MS no. 2105, fol. 153a; *GAL*, vol. 2, p. 82; Sabri K. Kawash, "Ibn Ḥajar al-'Asqalānī (A.D. 1372-1449): A Study of the Background, Education, and Career of an 'Ālim in Egypt," unpubl. diss., Princeton University, 1969, p. 196.

dox Islam on plague, based on the collation of the early *ḥadīth* literature, as well as the consideration of contemporary medical and theological views evolved during the Black Death.[4] The author classified his treatise as a work of *furū'* or "applied ethics"[5] (consisting of the systematic elaboration of canonical law in Islam). The treatise was written as a direct result of plague's reappearance during the author's lifetime. He tells us that he had drafted a work on the plague epidemic of 819/1416 but rewrote it much later. We know that Ibn Ḥajar himself was struck by plague when it occurred in Egypt in 848/1444.[6] On the night of Sunday, 5 Ṣafar/24 May, he felt a pain under his right arm, where a boil grew as large as a peach. It disappeared completely by the tenth of the same month.[7] Since the latest date of the work is 848/1444, the final revision may be dated within the four years before his death in 852/1449.[8] The plague treatise is divided into five chapters and an epilogue. The epilogue is an historical account of the occurrences of plague in Islamic history and is a common feature of the

[4] The plague treatises, in general, should be viewed within the context of an Islamic tradition of religio-legal learning. The medical traditions of the Prophet and his companions hold an important position in the history of Islamic medicine. This accounts for the remarkable amalgam of religio-legal scholarship and medical knowledge found in the works of the *'ulamā'*, known as "prophetic medicine" (*aṭ-ṭibb an-nabawī*). See the discussion of Ata, "Évolution de la médicine en turquie," p. 101, and Ullmann, pp. 17-20, 185-189. Muḥammad may have taken a number of his medical ideas from al-Ḥārith ibn al-Kaladah (d. ca. A.D. 634) of aṭ-Tā'if, who studied at Jundishāpūr and was known as "the doctor of the Arabs" (Ibn Abī Uṣaybi'ah, *'Uyūn al-anbā' fī ṭabaqāt al-aṭibbā'*, ed. by A. Müller [Cairo, 1882], vol. 1, pp. 109, 113).

[5] *Badhl*, fol. 109b.

[6] Most of the contemporary Arabic authors were personally affected by the plague epidemics. During the epidemic of 819/1416-1417, Ibn Hajar relates that two of his daughters died (*Inbā' al-ghumr*, British Museum Add. MS no. 7321, fol. 228a) and his eldest daughter, Zayn Khātūn, died in the epidemic of 833/1429-1430 (Kawash, "Ibn Ḥajar al-'Asqalānī," p. 59).

[7] É. M. Quatremère, *Histoire des Sultans Mamlouks de l'Égypte* (Paris, 1837-1845), vol. 1, p. 216.

[8] See Appendix 3.

plague treatises in the Middle East. A detailed examination of this work furnishes, in varying degrees, the normative conceptualization of plague and helps to explain, in part, the Muslim social response to the disease.

The first chapter discusses the early history of plague. The disease is considered a punishment by God on mankind before the advent of Islam.[9] The author draws on traditions derived from the Old Testament prophets to show God's heavy punishment in the form of plagues, particularly on the people of Israel.[10] For example, David's numbering of his people offended God, and in retribution for his presumption, David was given the choice of enduring seven years of famine, three months of flight before his enemies, or three days of pestilence. He chose the pestilence, and seven thousand people died.[11] The story is also related of God's punishment of the Pharaoh for not giving Moses and Aaron freedom to leave Egypt.[12] And finally, Ibn Ḥajar gives an account of God's chastisement of the Israelites by plague for their whoredom with the daughters of Moab.[13]

On the other hand, plague is considered a mercy and a martyrdom for the people of Muḥammad and a punishment for the infidel.[14] A number of pious traditions are cited to substantiate this claim, which is the major theological invention of the Muslim theologians and is, to my knowledge, unique in Semitic religions.[15] It avoids the difficulty of explaining an evil

[9] *Badhl*, fols. 3b-6a.

[10] *Ibid.*, fols. 7a-10b.

[11] *Ibid.*, fol. 7b. 1 Chron. 21.

[12] *Ibid.*, fol. 8a. Qur'ān 7:133-135. Exodus 9:8-11: "And the Lord said unto Moses and unto Aaron, Take to you handfuls of ashes of the furnace, and let Moses sprinkle it toward the heaven in the sight of Pharaoh. And it shall become small dust in all the land of Egypt, and shall be a boil breaking forth with blains upon men, and upon beasts, throughout the land of Egypt." It is a curious coincidence that the year of the plague of 'Amwās (A.H. 18) was called by the Arabs "the Year of the Ashes."

[13] *Ibid.*, fol. 8b. Qur'ān 2:59; Numbers 25:1-9.

[14] *Ibid.*, fols. 6a-7a.

[15] al-Bukhārī, *Le Recueil des traditions mahométanes*, vol. 2, p. 209, nos. 1 and 2; vol. 4, p. 60, nos. 5 and 6.

incompatible with God's nature. The primary emphasis, as the third chapter of the treatise makes clear, is the desirability of this martyrdom by plague.[16] In the customary list of the five Muslim martyrdoms, death by plague and by battle are always included;[17] they are equal in God's favor, and the believer is assured of reaching paradise.[18]

It is no accident that the descriptive terminology of plague is closely related to the terms of the actual *jihād* or holy war. The ideology of the *jihād* possibly served as a conscious and useful analogy for the Muslim jurists when they confronted the issue of plague. For example, in the account of 'Umar and the plague of 'Amwās the medieval scholars strongly disagreed with 'Umar's decision to withdraw Abū 'Ubaydah from the plague menace. They related the tradition of 'Ā'ishah, the Prophet's wife, that fleeing from plague was like fleeing from the army,[19] and whoever stayed in the time of plague was like a *murābiṭ*.[20]

The correlation between the holy war and plague is most clearly seen in the important tradition of the Prophet: "The destruction of my nation will be by piercing (*ṭa'n*) and plague (*ṭā'ūn*)." That is to say, the end of the Muslim people will be by martyrdom through battle and plague.[21] Another example of this equation is a tradition of the Prophet:

> The martyrs and those who died in their beds argue with our Lord about those who were killed by the plague. The martyrs say, our brothers died as we died. The deceased on their beds say, our brothers died on their beds as we died. Our Lord said: Consider their wounds which resemble the wounds of the slaughtered, and they are among them. And behold, their wounds had been similar; so they joined the martyrs.[22]

[16] *Badhl*, fols. 46b-63a.
[17] *Ibid.*, fols. 46b-49a.
[18] *Ibid.*, fols. 50a-54a.
[19] *Ibid.*, fol. 85a.
[20] *Ibid.*, fol. 86a.
[21] *Ibid.*, fols. 11b-12a. I have followed Ibn Ḥajar's interpretation of the *ḥadīth*.
[22] *Kitāb aṭ-ṭibb*, fol. 145b.

However, not all of the Muslim scholars considered plague as a mercy and a martyrdom. Ibn al-Wardī laments during the Black Death in Aleppo: "We ask God's forgiveness for our souls' bad inclination; the plague is surely part of His punishment." With an inconsistency which belies the tension between emotion and reason, Ibn al-Wardī claims as well that plague is a martyrdom and a reward for a Muslim despite his sins, while death by plague is a punishment for the disbelievers.[23] Ibn Abī Ḥajalah argues that the ultimate reason for plague is God's punishment of His people for their sins, such as adultery, usury, drinking alcohol, and so forth.[24] This certainly finds support in the historical accounts that relate the renewed enforcement of Muslim laws, particularly against alcohol and moral laxity, during periods of plague epidemics.[25]

A striking illustration of this idea of punishment took place during the plague epidemic of 841/1438 in Egypt. After the reading of the *Ṣaḥīḥ* of al-Bukhārī in the Citadel, Sultan Barsbay asked the assembled judges, jurists, and scholars whether men's sins were being punished by God with plague. One suggested that plague was caused by fornication and blatant prostitution. After vehement discussion, the sultan suggested prohibiting all women from going out into the streets. The next day, the council agreed on this measure, and a proclamation was made in Cairo, Fusṭāṭ, and the suburbs. A woman who left her house was consequently threatened with all kinds of maltreatment and even death. The sultan appointed a ruthless market inspector (who died a month later of plague) to enforce the prohibition, despite numerous complaints. After widespread suffering, the sultan proclaimed that female slaves could go to the markets for necessities, but their faces must be unveiled, so that no one could use the veil as a disguise. He also allowed old women to go out to the markets, and women

[23] *Risālat an-naba'*, p. 187.
[24] *Kitāb aṭ-ṭibb*, fols. 143b-144b.
[25] *Badhl*, fols. 6a-7a, 122b; *Daf' an-niqmah*, fols. 42a-43a; Ibn Ḥajar, *Inbā' al-ghumr*, vol. 1, p. 351; *as-Sulūk*, part 2, vol. 3, p. 777, and part 4, vol. 2, pp. 1031-1033; Sauvaget, "Décrets Mamelouks de Syrie," *Bulletin d'Études Orientales*, vol. 2 (Damascus, 1932), pp. 11-15, 24.

might go to the baths but not stay in them until nightfall. The plague increased, and the women were further distressed by not being permitted to attend the funerals of their children and relatives. Ibn Taghrī Birdī, a contemporary historian, comments that this decree was the result of the ineptitude of the sultan and the bad judgment of his officials, for "surely the virtuous woman is recognized even if she is in a tavern, and a harlot is recognized even if she is in the Sacred House."[26]

During this same epidemic, the sultan was dying, and he assembled the mamlūk army before him at the Duhayshah Gate, overlooking the Sultan's Park.[27] He cursed them for what they had done during his rule and said that God had sent plague epidemics in 833/1429-1430 and again in 841/1438 because of their crimes and corruption; as a result, large numbers of the mamlūks had perished. He then forgave them their misdeeds.[28] At this time, he reappointed our author, Ibn Ḥajar, to the office of Shāfi'ite grand *qāḍī* (judge) of Egypt because the sultan believed that the plague and his own illness resulted from selling this office to the previous incumbent.[29]

This belief in men's suffering and misfortune because of God's anger at their moral offenses is a very old one and was the preeminent medieval Christian interpretation, based on the Bible as well as on Greek and Roman literature.[30]

The second chapter of Ibn Ḥajar's treatise is devoted to the etymology of "plague" (*ṭā'ūn*)[31] and a description of the symptoms of the various forms of plague.[32] Ibn Ḥajar and

[26] *an-Nujūm*, Popper trans., vol. 18, pp. 146-147. This story appears in Ibn Ḥajar, *Inbā' al-ghumr*, British Museum MS no. 7321, fol. 332a, and in *as-Sulūk*, part 4, vol. 2, pp. 1031-1033.

[27] *Systematic Notes*, vol. 15, p. 22 and map no. 7.

[28] *an-Nujūm*, Popper trans., vol. 18, p. 153.

[29] Kawash, "Ibn Ḥajar al-'Asqalānī," p. 164.

[30] Seidel, "Die Lehre von der Kontagion bei den Arabern," p. 81; Hirst, pp. 6-16; Deaux, *The Black Death 1347*, pp. 8-17, 41; Ziegler, pp. 35-39, 260; Crawfurd, *Plague and Pestilence*, pp. 22-23; Millard Meiss, *Painting in Florence and Siena after the Black Death* (New York, 1964), pp. 75-78.

[31] See Appendix 2.

[32] *Badhl*, fols. 11b-16b.

other writers generally made a distinction between plague and other communicable diseases; the latter were referred to as *waba'*, "an epidemic" or "a pestilence."[33]

Unlike most of the Muslim and Christian writers on plague in the wake of the Black Death, Ibn Ḥajar attributes the immediate cause of plague almost exclusively to the jinn[34] rather than to the corruption of the atmosphere by a miasma; in one form or another, the idea of the miasma was the predominant theory of plague until the late nineteenth century.[35] In this instance, Ibn Abī Ḥajalah's treatise is more representative of the Muslim plague treatises in his presentation of miasma as the chief cause of plague, an ascription he derived from Ibn Sīnā and Ibn an-Nafīs.[36] Although Ibn Ḥajar is aware of the atmospheric theory, he is equally conscious of its defects. He reasonably asks why a plague miasma would appear in a place with a healthful climate; why it strikes one house and not its neighbor, or only one member of a household and not another; and why it attacks different parts of the body, unlike other diseases carried by the air.[37] The inability of the miasmatic theory to account satisfactorily for spatial irregularity in

[33] See Appendix 2.

[34] See *djinn* in Sir Hamilton Gibb and J. H. Kramers, *Shorter Encyclopaedia of Islam* (Leiden, 1953) and *genii* in T. P. Hughes, *A Dictionary of Islam* (London, 1896); Ernst Zbinden, *Die Djinn des Islam und der altorientalische geisterglaube* (Berne, 1953); B. A. Donaldson, *The Wild Rue* (London, 1938), chap. 3; Edward Westermarck, "The Belief in Spirits in Morocco," *Acta Academiae Aboensis Humaniora,* vol. 1, pp. 1-167. Von Kremer maintains that the idea of the jinn as the vehicle of plague had died out completely and was replaced by the idea of divine retribution in the later Middle Ages ("Ueber die grossen Seuchen," p. 102). This is clearly erroneous and specifically refuted by Ibn Ḥajar's discussion of the jinn and the magical practices and beliefs that existed in the later Middle Ages. See also *Daf' an-niqmah,* fols. 42a-55a, 71a.

[35] *Badhl,* fols. 15a-37a. See Seidel, "Die Lehre von der Kontagion bei den Arabern," p. 82 for a thirteenth-century example of pestilence being attributed to jinn.

[36] *Kitāb aṭ-ṭibb,* fols. 143a, 144b; and *Daf' an-niqmah,* fols. 55a-59b.

[37] *Badhl,* fol. 15b; see also *Taḥṣīl,* fols. 59b-63b.

the distribution of plague has always been the greatest weakness of this ancient hypothesis. Ibn Ḥajar believes that there is no contradiction between his explanation and the physicians' miasmatic interpretation, because both held that the disease is caused by a poisonous matter which excited the blood. However, our author asserts that this was the result of the internal piercing of the jinn. The basic tradition for his interpretation is the report of the Prophet:

> The destruction of my people is by the piercing and the plague. It was said: "Oh Prophet of God, this piercing we have known but what is the plague?" He said: "The pricking of your enemies is from the jinn and in everyone it is a martyrdom."[38]

The significance of the jinn as the agents of plague has ancient precedents in the Near East. Demons were accused of generating plagues in ancient Babylonia: Namtar, demon of pestilences, would periodically emerge from hell and roam the streets at night afflicting men.[39] The jinn and their poisonous arrows in Muslim literature—found in pre-Islamic poetry and in the Qur'ān[40]—are paralleled by the angel, in Christian literature and iconography, whose drawn sword is the specific device for striking mankind; its sheathing is the sign of the epidemic's termination.[41] From ancient to modern times, plague has been portrayed in the West by heavenly angels with swords, arrows, or fuming vessels; the iconography is usually derived from Biblical sources, especially David's vision of the angel with a drawn sword stretching over Jerusalem.[42] In 680, good and evil angels were said to have wandered through the streets of Pavia at night. At the command of the good angel, the evil angel pierced the doors of certain houses

[38] *Badhl*, fols. 17a-21b. Ibn Hajar examines all the versions and *isnāds* of this "interrupted" *ḥadīth*. See also Ullmann, p. 19.

[39] Hirst, p. 1.

[40] Especially Qur'ān 72; see Zbinden, *Die Djinn des Islam*, pp. 75-96.

[41] Crawfurd, *Plague and Pestilence*, pp. 10, 19, 91.

[42] 1 Chron. 21.

with a spear so that the inhabitants would fall ill of plague and die.[43] Similarly, during the siege of Kaffa in 1346, the beleaguered Christians saw the heavenly arrows strike the Mongols and cause the Black Death.

Although Islamic art lacks the vivid artistic representation of plague jinn, Ibn Abī Ḥajalah notes the belief in jinn at the time of a plague epidemic:

> In these days [Jumādā II, 764/March-April 1363] the entire story had recurred in dreams of the jinn with lances in their hands with which they pierce mankind. Some people had seen them doing this when they awoke, and more than one had reported this to me.[44]

Ibn al-Khaṭīb speaks of "the sword of the plague" over the people of Andalusia.[45] Concerning the plague of 864/1459-1460 in Egypt, Ibn Taghrī Birdī states: "Death was sweeping them away and the blessings of God were upon our master Izrā'il [the angel of death]."[46]

The popular belief in the jinn as the agents of plague is well attested by the common man's magical practices and tales. One legend relates the story of a peasant of Bilbais, in Lower Egypt, who mysteriously visited the jinn in the underworld, where they were preparing their arrows of plague. He was told that one-third of the inhabitants of Bilbais would be destroyed by plague, but not himself and his family. When he returned to his village, he found that the jinn had inflicted plague on its people, as he had been told.[47] The same belief in jinn was observed in Morocco at the beginning of this century; the jinn were held responsible for plague and other epidemics because of their shooting poisoned arrows at their victims.[48]

[43] Crawfurd, *Plague and Pestilence,* p. 95.

[44] *Kitāb aṭ-ṭibb,* fol. 145b.

[45] *Muqni'at,* fol. 42b.

[46] *an-Nujūm,* Popper trans., vol. 22, p. 95.

[47] René Basset, *Mille et un contes, récits de légendes Arabes* (Paris, 1924), vol. 1, pp. 123-125.

[48] Westermarck, *Ritual and Belief in Morocco* (London, 1926), vol. 1, p. 271.

The fourth chapter of Ibn Ḥajar's treatise concerns the prohibition against leaving a land that has been stricken by plague or entering a plague-stricken land.[49] Ibn Ḥajar draws support for this proscription from the story of 'Umar and Abū 'Ubaydah, in spite of the evacuation of the army from 'Amwās. The author disapproves both of the analogy of as-Subkī that flight was justified, as one would flee an enemy or lion he could not face,[50] and of the analogy of az-Zarkashī[51] that one was justified in fleeing from lepers.[52] Most of the commentators, however, agreed with Ibn Ḥajar about the prohibition against fleeing; for example, Ibn Abī Ḥajalah states that it was necessary to remain at home, for otherwise the epidemic would only increase in intensity and scope.[53] In contrast to the Muslim interdiction, flight was universally counseled by the European Christian tractators.[54]

Subsequently, Ibn Ḥajar presents the orthodox view that there is no infection. Pestilence must be from God alone. Following one tradition, a bedouin asked the Prophet: "Oh Envoy of God, how do you explain that my camels were as healthy as gazelles, and then a mangy camel comes, mixes with them, and makes them mangy?" Rejecting the implied belief in contagion-infection, the Prophet answered: "Who infected the first camel?"[55] Muḥammad is, furthermore, supposed to have denied the pre-Islamic Arab belief in infection.[56] The orthodox position is summed up by Ibn Ḥajar in the *ḥadīth*: "No contagion, no augury, no ill omen."[57]

The last chapter of the treatise deals with what is prescribed

[49] al-Bukhārī, *Le Recueil des traditions mahométanes*, vol. 4, p. 59, no. 1; p. 60, no. 3.

[50] *Badhl*, fol. 91b.

[51] *Ibid.*, fol. 92a.

[52] "Flee before the lepers as you flee before the lions" (al-Bukhārī, *Le Recueil des traditions mahométanes*, vol. 4, p. 55).

[53] *Daf' an-niqmah*, fol. 85a.

[54] Campbell, p. 65.

[55] *Badhl*, fol. 93b. See al-Bukhārī, *Le Recueil des traditions mahométanes*, vol. 4, p. 55.

[56] *Badhl*, fol. 101a.

[57] *Ibid.*, fols. 96a, 101b: *lā 'adwā wa lā ṭīrah wa lā hāmah.* See Ullmann, p. 243, n. 6.

for the Muslim once plague has occurred.[58] Ibn Ḥajar advises prayer and repentance, in groups and individually, for the lifting of the epidemic. All the plague treatises recommend prayer and offer formulae for it, particularly specific verses from the Qur'ān. There is some disagreement among the legal schools about the form of the supplicatory prayers. Ibn Ḥajar did not initially approve of the prayer ritual for the raising of plague based on the ritual for rain (*ṣalāt al-istisqā'*), which consisted of fasting and going out into the desert in procession to pray. He considered it an innovation when the ritual took place at the time of the Black Death in Damascus, without any precedent in *ḥadīth*.[59] Yet during the great plague of 833/1429-1430, Ibn Ḥajar agreed to its legality with the other religious teachers in Egypt.[60] It became a common practice in Egypt in the fourteenth and fifteenth centuries.[61] In addition, Ibn Ḥajar does not approve of the visions of the Prophet and the recommended prayers that were allegedly received by a number of Muslims during the plague epidemics.[62]

Ibn Ḥajar then gives a perfunctory list of medical treatments[63] and a number of prayer formulae for the afflicted (one of which is remarkably similar to the Lord's Prayer).[64] Altogether, he recommends patience,[65] piety, and the visiting of the sick. Furthermore, Muslims are not to curse one another with plague.[66] The prohibition seems to indicate simply that it was not an uncommon curse.[67] In present-day Cairo, one Egyptian may say to another: "kubbah"—"a plague on you," and the other may reply: "kubbatyn" —"two plague boils on you!"

[58] *Badhl*, fols. 101b-120a.

[59] *Ibid.*, fols. 108b-109a, 110a.

[60] *Ibid.*, fol. 109a.

[61] The ritual is fully described in *as-Sulūk*, part 2, vol. 3, pp. 787-788; *al-Bidāyah*, vol. 14, p. 226; and *Daf' an-niqmah*, fol. 75b.

[62] *Badhl*, fols. 110b-111a.

[63] *Ibid.*, fols. 113b-114a.

[64] *Ibid.*, fol. 116a.

[65] See al-Bukhārī, *Le Recueil des traditions mahométanes*, vol. 4, p. 60, no. 1.

[66] *Badhl*, fol. 103b.

[67] For example, see the curse of plague recorded from Tangiers by Westermarck, *Ritual and Belief in Morocco*, vol. 1, p. 481.

In this final chapter of his treatise, Ibn Ḥajar includes a discussion of Shaykh Walī ad-Dīn al-Malawī's essay *Ḥall al-ḥibā'*.[68] Al-Malawī questions the utility of beseeching God to raise plague and nicely plays the devil's advocate to much of Ibn Ḥajar's academic interpretation of plague. For, as al-Malawī argues, there is an obvious contradiction in praying for the lifting of plague if it is a martyrdom and a mercy from God. Is such prayer not a fleeing from what has been predestined? Is such prayer not opposed to the Prophet's desire for his nation? Although Ibn Ḥajar answers the questions, they legitimately pull his views back to reality.

Another plague treatise quotes al-Ghazzalī's resolution of this theological problem posed by al-Malawī. Al-Ghazzalī, one of the great theologians of Islam (d. 1111), argues that prayer to repulse plague is *part* of what has been predestined by God along with plague itself. He uses the metaphor of an arrow whose head is prayer and whose shaft is the epidemic disease. In other words, even if one accepts divine predestination, he does not go unarmed into battle.[69]

In sum, Ibn Ḥajar's plague treatise is only one example of the many attempts that were made in the wake of the Black Death to harmonize the contradictory *ḥadīths* concerning plague and infection, which date from the theological discussions of the ninth century, and to provide a thorough religious interpretation of plague for co-religionists.

C. MAGICAL BELIEFS AND PRACTICES

In general, the magical beliefs and practices indicate a common need to supplement or replace inadequate medical knowledge with supernatural devices for protection and relief from plague. These beliefs and practices may be said to be a popular extension of the Muslim religion: in most cases, we find that the incantations and charms are drawn primarily from traditional Islamic sources, as Ibn Ḥajar's treatise demonstrates. The use of magic actually reinforces the contention that religious influence was paramount in any attempt to under-

[68] *Badhl*, fols. 103b-104a.

[69] Tāshköprüzāde, fol. 40b.

stand the nature of plague and combat its effects: God was ultimately responsible for sending the disease and consequently was the only one who could remove it.

Magic played a significant role in the popular response to the Black Death. Similar to the medical discussions of plague, the recommendations of magic in the plague treatises must reflect, to a great extent, the actual practice of many Muslims, regardless of the limited historical observations of its use. Islam had inherited through late Judaism and Christianity that most fateful legacy of Zoroastrian Persia: a belief in the absolute division of the spiritual world between good and evil powers, between angels and demons. We have only to be reminded that the success of early Christianity was due principally to its attacks on men's invisible enemies, the demons, through exorcism and miracles of healing.[1] The spread of Islam, at least initially, cannot be similarly explained, but Islam became intimately associated with popular magical beliefs and practices during the medieval period. To the problem of evil, the Muslim belief in jinn offered an answer designed to relieve nameless anxiety; Muslims focused this anxiety on the jinn, and at the same time Islam offered a remedy for it. Thus, the magical practices directed against plague were not unique phenomena; they were only a part of a vast body of supernatural beliefs and practices that surrounded and sustained men's lives in a hostile world.

The magical beliefs took the form of specific prayers or incantations (which should be said at a certain time and in a certain manner) and magical objects, such as inscriptions and talismans—a Greek word coming into English through Arabic.[2] Many of these esoteric practices are related to "letter

[1] Peter Brown, *The World of Late Antiquity:* A.D. *150-750* (London, 1971), p. 55.

[2] The only example of an amulet specifically directed against an epidemic, to my knowledge, is one illustrated in Rudolf Kriss and Hubert Kriss-Heinrich, *Volksglaube im Bereich des Islam* (Wiesbaden, 1960-1962), vol. 2, plate 78 nos. 1A and 1R; description, p. 93. The common use of amulets against plague and other maladies is noted, but no examples are given in M. Reinaud, *Description des monumens musulmans de cabinet de M. Le Duc de Blacas* (Paris, 1828), vol. 1, p. 62.

magic,"[3] which is the use of the Arabic language against evil; the sacredness of Arabic and its magical qualities were "early and inseparable properties of writing."[4] However, Ibn Khaldūn, who probably witnessed a number of such exorcisms[5] during the Black Death, gives a salutory warning to whoever wishes to understand letter magic: "It is an unfathomable subject with innumerable problems."[6] For this reason, the object of the following discussion is merely to describe a number of the magical instructions related directly to plague, rather than to hazard an interpretation of their meaning.[7] Again, the value of such description is that it signifies practices that were an important element, together with strictly medical and religious activities, in men's reaction to plague.

The advocacy of supplicatory prayers with suggested texts and cryptograms is a common feature of many plague treatises for both the prevention and alleviation of plague.[8] A particularly full exposition of such practices is to be found in the sixteenth-century plague tract, *Majmū'at ash-shifā' li-adwiyat*

[3] See *EI*²: "Ḥurūf" (T. Fahd).

[4] Rosenthal, *Four Essays on Art and Literature in Islam*, p. 53.

[5] See *EI*²: "Djafr" (T. Fahd).

[6] *The Muqaddimah*, vol. 3, p. 172. The section on magic and sorcery (vol. 3, pp. 156-226) is an excellent introduction to these occult beliefs both because of its clarity and because it was written during the period immediately following the Black Death. See also Kriss, *Volksglaube*, especially vol. 2, chap. 2; James Robson, "Magic Cures in Popular Islam," *Moslem World*, vol. 24 (1934), pp. 33-43 (based primarily on Ahmad ad-Dayrabī [d. 1151/1738], *Kitāb al-mujarrabāt* [Cairo, n.d.]); Lane, *Arabian Society in the Middle Ages*, pp. 80-96; Ullmann, pp. 251-254, and *Die Natur- und Geheimwissenschaften im Islam* (Leiden, 1972), chap. 6 (the author notes especially on p. 389 the use of amulets to expel plague from inhabited places advocated by ar-Rāzī in his *Kitāb as-sirr al-maktūm fī mukhāṭabat an-nujūm*).

[7] Arabic magic has not been adequately studied. Such investigation, in turn, must await the systematic study of pre-Islamic magic, particularly in Egypt the pharaonic magical texts; see J. F. Borghouts, "Magical Texts," *Textes et Langages de l'Égypte Pharaonique*, IFAO, vol. 64, no. 3 (Cairo, 1972), pp. 7-19.

[8] I have been unable to see the work by Ibn Kamāl Pāshā, *Rāhat al-arwāh fī daf' 'āhāt al-ashbāh*, which is reported to contain a large number of prayers and magical practices (Ullmann, p. 248).

al-wabā', by Ṭāshköprüzāde.[9] At the beginning, the author warns the reader that he should not neglect the customary prayers in favor of the specific magical prayers and rituals that the treatise suggests. One should clean one's body and house, give alms, and settle any debts to assist the prayers against the disease. It is advised that a Muslim should repeat the special prayers according to the number of words in the prayer; and if more prayers were needed, the prayer should be repeated according to the number of letters in the prayer. Devotions were best said at dawn and on Friday at suitable places.[10]

These prayers and inscriptions frequently employed the divine names of God (*al-asmā' al-ḥusnā'*),[11] which have occult properties. Most of the Arabic authors have drawn their information directly from the major work on the magical use of these divine names, *Shams al-ma'ārif al-kubrā*, by Aḥmad ibn 'Alī al-Būnī (d. ca. 622/1225).[12] Al-Būnī was one of the most important Muslim writers on occult sciences and is still employed by present-day exorcists. He furnishes the forms for magic squares, cabalistic letters, and talismanic signs which may be employed against plague.

An example from al-Būnī's manual may be helpful. Two of the divine names of God, "the Giver of life and death" (*al-mumīt wal-muḥyī*), al-Būnī states are particularly effective in warding off plague.[13] The two names should be recited or written on a square made of gold, silver, or parchment. The

[9] Fols. 37b-41b. For a comparable European plague treatise that contains magical remedies, see the dual work on pestilence and poisons in the *Summa* of Antonius Guaynerius, written shortly before 1444 (Thorndike, *The History of Magic*, vol. 4, pp. 215-231).

[10] Ṭāshköprüzāde, fols. 38b-39b.

[11] See *EI*[2] (L. Gardet); Kriss, *Volksglaube*, vol. 2, pp. 68-91; E. W. Lane, *An Account of the Manners and Customs of the Modern Egyptians* (London, 1895), p. 257.

[12] Cairo, n.d. *GAL*, vol. 1, p. 498; Ullmann, p. 249. A later source than al-Būnī for magical practices that was cited in plague treatises was al-Bisṭāmī (d. 858/1454): *Bahr al-wuqūf fī 'ilm al-hurūf*, and *Shams al-āfāq fī 'ilm al-hurūf wal-aufāq* (*GAL*, vol. 2, p. 232, nos. 20 and 21).

[13] *Shams al-ma'ārif al-kubrā*, part 4, pp. 74-75.

author supplies the following cryptogram (Fig. 1), composed of the letters of the two divine names in addition to the prayer which should be recited using God's names.

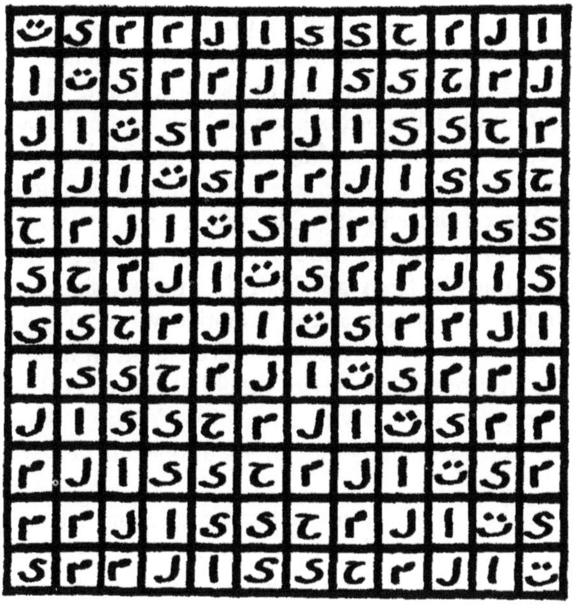

Figure 1.

Most of the recommended prayers in the plague treatises are in the common form of "seeking refuge" (*isti'ādhah, iltijā'ah*) with God, based on portions of the Qur'ān, which are felt to be efficacious against disease or hardship.[14] Naturally, the Qur'ān was the primary source for such prayers and magical devices. The basis for the belief that the Qur'ān was itself a cure against illness is given in the Qur'ān: "We send down [verses of] the Qur'ān which is a healing [*shifā'*] and a mercy to the believer."[15]

[14] See Jan Knappert, *Swahili Islamic Poetry* (Leiden, 1971), vol. 1, p. 87, and C. E. Padwick, *Muslim Devotions* (London, 1961), chap. 6.
[15] Qur'ān 17:82.

A handbook for the appropriate use of short Qur'ānic verses for healing was *ad-Dā' wad-dawā'* by Shams ad-Dīn al-Jauzīyah az-Zar'ī (d. 751/1350).[16] Certain *sūrahs* or chapters of the Qur'ān are specifically mentioned. For example, it was beneficial to read after every obligatory prayer the *sūrat al-ikhlāṣ*[17] eleven times with enthusiasm and *al-mu'awwidhatayn*[18] and the *sūrat al-kāfirīn*[19] once in the proper succession. Then one was to spit on the palm of his hand and wipe it on his body.[20] Ibn Ḥajar recommended reading the verse entitled *al-kursī* or "Throne Verse"[21] in a house for three consecutive nights, to prevent plague from entering. He also advised the repetition of *subḥānallāh* ("Glory to God") in treating plague victims, according to advice from ash-Shāfi'ī.[22] Further, six Qur'ānic verses known collectively as the "curative verses" (*āyāt ash-shifā'*) were considered especially effective in warding off sickness or disease.[23] These verses should be recited at the time of a plague epidemic,[24] as well as the *sūrat Yūnus*,[25] the *sūrat al-an'ām*,[26] and particularly the *fātiḥah* or opening verse of the Qur'ān.[27]

Many of these verses were used for inscriptions on amulets and talismans, besides the divine names. The *fātiḥah* and other verses were highly recommended for being written on the inner surface of earthenware cups and bowls. After water had been placed in the vessel and the verse written in ink had dissolved, the water had magical qualities against plague if it

[16] *GAL*, vol. 2, p. 106; *Supplement*, vol. 2, p. 127.

[17] Qur'ān 112.

[18] The two verses from the Qur'ān 113 and 114: "Say: 'I take refuge with the Lord of the Daybreak,'" and "Say: 'I take refuge with the Lord of the people.'"

[19] Qur'ān 109.

[20] Ṭāshköprüzāde, fols. 41b-42a.

[21] Qur'ān 2:255.

[22] *Badhl*, fols. 40a-44b.

[23] Lane, *Manners and Customs*, pp. 260-261.

[24] Tāshköprüzāde, fol. 41b.

[25] Qur'ān 10. Ṭāshköprüzāde, fol. 46b; Ibn Haydūr, *Risālah fī l-amrāḍ*, fol. 104b.

[26] Qur'ān 6. Tāshköprüzāde, fol. 43a.

[27] Ṭāshköprüzāde, fol. 42b.

were drunk or used for bathing.[28] Some of the religious teachers said that when someone wrote the *fātiḥah* on paper at the hour of Venus and washed it in water and then sprinkled it on the face of the sick, the patient would be cured of the disease.[29]

Typical of the recommendation of such prayers from the Qur'ān is the advice taken from Shihāb ad-Dīn 'Umar as-Suhrawardī: "I heard that the reading of the *sūrat al-burūj*[30] at the noon prayer saves one from the plague boils [*damāmīl*], and whoever recited the *salām* aloud in the time of an epidemic twenty-eight times every day is safe from the plagues."[31] The complete reading of the Qur'ān itself during a week, beginning on a Friday and ending on the following Thursday, was strongly suggested.[32]

A large number of prayers to avert plague were taken from non-Qur'ānic sources. Some were derived from the sayings of the Prophet and his companions, as well as from later scholars and religious men such as ash-Shāfi'ī. It is evident that many of the special prayers originated from specific outbreaks of plague in the period following the Plague of Justinian.[33] The prayer of the Persian *ḥadīth* scholar aṣ-Ṣābūnī, who died of plague in 449/1057, is representative.[34] Aṣ-Ṣābūnī saw the Prophet in a dream and complained to him about the disease. God gave him a prayer to recite over water placed in a new cup and instructed him to drink the water when the epidemic occurred.[35] A number of similar prayers are reported to be the result of seeing the Prophet in a vision or dream at the time of the Black Death.

A prayer commonly used during the Black Death was the following:

28 *Ibid.*, fol. 42b; see Lane, *Manners and Customs*, pp. 263-264.

29 Ṭāshköprüzāde, fol. 42b.

30 Qur'ān 85.

31 Ṭāshköprüzāde, fol. 42a.

32 *Ibid.*, fol. 43a.

33 *Ibid.*, fols. 46b, 50a.

34 *GAL*, vol. 1, p. 362.

35 Ṭāshköprüzāde, fols. 46b-47a is followed by a large number of prayers (fols. 47a-56b).

> Oh God, allay the fearful stroke of the lord of al-Jabarūt[36] by Thy descending kindness which comes from the abundance of heaven, so that we may cling to the coat-tails of Your kindness. We seek refuge with You from the events of Your power. You are the omnipotent and universal power. There is no power and strength save in God Almighty.[37]

This should be said every day during a plague epidemic. Ibn Haydūr in his plague treatise instructed his reader to write this prayer on strips of paper and attach them to the walls of one's house so that plague would not strike his home.[38]

Other short prayers usually begin by invoking God by one of His divine names, as was mentioned in the discussion of al-Būnī. These prayers should be repeated a specified number of times every day. For example, whoever said: "The Eternal, there is no destruction and cessation of His kingdom" every day 136 times would be saved from the disease.[39] Whoever repeated the various names of God, such as "the Preserving" every day 898 times or "the Vigilant" 312 times, would be safe. If a Muslim were devout and repeated "the Subduer" over the ill 2142 times, plague would depart.[40] The divine name "the Believer" was considered by some to be the most beneficial during a plague epidemic and should be repeated 136 times a day, but if necessary 299 times a day. Further, it was advisable to put this word into a square and engrave it on a square piece of silver, and the talisman would ward off the evil when it was carried.[41] Likewise, an early eighteenth-century Egyptian plague tract commends the following talismans (Figs. 2 and

[36] See *EI*²: " 'ālam" (L. Gardet).

[37] Ṭāshköprüzāde, fols. 45b, 46a; Lutfallāh aṭ-Ṭuqātī, *Risālah fī tadʿif al-madhbah*, Istanbul MS no. 3596, fol. 8b; *as-Sulūk*, part 2, vol. 3, p. 780; Ibn Haydūr, *Risālah fī l-amrāḍ*, fol. 104a gives a longer version of the same prayer and comments that it is a famous prayer related from the Prophet.

[38] *Risālah fī l-amrāḍ*, fol. 104a.

[39] Lutfallāh aṭ-Ṭuqātī, *Risālah fī tadʿif al-madhbah*, fols. 8b-9a.

[40] *Ibid.*, fol. 9a.

[41] Tāshköprüzāde, fol. 44a.

يا مقتدر	يا رقيب
يا عظيم	يا خلاق

Figure 2

3) with the names of God; carrying them would guard the wearer against plague. The second (Fig. 3) should be drawn on Tuesday before the noon prayer.[42]

Other beatific names were used in magical practices. The name "the Healer" (*ash-shāfī*) should be written on a piece of parchment or the skin of a gourd, placed in violet ointment

يا مغيث	يا رقيب
يا عليم	يا خلاق

Figure 3

and then hung in the sun for forty days. At the same time the name should be recited every day 391 times over this ointment. Then, whoever was smeared with the ointment would be safe from plague during the year.[43] Another example of using the divine name "the Healer" is a chronogram placed on a square during the second hour of Sunday (Fig. 4):

[42] as-Saḥalāwī, *Risālah taṭhīr*, p. 4.

[43] Ṭāshköprüzāde, fol. 44a. This treatise gives a large number of divine names with their properties and the manner of using them similar to what has been described above (fols. 44b-45b).

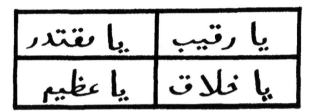

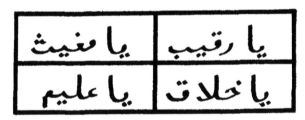

ى	ف	ا	ش
302	3	79	11
78	8	302	3
4	301	9	8

Figure 4

It should be washed away with water and the water given to anyone who was ill with plague.[44] If one wrote "God is gentle to His servants" (*Allāh laṭīf bi-ʿibādihi*) on a glass cup during the time of prayer, washed it off with water, and gave a *mithqāl* weight of the water to the plague victim to drink, he would be saved (Fig. 5).[45]

Ibn Haydūr relates other magical practices to avert plague by writing various signs and letters on cups, filling them with water, and then drinking the water in which the incantation had been dissolved. For example, the following design (incomplete in the manuscript) should contain twenty *ḥā*'s and five *hā*'s (Fig. 6):[46]

[44] *Ibid.*, fol. 45b. In this and subsequent diagrams the original numbers are given in Western "Arabic" numerals.

[45] *Ibid.*, fol. 47b.

[46] *Risālah fī l-amrāḍ*, fol. 103a.

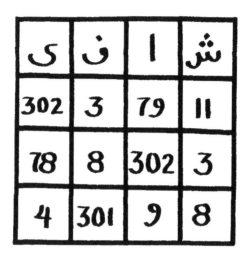

ده	بعبا	لطيف	الله
65	13	74	10
77	13	74	127
128	63	13	116

Figure 5

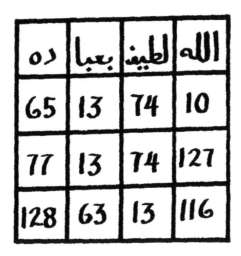

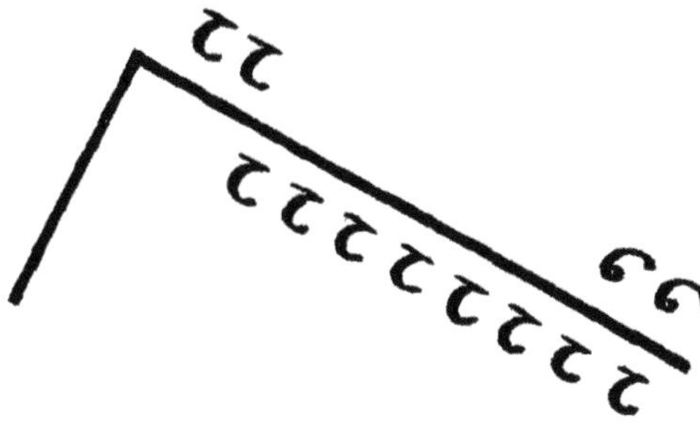

Figure 6

Similarly, the author recommends, during an unspecified epidemic of plague that was then occurring, this triangular form with fourteen *alifs*, seven *ḥā*'s, seven *nūns*, and two *mīms* (Fig. 7):[47]

[47] *Ibid.*, fol. 103b.

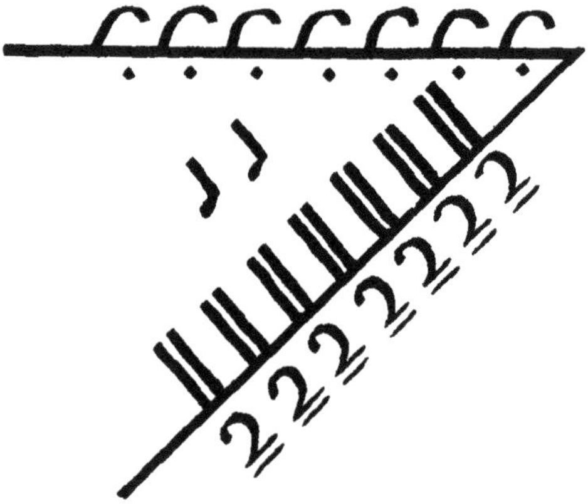

Figure 7

Such incantations were used in still other ways. Frequently a magical sign was made on a piece of bread, and it was swallowed in order to ward off plague.[48] In other cases, a piece of paper or parchment with the incantation was burned, and the fumes were considered beneficial to inhale.[49] One plague treatise quotes al-Būnī concerning the two names of God, "the Guardian, the Powerful" (*al-muqtadir, ar-raqīb*). If these two names were engraved on the stone of a ring in this manner:

Figure 8

[48] al-Jazā'irī, *Kitāb masḳin ash-shujūn fī huḳm al-firār min aṭ-ṭā'ūn*, Berlin MS no. 6377 (Ahlwardt), fol. 149.

[49] See the description of these practices for various illnesses in M. Galal, "Essai d'observations sur les rites funéraires en Égypte actuelle," *REI* (1937), pp. 136-145; see also Westermarck, *Ritual and Belief in Morocco*, vol. 1, chap. 5.

(combining the letters of the two names alternatively), plague would not befall the wearer as long as he lived.[50]

The plague treatise of Ibn Haydūr is devoted primarily to these various ways of using the "secrets of letters" in treating plague, in addition to prayers and medical advice. At the beginning of his interesting discussion of letter magic, Ibn Haydūr relates[51] that his teacher informed him that one night in the year 764/1362-1363 he had gone to bed and thought about the epidemic of plague that was rampant in this year. He slept badly because of the distress caused by the epidemic. In his sleep, he saw a man take a small book from his own library and bring it to him. The man laid his hand on the last line on the right side of a page of the book and said: "These names will intercede for you during the epidemic and read them in this manner—'Oh Living One, Oh Patient One, Oh Loving One, Oh Wise One.'"[52] Then the shaykh awoke and opened the book he had recognized in the dream and, looking at the last line of every right-hand page, found the passage. When it was morning, he told his friends about the dream. Among them was Ḥājj Rashīd al-Ḥabishī al-Mashriqī,[53] who, when he heard the recitation of the names of God in this manner, said that these names were engraved on rings among the people in the East but with the addition of the letter *ḥā'*.[54] There follow in the manuscript three designs (Figs. 9, 10, & 11) for this engraved inscription. Figs. 10 and 11 differ from Fig. 9 in the juxtaposition of God's names.

The stone engraved in this way would guard a person against the burning fever that accompanied plague, if he drank

[50] Luṭfallāh aṭ-Ṭuqāṭī, *Risālah fī tadʿīf al-madhbaḥ*, fol. 9a; the same quotation is found in Ṭāshköprüzāde, fol. 44a.

[51] *Risālah fī l-amrāḍ*, fol. 101b-102b.

[52] *Yā hayā—yā halīm—yā hanān—yā hakīm.*

[53] He may be identified with the mystic Jamāl ad-Dīn al-Ḥabishī, d. 782/1382 (*GAL*, vol. 2, p. 189).

[54] The same description of the engraved ring is repeated on fol. 103a of Ibn Haydūr's treatise.

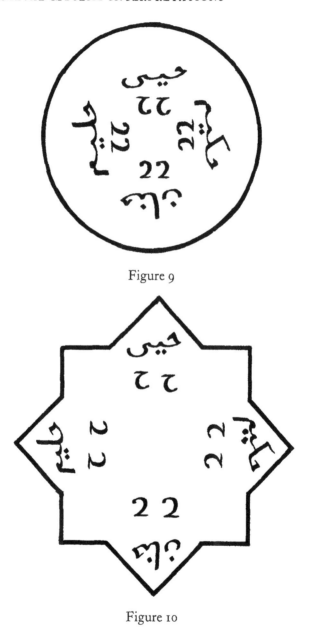

Figure 9

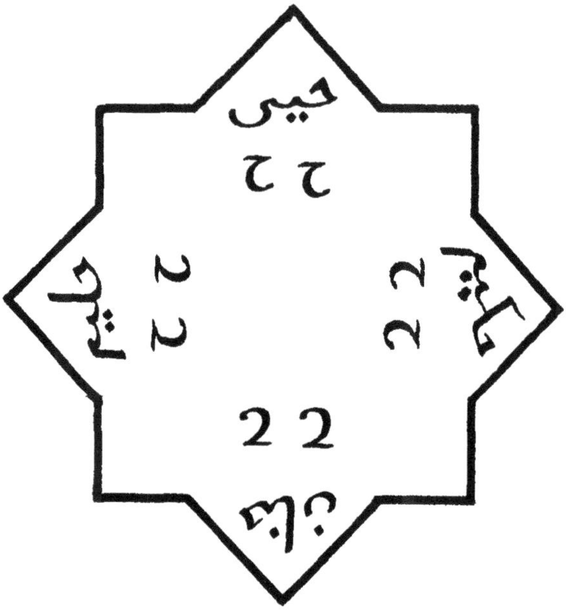

Figure 10

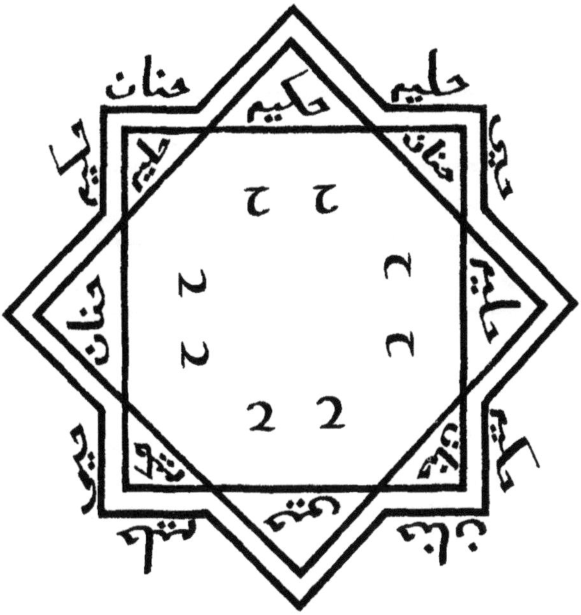

Figure 11

water in which the ring had been submerged. One of the conditions of the seal was that it must not be worn on Saturday or Monday. Ibn Haydūr explains that this was because of the coldness of the two stars, Saturn and the moon, ascribed to these two days. Among other properties of such a ring or the recitation of these names of God was its effectiveness in alleviating the severe heat in the summer and the reduction of sexual powers.[55]

In a similar manner, Ṭāshköprüzāde describes in his plague treatise an engraved ring that warded off plague from its wearer.[56] Using the name of God, "the Powerful" (*al-muqtadir*), the ring should be inscribed in the following manner (Fig. 12):

[55] *Risālah fī l-amrāḍ*, fols. 103a-103b.
[56] Ṭāshköprüzāde, fols. 44b-45a.

ر	د	ث	ق	م
ث	ق	م	ر	د
م	ر	د	ث	ق
د	ث	ق	م	ر

Figure 12

The wearing of a sapphire in a ring or necklace is frequently mentioned as an effective charm against plague. This property of sapphire is usually related on the authority of Plato and Aristotle.[57] Ibn al-Wardī tells us specifically that rubies were worn to guard against the Black Death in Aleppo.[58]

The Andalusian physician, ash-Shaqūrī, states that if a piece of elephant tusk were hung around the neck of a child, the child would be safe from plague. On the authority of Ibn Zuhr al-Ishbīlī's *Khawāṣṣ al-ḥayawān*,[59] ash-Shaqūrī asserts that if a piece of the herb doronicum were hung inside a house, plague would not befall the inhabitants. And from a work by the famous doctor ar-Rāzī about plague: if a man wore a ring made of mixed fresh myrtle on his little finger, his plague boils would be quieted. Some people claimed that if the herb eryngium were put on the buboes, it would pickle them.[60]

[57] ash-Shaqūrī, *Taḥqīq an-naba'*, fol. 110b; Ṭāshköprüzāde, fol. 35b. "Of the characteristics of sapphire: whoever puts on a necklace of the stone or puts on a ring of sapphire, it is his protection against the plague's striking him in a land where plague has occurred among others, the nobility, and the leaders of the people." (Shihāb ad-Dīn Abū l-'Abbās at-Tīfāshī [d. 651/1253], *Azhār al-afkār fī jawāhir al-ahjār*, Dār al-Kutub al-Miṣrīyah microfilm copy of Topkapī Sarī MS, p. 19 [*GAL*, vol. 1, p. 495]).

[58] *Risālat an-naba'*, p. 186.

[59] *GAL*, vol. 1, p. 486.

[60] ash-Shaqūrī, *Taḥqīq an-naba'*, fols. 110b-111a.

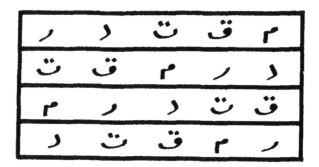

From al-Būnī's *'Ilm al-hudā*,[61] there is a recommendation that if a man engraved on the door of his house the beatific names, "the Eternal, the Creator," no one in the house would die of plague.[62] Likewise, if "the Life" were written on one's house eighteen times in the first hour of Friday, the inhabitants of the house would be safe from plague.[63] 'Abd ar-Raḥmān al-Bisṭāmī (d. 858/1454)[64] relates from the religious teachers that if God's name, "the Eternal" (*al-bāqī*), were painted in four squares in the following form (Fig. 13) on the outside of a house or wall, it protected the inhabitants from

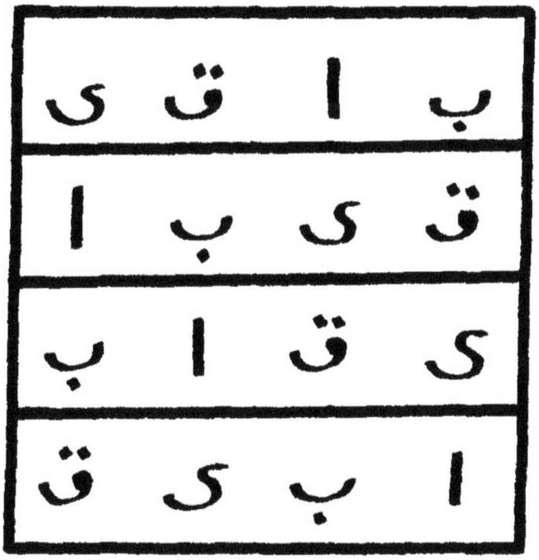

Figure 13

[61] Cited in Ṭāshköprüzāde, fol. 44a; *GAL*, vol. 1, p. 497, no. 5.

[62] Luṭfallāh aṭ-Ṭuqātī, *Risālah fī taḍ'īf al-madhbah*, fol. 9a.

[63] *Ibid.* These practices recall the English custom of painting blue, and later red, crosses on plague-stricken houses and the inscription: "Lord have mercy upon us." (Shrewsbury, *A History of Bubonic Plague*, p. 204 *et passim.*)

[64] *GAL*, vol. 2, p. 231.

plague. It was said that it had been painted on the house of the caliph in Baghdad, and protected him for eighty years.[65]

Like the use of the divine names for magical practice, there were the magical names of the "Seven Sleepers" (*aṣḥāb al-kahf*) and their dog, Qiṭmīr, which could be engraved on a talisman or written on the body.[66] One plague treatise recommends this cryptogram (Fig. 14):[67]

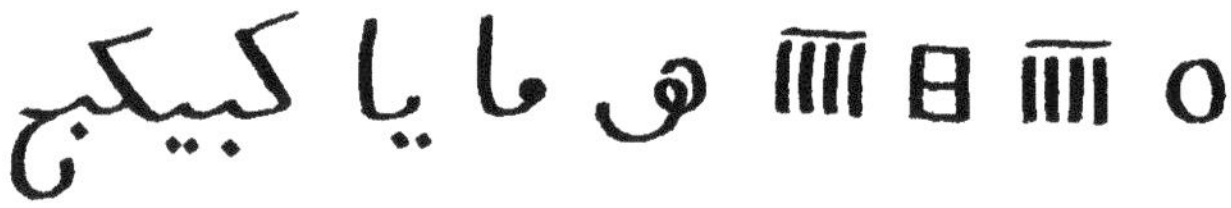

Figure 14

The following set of symbols is found in a plague treatise written during the plague epidemic of 1125/1713-1714 in Egypt (Fig. 15):[68]

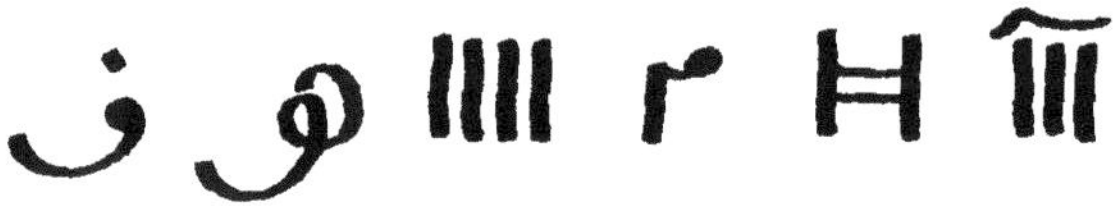

Figure 15

Obviously, the cryptograms show a great variety, being composed of words, letters, numbers, symbols, or any combination of these. As in the latter two examples, their symbolism

[65] Tāshköprüzāde, fol. 45a.

[66] *EI*²: "asḥāb al-kahf" (R. Paret); Louis Massignon, "Les 'Sept Dormants' Apocalypses d'Islam," *Opera Minora*, vol. 3, pp. 104-180, particularly pp. 146-147. Concerning their use in amulets, see Kriss, *Volksglaube*, vol. 2, pp. 82-84, and S. Seligmann, "Das Sieben schäfer-Amulett," *Der Islam*, vol. 5 (1914), pp. 370-388; Lane, *Manners and Customs*, pp. 257-258.

[67] Ṭāshköprüzāde, fol. 53b. The use of this cryptogram is taken from Ḥāfiẓ ad-Dīn an-Nasafī, d. 710/1310 (*GAL*, vol. 2, p. 196).

[68] as-Saḥalāwī, *Risālah taṭhīr*, p. 3.

is often not readily apparent. In some instances, there is a perfect square in which the sum is always the same whether the numbers are added horizontally, vertically, or diagonally, or when any group of four contiguous numbers are added together. For example, the two following "magic squares"[69] are presented in one plague treatise (Figs. 16 and 17):[70]

406	409	412	398
411	399	405	410
400		407	404
408	403	401	413

414

Figure 16

The instructions state that when the quadrants were completed by the inclusion of the number outside the diagram the square would avert the plague. In the first case, any sequence gives the sum of 1625 and in the second, 1635. These magic quadrants may have been used in numerous ways, but it is certain that they were often inscribed on metal amulets.[71]

[69] See Kriss, *Volksglaube*, vol. 2, pp. 84ff.
[70] Lutfallāh at-Tuqātī, *Risālah fī tad'if al-madhbah*, fol. 8b.
[71] See examples of this type in Kriss, *Volksglaube*, vol. 2, plate 79.

408	411	418	401
414	402	407	412
403		409	406
410	405	406	416

417

Figure 17

Related to such popular prophylaxes may be the unusual story given by as-Suyūṭī (which he took from Ibn Abī d-Dunyā's *Kitāb al-i'tibār*) of two similar reports about the death of Ayyūb, the son of Caliph Sulaymān ibn 'Abd al-Malik, in 98/717. According to one report, Abū l-Abṭāl told Ibn Abī d-Dunyā:

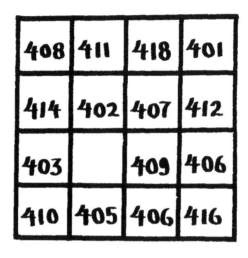

> I was sent to 'Abd al-Malik and with me were six loads of musk from Khurāsān. I passed by the house of Ayyūb ibn Sulayman, and I was admitted and walked through the rooms in which all the clothing and carpets were white. I entered another house, and it was yellow and what was within it was the same. I was admitted into a red house, and everything in it was also red. Then, I was admitted to a green house, and all was green inside. When I was with

> Ayyūb, who was on the throne, the people overtook me and devoured the musk I had brought. I passed by the house of Ayyūb after seventeen days and, behold, the house was boarded up. I asked what had happened, and they said that plague had struck them.[72]

There is a similar report of a man who whitewashed his furniture and dyed his muslin yellow in Ibn Abī Ḥajalah's account of the plague during 761/1359-1360.[73] These reports may indicate a domestic practice aimed at plague prevention that is not mentioned specifically in the treatises but that may have had a magical significance. The account of Abū l-Abṭāl does, however, attest to the strong demand for scents to improve the pestilential air during a plague epidemic, for musk is a basic ingredient of perfumes.

Among a number of random superstitions associated with plague was the belief that when pigeons roosted in a house, the inhabitants were safe from the plague miasma. The use of *kuḥl* (powdered antimony sulfide) was suggested for one's eyes to ward off the evil jinn, who were thought to bring plague. And it was supposed to have been remarked by the Prophet that whoever passed his comb through his eyebrows was safe from plague.[74]

Finally, Evliyā Çelebī, the noted traveler and Ottoman historian, recorded a number of plague epidemics during his lifetime (d. ca. 1093/1682); he states that there once existed in Constantinople a tall column of marble at the present site of the baths of Bāyazīd II (1481-1512). According to popular belief, the column had magical power to prevent plague from entering the capital. Plague was said to have entered Constantinople on the day that Bāyazīd removed this column in order

[72] *Mā rawāhu l-wā'ūn*, pp. 151-152.

[73] *Daf' an-niqmah*, fol. 84b.

[74] *Badhl*, fol. 39b; Tāshköprüzāde, fol. 33b. The last belief is reported on the authority of Abū Nu'aym al-Isfahānī (d. 430/1038), probably from his *Tibb an-nabī* (*GAL*, vol. 1, p. 362).

to build the baths. The first victim of plague was the son of the sultan, and disease had recurred in the city since that day.[75]

In whatever way men viewed the disease and tried to deal with its threat to human life, the Black Death was able to follow its inexorable course. Into a populous and prosperous age, the Black Death introduced a sudden decline in population, succeeded by irregular but continual retardations of population caused by recurrent plague epidemics.

[75] Quoted in Suhëyl Ünver, "Sur l'histoire de la peste en Turquie," p. 480. See the translation by Hammer-Purgstall, *Narrative of Travels in Europe, Asia and Africa in the Seventeenth Century by Evliya Efendi* (London, 1834, 1968 reprint), p. 18.

V

THE DEMOGRAPHIC EFFECTS OF PLAGUE IN EGYPT AND SYRIA

A. THE POLITICAL AND SOCIAL CONTEXT

The Black Death spread throughout the Muslim lands of the Middle East and the southern Mediterranean littoral, but we are best informed about Muslim society and its response to the pandemic in Egypt and Syria. The relatively full documentation for Egypt and Syria dictates our focusing on the decline of population and the discernible effects of the pandemic in this region of the Middle East. In the middle of the fourteenth century, Egypt and Syria had been ruled for almost a century by a military oligarchy of freed slave corps, known as *mamlūks*. A brief description of the state of Egypt and Syria before the Black Death, mainly in terms of its most outstanding characteristic, the mamlūk élite, furnishes the essential context for understanding the detailed consequences of dramatic depopulation.[1]

Mamlūks were white male slaves who had been imported from the Eurasian steppelands into the Middle East since the early ninth century in order to form reliable and skilled cavalry regiments. The political leaders attempted to preserve in the mamlūk corps the martial virtues of the steppe peoples,

[1] For general historical surveys of the Mamlūk Sultanate, see chap. 1, n. 6. The description of the mamlūk institution is based on the monographic studies of David Ayalon (Neustadt) cited in the Bibliography, especially *L'Esclavage du Mamelouk* in *Oriental Notes and Studies* published by the Israel Oriental Society, no. 1 (Jerusalem, 1951). For a medieval estimation of the mamlūk army, see al-Jāḥiẓ, "The Merits of the Turks and of the Imperial Army as a Whole," *The Life and Works of Jāhiẓ*, ed. by Charles Pellat (Berkeley and Los Angeles, 1969), pp. 91-97.

while substituting an efficient and unified form of organization for the tribal formation—an uneasy marriage between the steppe and the sown. From having been a type of military organization, the mamlūk corps rapidly gained political control over civilian governments; this preponderance of the military class was to characterize Muslim polity throughout the medieval period.[2]

Naturally, the mamlūk organization in its various aspects lacked an absolute institutional uniformity, adapting as it did from the ninth century to the different conditions existing in the medieval epigone of the 'Abbāsid Empire.[3] However, it was brought to fruition in Egypt and Syria by Saladin (d. 589/1193) and the Ayyūbid dynasty that he founded.[4] Saladin based his power on a mamlūk army and the reorganization of Egypt's financial structure. The army received its payment by the granting of *iqṭā*'s or land grants, an idea borrowed, along with the mamlūk system, from the military organization of the Seljuk principalities in the East.[5] With heavily armored Kurdish and Turkish mamlūks, Saladin was able to create a political unity between Egypt and his Syrian possessions, making it the strongest power in the eastern Mediterranean.

Following the increased militarization of the Egyptian government and society, which enabled Saladin successfully to confront the Crusaders and his Muslim antagonists in Syria,

[2] The mamlūk army is a major subject in the instructive treatise by the great Seljuk statesman, Niẓām al-Mulk, on the conduct of government, the *Siyāsatnāmeh* (ed. with French trans. by C. Schefer, Paris, 1891-1893; English trans. by H. Darke, London, 1960), chaps. 26 and 27 especially.

[3] For a modern analysis of the role of the mamlūk corps in one medieval dynasty, see the excellent study of C. E. Bosworth, *The Ghaznavids* (Edinburgh, 1963).

[4] Ehrenkreutz, *Saladin*, p. 12.

[5] Sir Hamilton Gibb, "The Armies of Saladin," *Cahiers d'Histoire Égyptéenne*, series 3, fasc. 4 (Cairo, 1951), pp. 304-320, and "The Achievement of Saladin," *Bulletin of the John Rylands Library*, vol. 35, no. 1 (Manchester, 1952), pp. 44-60; both articles are reprinted in *Studies on the Civilization of Islam*, ed. by S. J. Shaw and W. R. Polk (Boston, 1968), pp. 74-90 and pp. 91-107 respectively.

the mamlūk organization reached the apogee of its development in the middle of the thirteenth century. As the challenge of the Crusaders had evoked the brilliant leadership of Saladin and then receded, the advance of the Mongols in the mid-thirteenth century gave the mamlūk army the opportunity to prove its capacity for leadership; its victory over the Mongols in 1260 also gave it its claim to legitimate rule. The distinct corps of Turks was able to establish at this time a state that was ruled exclusively by mamlūks and in their own interests. The mamlūks were thus an élite that held all of the highest executive and military posts.

These élite personnel were usually sold as young slaves in Cairo, where the majority were purchased by the sultan and housed in government barracks. The future mamlūks were supervised with severe discipline by palace eunuchs. They were effectively cut off in this way from all of their earlier connections: the environment of the steppe, their tribe and religion, and their own families. The mamlūk training began with a basic Muslim education and conversion to Islam; this was followed by a rigorous military training in the garrison complex. The training in military arts was essential to the mamlūk. The *furūsīyah* exercises or paramilitary sports were the privilege of the mamlūk caste. After this training and the slaves' attainment of manhood, they were formally manumitted in groups of several hundred by the sultan, who gave them horses and accouterments during a passing-out ceremony at the Cairo Citadel.

The adult mamlūk was then a freedman and a trained soldier, who was eligible to rise to important military and executive offices according to his personal ability, his performance on the battlefield, and his loyal service to his previous master. The freedman still owed complete loyalty to his former master and to his senior and fellow mamlūks; a firm bond attached him especially to his former owner in domestic matters as well as in politics and warfare. The relationship approached kinship more closely than servitude.

A number of characteristics of the mamlūk sharply distin-

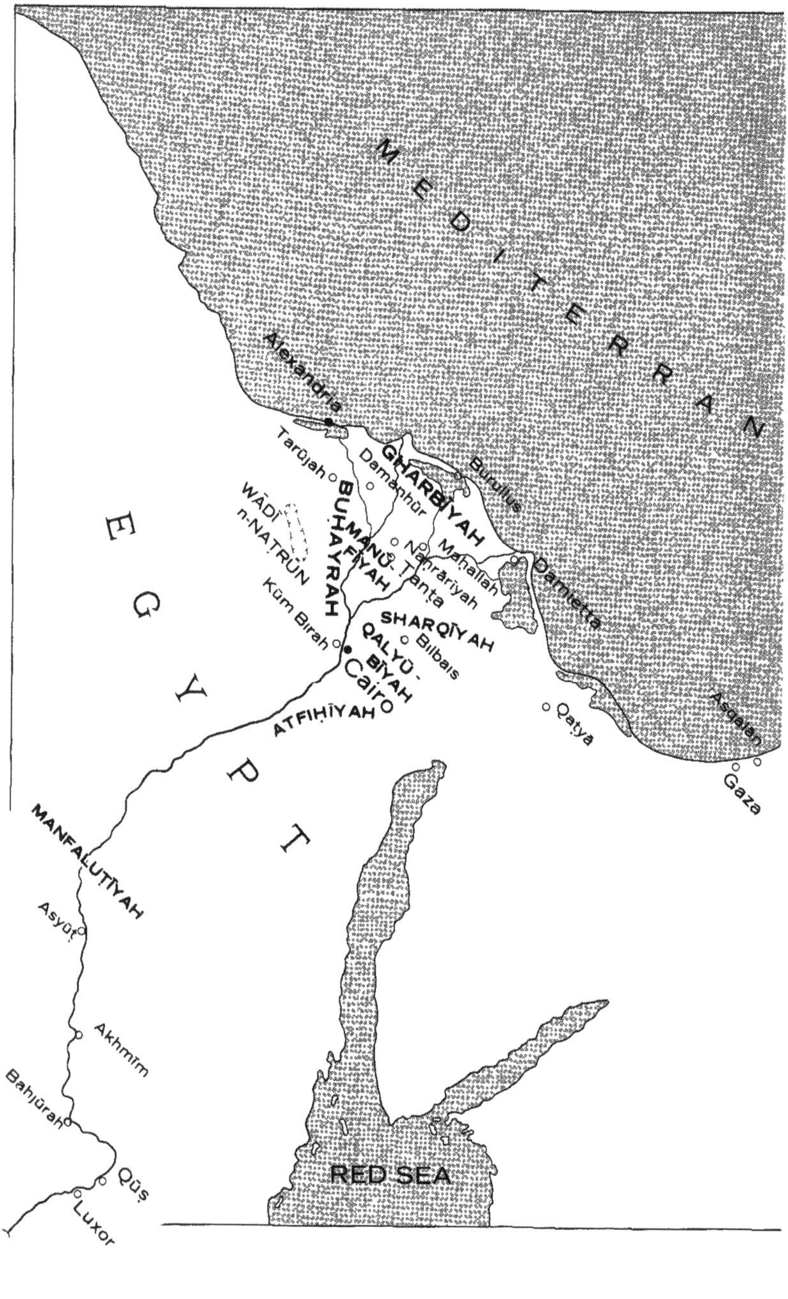

MEDITERRAN
Alexandria
Tarūjah
Damanhūr
GHARBĪYAH
Burullus
WĀDĪ n-NAṬRŪN
BUḤAYRAH
MANŪFĪYAH
Nahrārīyah
Ṭanṭa
Maḥallah
Damietta
EGYPT
Kūm Birah
SHARQĪYAH
QALYŪBĪYAH
Bilbais
Cairo
ATFIḤĪYAH
Qaṭya
Asqalān
Gaza
MANFALŪṬĪYAH
Asyūṭ
Akhmīm
Bahjūrah
Qūṣ
Luxor
RED SEA

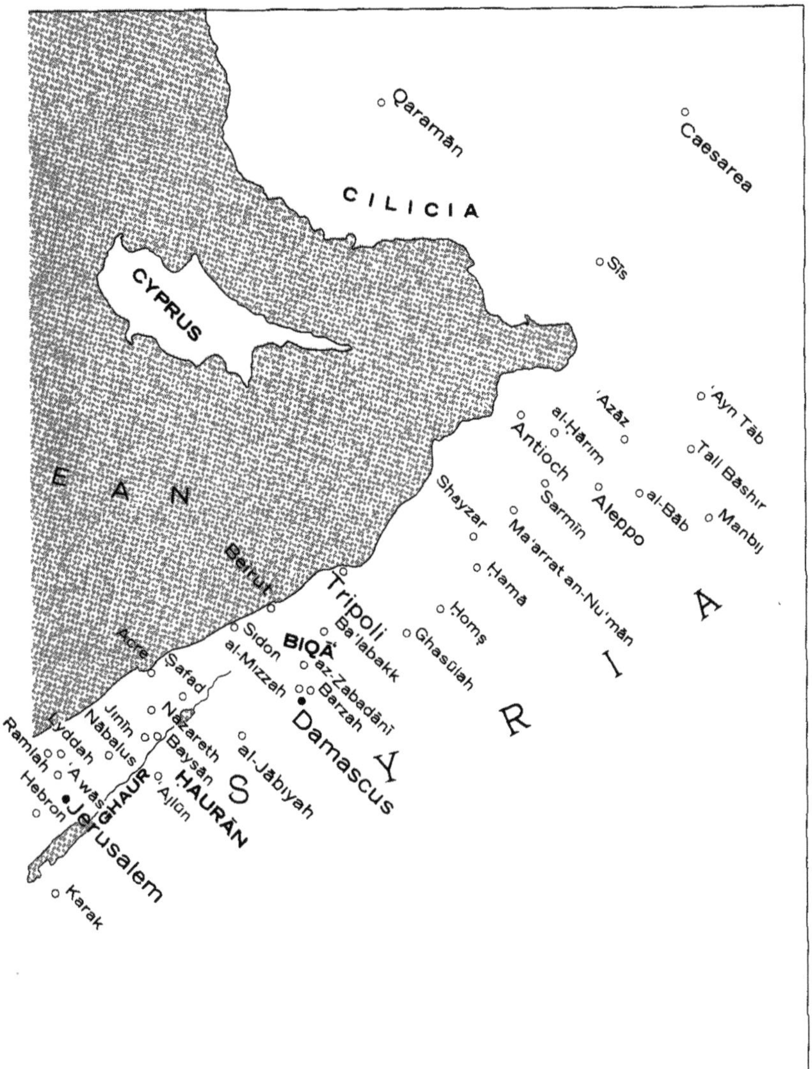

The Mamlūk Empire of Egypt and Syria
1250 – 1517

guished him from the native Egyptian. A non-Muslim by birth, the mamlūk maintained his non-Arabic name even after conversion. The foreign name was far from being a stigma; on the contrary, it was a sign of social superiority. The mamlūks commonly spoke a dialect of Turkish among themselves and frequently remained illiterate in Arabic. While the mamlūk regime allowed all four major orthodox schools of Muslim Law in their domain, the mamlūks were subject to an uncodified system of political law (*siyāsah*); its origin is ascribed to the law (*yāsā*) of Jenghis Khan and was administered by one of the military officials, with final recourse to the sultan himself. Moreover, mamlūk privileges were numerous; they included special dress, coats-of-arms, reserved offices, and tax exemptions. The mamlūks, generally, married Turkish slave-girls or daughters of other mamlūks.

The adept mamlūk had an unlimited scope for his personal ambition; he was able to gain enormous wealth, acquire his own loyal mamlūk contingent, and realistically hope to rise ultimately to the sultanate. The mamlūk amir or colonel was continually conciliated by the sultan with the bestowal of appanages, honors, and unstinted largesse to encourage the amir's support. The principal deterrent to the sultan's overthrow was the strength and loyalty of the royal mamlūks and his ability to manipulate the amirs' jealousies. The danger of a coalition of the amirs continually threatened the sultan's reign; the political machinations of the mamlūks did insure the rule of a strong leader, but at the expense of political stability and considerable human suffering. Such a period of political instability occurred following the death of Sultan an-Nāṣir in 741/1340. His prolonged reign did not insure the peaceful transference of political leadership. While the sons and grandsons of an-Nāṣir claimed the sultanate for the next forty years, the mamlūk factions contended with one another in a turbulent struggle for actual control of the state. At the time of the Black Death, one of his sons, al-Ḥasan (reigns: 748-752/1347-1351, 755-762/1354-1361), ruled as sultan but was actually a figurehead for the powerful mamlūk princes.[6]

[6] *Muslim Cities*, pp. 20-21.

In addition to consolidating the mamlūk organization, Saladin set the general pattern of Muslim society for succeeding centuries in Egypt and Syria by restoring *sunnī* or orthodox Islam. Confronted by the pagan Mongols and the remnant Crusader state, Baybars (658-676/1260-1277), the founder of the Mamlūk Sultanate, reaffirmed this religious orthodoxy. When Baghdad and the caliphate were destroyed by the Mongols in 1258, the center of Islamic learning shifted permanently to Cairo. Religious leadership was also transferred to Cairo when Baybars brought a descendant of the 'Abbāsid family to Egypt and established the caliphate in Cairo in 1261.

As a part of this religious revival, the mamlūks continued to assail the Crusader state. The mamlūks successfully eliminated the remaining Crusader kingdom in the Middle East by the late thirteenth century. The success of the mamlūk regime against the Crusaders and the pagan Mongols culminated in massive conversions to Islam and the final eclipse of Oriental Christianity in the thirteenth century.

Saladin also ushered in a period of increasing economic prosperity and sustained population growth that lasted until the time of the Black Death. This well-being was reflected in the considerable expansion and embellishment of Cairo. The population of Egypt as a whole appears to have risen rapidly from the end of the twelfth century, according to the land tax records. It has been estimated that the population grew from about 2.4 million at the time of Saladin to approximately 4 million prior to the Black Death in the middle of the fourteenth century,[7] although these figures probably underestimate the actual population levels. In general, this population increase follows the pattern of demographic growth in medieval Europe; however, European population experienced a marked retardation of growth during the half-century before the Black Death.[8] It is still premature to outline the nature of Middle Eastern population with the same assurance, be-

[7] Russell, "The Population of Medieval Egypt," p. 76.

[8] The Macedonian peasant population of the Byzantine Empire also seems to have been declining in the first half of the fourteenth century (communication of Professor Angeliki E. Laiou, November 13, 1973).

cause of the lack of demographic studies of the area. Yet the pacification and the large-scale colonization of Syria, favorable ecological conditions (except for the pestilence and famine of 1295-1296 and an earthquake in 1303), and political and economic stability were conducive to population increase through the first half of the fourteenth century.

The half-century before the Black Death was a period of political security and peace in Egypt and Syria under the long reign of an-Nāṣir, who ruled with two interruptions from 696/1294 until 741/1340. His political leadership encouraged long-term tenure of office, establishment of ties between the mamlūk regime and the native population, and investment. The surplus wealth from investment together with regard for the popular welfare produced urban and rural improvements and numerous endowments, which supported the religious, educational, and philanthropic life of urban communities. The reorganization of the *iqṭā'* or land-grant system between 1313 and 1324 contributed to the economic stability of the state by regulating the pay of the mamlūks and the duties of the taxpayers. This fiscal regularity was reflected in the exceptional monetary stability of the half-century; general prosperity was supported by the constancy of gold and silver values and of the prices of basic food commodities.[9]

Furthermore, the early sultanate fostered international trade between the Orient and Europe, and domestic industry. European merchants were excluded from the Indian Ocean, but they played an increasingly active part in the transit trade from Egypt. In Egypt and Syria, the mamlūks, like earlier regimes, held important sectors of both production and commerce under state control, such as sugar cultivation and the trade in

[9] *Muslim Cities*, p. 16. The following survey of mamlūk social history relies heavily upon the studies by Ira Lapidus: *Muslim Cities*, and "Muslim Cities and Islamic Societies," in *Middle Eastern Cities*, ed. by Ira Lapidus (Berkeley and Los Angeles, 1969), pp. 47-79. For a detailed descriptive account of traditional Muslim urban life, see Lane, *Manners and Customs*, and *Arabian Society in the Middle Ages*, ed. by Stanley Lane-Poole.

metals and timber, which were strategic military supplies. The governmental control by the mamlūk regime did not cause serious economic dislocation until the fifteenth century, when the controls were extended over a rapidly contracting economy.

Besides the mamlūks' control of certain domestic industries, luxury crafts flourished especially in Cairo and Damascus, in response to the mamlūks' desire for refinement and display. The metalwork and ceramics, glass and weaving that have survived attest to the remarkable standard of living that the mamlūks enjoyed. The domestic life of the mamlūk amirs is reflected in *A Thousand and One Nights*; whatever were the origins and scenes of the stories, the manners and customs were drawn from mamlūk society when the narrative took its final form and was written down. The reports of the almost fabulous prodigality of the mamlūk amirs and their construction of more than thirty mosques in Cairo during an-Nāṣir's reign reveal their vast financial resources; parenthetically, the additional mosques may also denote the needs of an enlarged urban population. The buildings of the mamlūk princes were paralleled by the large-scale public works undertaken by the sultan. The elaborate household and splendid court ceremonies, the athletic exercises and royal processions of the sultan were imitated by the households of the amirs.

Thus, the large households were important consumers of goods and services. In addition, the military corps extended their political control over the financial resources of the state, particularly the vital agricultural sector of the economy. The mamlūks entered actively into the urban economy by their sale of grain supplies, investment in real estate, and direction of labor and scarce building materials. The mamlūks' financial success in these ventures was made possible, if not assured, by the exploitation of their political offices. "The mamlūk household was a means of transforming public into private powers and state authority into personal superiority."[10] It is difficult to escape the conclusion that there existed a sharp division separating this alien ruling oligarchy, with its effective polit-

[10] *Muslim Cities*, pp. 48-50.

ical and economic power, from the rest of society; policy, power, and position were the prerogatives of the military élite.

The commanding military-political position of the mamlūk élite was imposed on the economic and social life of Egyptian and Syrian society. In a traditional society that lacked the concept of public or municipal agencies, as individuals, the members of this ruling class assumed responsibility for what we would consider public concerns. The mamlūks were patrons of art, schools, and mosques; builders of roads, bridges, and markets; and overseers of "public works," morality, and charity. The fulfillment of these communal needs depended on the self-interest and sense of duty of the mamlūks, their desire for legitimation by the people, and their financial capacity. In this privatization of power, characteristic of traditional society but more intense in a military oligarchy, the early indoctrination of the mamlūks in the garrison schools was highly significant; they were introduced to the customs and expectations of the native Muslim people and to their part in carrying on public affairs for which there was no regular provision in the government.[11]

The major cities were the homes of the mamlūks, their government and garrisons; the centers of religious life, including schools and *ṣūfī* confraternities; the seats of justice; and the sites of large markets and specialized crafts. What characteristics distinguish the pre-industrial city from the countryside in the Middle East is a controversial question, yet there was a perceptible imbalance between the two, which the mamlūk regime accentuated by their residence in the cities.[12] Agrarian production flowed into the urban areas largely as income from the *iqṭā*'s; in return, there was apparently very little corresponding movement of urban goods and services to the countryside. Parallel to this economic pattern, there was a constant but fluctuating movement of population toward the urban centers. Medieval cities, in general, could not sup-

[11] *Ibid.*, pp. 44-78.

[12] Lapidus, "Muslim Cities and Islamic Societies," pp. 47-79.

port their own populations without continual immigration, facilitated by socio-religious bonds between the cities and rural communities.

These bonds were conspicuous in the cities, where kinship groups and village affiliations might determine the immigrants' settlement in urban quarters as well as occupation, clientage, and religious and ethnic identity. With regard to the latter, religious and racial distinctions in Egypt and Syria by the late Middle Ages had largely given way to the overwhelming predominance of Islam and the Arabic language and to extensive racial amalgamation through intermarriage, which should be considered a major factor in the general lack of racial prejudice in social relations.[13]

The quarter served as an important basis of communal association and as an essential administrative unit. Cutting across quarter boundaries, Professor Lapidus has distinguished fraternal associations of *ṣūfī* brotherhoods, weak professional groupings, youth clubs, and criminal gangs. But these solidarities were peripheral to the rest of society and failed to integrate the entire community. The true cohesiveness of the city was based on fluid and complex patterns of social relationships—reflected in the amorphous physical nature of Muslim cities in the Middle East—led by the *'ulamā'*, the religious scholars. Originally a religious élite entrusted with the preservation and application of Muslim Law, the *'ulamā'* had assumed alongside the development of the mamlūk military institution, a number of the civilian functions of the older administrative and land-owning classes. In this manner, they became in the later Middle Ages an administrative and social élite.

The *'ulamā'* served as mediators between the mamlūk establishment and the common people and attempted to accommodate and coordinate as far as possible their diverse interests and goals. On the part of the local community, the *'ulamā'* sought to protect Muslim religious and educational values, to gain financial support from the mamlūks for communal

[13] Cf. Bernard Lewis, *Race and Color in Islam* (New York, 1971).

services, and to defend commercial activity. On the part of the mamlūk class, they served as the knowledgeable infrastructure—what we would normally associate with bureaucratic, judicial, and sometimes parliamentary functions—on which the mamlūk regime relied, and as the promoters of social order. Within this scheme of urban social relations, the *'ulamā'* played a prominent role in directing communal activity during the Black Death and later epidemics.

In the broad view, therefore, Egypt and Syria witnessed in the later Middle Ages the successful implantation of an alien military élite that was the center of a diffuse system of social and political relations with the native population. The mamlūk corps was largely the creation of Saladin, and they were faithful to their progenitor not only by augmenting the mamlūk military organization but also by the continuance of his religious policy, the defense of Egypt and Syria from foreign aggression, and the fostering of internal economic growth. Into this society, however, the Black Death and recurrent plague epidemics introduced a significant decline in population, particularly among the vital mamlūk army, and greatly modified the nature of Egyptian-Syrian society. After the remarkable prosperity and growth of the early Mamlūk Sultanate, this society began a precipitous decline from the middle of the fourteenth century that lasted at least until the early sixteenth century. Before proceeding to the social and economic consequences of depopulation caused by plague, it is necessary to describe the manner in which the Black Death reduced and impoverished the people in the countryside and the major cities.

B. RURAL DEPOPULATION

The Black Death reached Egypt during the autumn of 748/1347 and then slowly spread throughout Lower Egypt from the beginning of Muḥarram 749/April 1348. The epidemic reached its peak during the months of Sha'bān, Ramaḍān, and

Shawwāl 749/October 1348 to January 1349, and ceased in the middle of Dhū l-Qa'dah/the beginning of February.[1] The first Egyptian city to be struck by plague was Alexandria, and we might expect this if we assume that the pandemic was transmitted by the important trade from the Crimea.[2]

From Alexandria, the Black Death radiated throughout the Delta, southeastward to the entire province of Buḥayrah, where the taxes (*ḍamānāt* and *mūjibāt*) were not collected because of the number of deaths; the cities of Damanhūr and Tarūjah are specifically reported as being subjected to plague.[3] Eastward, plague advanced through the province of Gharbīyah. In the important provincial capital of Maḥallah, in the center of the Delta, the death rate was so great that the prefect of the city was no longer able to receive plaintiffs in legal cases; the judges, whose signatures were necessary for the validation of wills, could procure honest witnesses only with great difficulty. Officials were sent to the various villages of

[1] *as-Sulūk*, part 2, vol. 3, p. 772. The important description of the Black Death in the Middle East by al-Maqrīzī (*ibid.*, pp. 772-791) has been translated by Gaston Wiet ("La Grande Peste Noire"). Wiet notes that Ibn Taghrī Birdī copied the account from al-Maqrīzī except for a final reflection by Ibn Taghrī Birdī in his *an-Nujūm* (ed. by Popper, vol. 5, pp. 62-76; Cairo ed., vol. 10, pp. 195-213). Besides the collation of the two texts and this final reflection of Ibn Taghrī Birdī, Wiet has added a brief translation of excerpts from Ibn Kathīr (*al-Bidāyah*, vol. 14, pp. 225-230) and Ibn Iyās (*Badā'i' az-zuhūr*, Būlāq ed., vol. 1, pp. 191-192) concerning the Black Death.

[2] Gaston Wiet, *L'Égypte musulmane de la conquête Arabe à la conquête Ottoman*, vol. 2, part 2 of *Précis de l'histoire d'Égypte par divers historiens et archéologues* (Cairo, 1932), p. 241. Although the information from Alexandria is not as abundant as for Cairo, we may surmise that Alexandria, being particularly exposed to the importation of foreign diseases, suffered appreciably from the Black Death and its recurrences. Paul Kahle has, perhaps, placed too great an emphasis on the Cypriot attack led by Peter de Lusignan on Alexandria in 1365 to account for the marked deterioration of the city in the late fourteenth century ("Die Katastrophe der Mittelalterlichen Alexandria," *Mélanges Maspéro*, vol. 3 [1940], p. 139).

[3] See "La Grande Peste Noire," p. 372, ns. 14 and 15.

this province to gather important sums, probably the *kharāj* or land tax, but were able to collect only 60,000 *dirhems*.[4]

Along the Mediterranean coast of Gharbīyah province, plague struck particularly the towns of Burullus, Nastirāwah,[5] and Damietta,[6] where large numbers of fishermen died. As in most accounts of the Black Death in Europe, there are frequent reports in the Arabic sources of dead animals that were believed to have perished from the same pestilential miasma. The description of buboes found on the heads of fish that were caught in these three cities is fantastic,[7] but the repeated statements of zoological mortality raise the perplexing problem of whether or not the fishes' death was due to plague. In this case, plague may have indirectly caused their destruction through the pollution of lakes and rivers with bodies of dead men and animals.

It is natural that there would be reports of the plague epizootic among certain animals in the countryside, and various authors mention the plague bubo found on their bodies. For example, Ibn Iyās states:

> The country was not far from being ruined. The piercing [of the plague] also occurred to cats, dogs, and savage beasts. One found in the desert the bodies of savage animals with the bubos under their arms. It was the same with horses, camels, asses, and all the beasts in general, including birds, even the ostriches.[8]

An observer of the Black Death in Damascus suggests the same epizootic: "There died in this plague birds, wild animals, cats, and other animals with a tumor under their arms."[9] As

[4] *as-Sulūk*, part 2, vol. 3, p. 778. The total revenue of Gharbīyah province in 1315 is estimated at 2,182,933 *dīnārs* (Russell, "Population of Medieval Egypt," p. 77).

[5] See Muḥammad Ramzī, *al-Qāmūs al-jughrāfī* (Cairo, 1953-1968), vol. 1, pp. 459-460.

[6] *as-Sulūk*, part 2, vol. 3, pp. 778-779.

[7] *Ibid.*; al-Maqrīzī mentions fish with plague buboes being drawn from the lakes at Damietta, Nashirāwah, and Sakhā (p. 785).

[8] Ibn Iyās, vol. 1, p. 191.

[9] *Daf' an-niqmah*, fol. 75a.

in the ancient account of the "Athenian Plague" by Thucydides, the destruction of birds of prey is often described in Arabic sources; it is most probable that these birds were infected by ingestion or by the fleas of animals that had died of plague. We know that the mamlūk sultan fled from Cairo to Siryāqūs, a country retreat northeast of Cairo, during the Black Death and later epidemics. The local population had complained in the past about the large number of kites and crows that had scavenged among the discarded refuse of the court. While the sultan stayed there during the month of Ramaḍān 749/December 1348, however, no one saw any birds.[10]

Al-Maqrīzī describes the general destruction of animals in the following manner:

> The falcons of the chase, when released by the falconers, overtook the savage geese or other birds; on the prey was always found a bubo [*kubbah*] about the size of a hazelnut. Numerous dead birds were found in the fields—crows, kites, and many other birds of all kinds. When they were plucked, one found the traces of the bubo. Cats died until practically no more were seen. According to the information that arrived constantly from the Ghaur [the Jordan Valley], from Baysān, and from other neighboring villages, lions, wolves, hares, camels, wild asses, wild boars, and other savage beasts all lay dead and on them was the trace of the bubo.[11]

There may be some truth, therefore, in al-Maqrīzī's general conclusion that plague "encompassed not only all mankind but also the fish of the sea, the birds in the sky, and the savage beasts."[12]

[10] *as-Sulūk*, part 2, vol. 3, p. 785.

[11] *Ibid.*, p. 784.

[12] *Ibid.*, p. 773. The author also cites the death of beasts of burden and cattle in the regions of Qaramān and Caesarea in Anatolia (p. 774); beasts of burden, sheep, and cattle in North Africa (p. 777); beasts in Damietta (p. 779); work animals in Buḥayrah province (p. 777); oxen in Gaza (p. 775); cattle and oxen in Khaysīyah (p. 779, see

However, there is a curious failure in the Middle Eastern sources, as there is in the European accounts, to mention the extermination of plague-carrying rodents, although rats were plentiful and were a common domestic nuisance. In a discussion of the differences in the standards of living within a Muslim city at this time, Ibn Khaldūn remarks:

> The premises and courtyards of the houses of the prosperous and wealthy [inhabitants of the town], who set a good table and where grain and bread-crumbs lie scattered around, are frequented by swarms of ants and insects. There are many large rats in their cellars, and cats repair to them.[13]

There can be little doubt that rats were present and served as the effective carriers of the disease in the mid-fourteenth century.[14] Parenthetically, the high plague mortality among

---

also "La Grande Peste Noire," p. 374, n. 18). Similar accounts of probable epizootics occur during the later plague epidemics: A.H. 833 (*an-Nujūm*, Popper trans., vol. 18, pp. 70, 73; Ibn Ḥajar, *Inbā' al-ghumr*, vol. 3, p. 438; *as-Sulūk*, part 4, vol. 2, p. 821 *et passim*); A.H. 841 (*as-Sulūk*, part 4, vol. 2, p. 1031 *et passim*); A.H. 897-898 (al-Manṣūrī, Dār al-Kutub al-Miṣrīyah MS no. 102 *majāmī' m*, fols. 103b-104a).

[13] *The Muqaddimah*, vol. 2, p. 275.

[14] The following summary concerning rats is taken from Hassanein Rabie, "Some Technical Aspects of Agriculture in Medieval Egypt," paper delivered at the Princeton Conference on the Economic History of the Near East (June 16-20, 1974), pp. 42-44: "Rats caused extensive damage to the agriculture of medieval Egypt. . . . From the Mamlūk Period there are ample accounts of the devastation which occurred in 696/1297 as a result of rats, whose number increased greatly in Egypt just before the time of harvest. According to the contemporary historian Baybars al-Mansūrī and others, packs of these rats had a race with the *fallāhīn* in the fields, and the peasants were able to save only a small portion of their crops. Ibn Abī al-Faḍā'il states that rats during that infestation destroyed the crops of about fifty *faddāns* in the course of one night in one village. Although one might accept such figures with some reservation, there was a similar occurrence in 715/1315 when rats attacked the fields in Upper Egypt. Some officials in the village of Umm al-Quṣūr in the Manfalūtiyya province killed a multitude of rats. According to Ibn Taghrī Birdī when these officials wanted to estimate the number of these dead rats, they used a grain measure.

humans and the inconspicuous rodent mortality argue for the predominance of infectious pneumonic plague during the Black Death.

The general destruction of animals may be explained in a number of ways. Some animals are known by modern clinical tests to be resistant to plague infection,[15] but the intensity of the Black Death may have caused infection in otherwise unsuspectible but passive transmitters of rodent fleas. There is also the possibility that this plague may have differed biologically from the modern plague bacillus and may have been more virulent among animals.[16] Moreover, the Black Death may have been accompanied by a separate cattle murrain.

This widespread destruction, especially of work animals, must have contributed to a reduction of cultivation. Considering the important role of particularly the *jāmūs* or ox to traditional agriculture, their costly replacement would have increased the indebtedness and the general personal hardship of the peasantry. The loss of cattle and beasts of burden is

---

They found that in seven days they had killed the volume of 326 2/3 *irdabbs*. A report was written by them to be sent to Sultan al-Nāṣir Muhammad in Cairo. Al-Maqrīzī, who puts the figure at the amount of 316 2/3 *irdabbs,* states that when these officials tried to count the number of dead rats in a single *irdabb,* they found 8,400 rats in the *irdabb* and 1,400 rats in each *wayba* (one-sixth of an *irdabb*). The province of Manfalūṭ suffered another invasion of rats in 738/1337-8 which destroyed the crops in the fields and that stored in the granaries. Within one night a quarter of a whole granary was destroyed by rats. Two groups of *fallahīn* in turn spent all night, with torches, and all day killing them. There were about sixty thousand *irdabbs* of beans lost for Sultan al-Nāṣir ibn Qalāwūn in Manfalūṭ alone as a result of the rat incursion of that year. Damage to crops by rats is continuously mentioned in sources for later periods. For example, in 818/1416, during the reign of Sultan al-Mu'ayyad Shaykh, the rats destroyed the plants of Lower Egypt and as a result the grain supply decreased in the markets. The Sultan and the amirs tried to bring grain from Upper Egypt, but the inhabitants of the *Ṣaʿīd* were reluctant to sell grain unless they could increase prices greatly."

15 Pollitzer, *Plague*, pp. 305-307.

16 Langer, "The Black Death," p. 114.

specifically mentioned during the Black Death, as for example in Bilbais, where the majority of the dromedaries of the mamlūk sultan and the amirs perished.[17]

Bilbais, an important caravan station on the route from Cairo to Palestine, illustrates what occurred in the provincial towns during the pandemic. The roads were covered with bodies, and corpses were thrown against the walls of the great mosque, where dogs devoured them. (During the Black Death in Damascus, the governor ordered the execution of all the dogs in the city, presumably for this reason.[18]) The people living in tents around Bilbais perished with their flocks and dogs, and the waterwheels in the countryside were stilled. The markets of Bilbais were deserted, for few would stay in the city. No muezzin was left to call the people to prayer, and a number of the inhabitants emigrated to Cairo. The population of this province (Sharqīyah) was unable to harvest their crops because of the high mortality rate among the peasantry and their flight from the land where plague had struck at the beginning of the summer (Rabī' II, 749/June 1348).[19]

Most of the cultivation of Burullus was similarly abandoned. Although the chroniclers imply that the miasma affected agricultural products as it did men and animals, it is reasonable to assume that agriculture was simply neglected by the peasants because of their diminished number. For example, the gardens and irrigation system at Damietta were abandoned. The fruit trees of this city dried up, following the death of their owners and the work animals.[20] Because of the depopulation, the demand for and supply of agricultural products were reduced. For instance, no one would buy green clover or send his horses to graze in the countryside any longer; the pandemic caused the ruin of the royal properties in the suburbs

[17] *as-Sulūk*, part 2, vol. 3, p. 779.

[18] *al-Bidāyah*, vol. 14, p. 227. See also Henri Laoust, trans., *Les Gouverneurs de Damas sous les Mamlouks et les Premiers Ottomans (658-1156/1260-1744): Traduction des Annales d'Ibn Tūlūn et d'Ibn Ghum'a* (Damascus, 1952), p. 11.

[19] *as-Sulūk*, part 2, vol. 3, p. 779.

[20] *Ibid.*

of Cairo (Maṭarīyah, Khuṣūṣ, Siryāqūs, and Bahtīt).[21] Likewise, in the regions of Nāy and Ṭanā in the district of Qalyūb, 1500 *faddans*[22] were abandoned when no one sent animals there for grazing, and the manufacture of dried clover was discontinued.[23]

Depopulation was not confined to the Delta, but appears to have been even more severe in Upper Egypt, where plague seized the people from the end of 749/February 1349.[24] The upper Nile Valley was virtually deserted, despite the vast area of normally cultivated lands. In the region of Asyūṭ, the land tax was customarily gathered from about 6,000 people, but during the Black Death the tax was collected from only 116. Some areas, such as Aswān, were lightly affected; only eleven deaths were counted.[25] For this reason, the pandemic appeared capricious to contemporary observers. We are told that the Black Death similarly bypassed the Syrian towns of Ma'arrat an-Nu'mān, Shayzar, and al-Ḥārim.[26] However, in most of

[21] "In winter the royal mamlūks and the amirs of Cairo received instead of barley, strips of the great royal pasturage in the neighborhood of Gizah sown with clover and lucern-grass, and denoted in Arabic as *ar-rabī'* and in Turkish as *otlāq*." (Poliak, *Feudalism*, p. 5)

[22] A *faddan* was equivalent to about 1.35 acres during the Mamlūk Period; see *Systematic Notes*, vol. 16, p. 37.

[23] *as-Sulūk*, part 2, vol. 3, pp. 785-786.

[24] Because of the complexity of plague pathology, it is difficult to determine what may have accounted for the high mortality rate that all observers noted was very severe in Upper Egypt. One curious factor, however, may have been directly responsible for such a high death rate. Hassan Fathy, the distinguished Egyptian architect, has noted that the villages of Upper Egypt are usually built on mounds raised above flood level to avoid the large cracks in the earth caused when the flood waters recede. "The mounds, though, have their own problems, one of which is that, as the waters rise, all the vermin of the fields—rats, mice, snakes, and insects take refuge in the village, bringing a variety of diseases with them." (*Architecture for the Poor* [Chicago, 1973], p. 179)

[25] *as-Sulūk*, part 2, vol. 3, pp. 784-786.

[26] *Ibid.*, p. 775; possibly copied from *Risālat an-naba'*, p. 185. During the severe plague of A.H. 864, a number of villages were not affected in a similar manner, which perplexed Ibn Taghrī Birdī (*an-Nujūm*, Popper trans., vol. 22, p. 91).

Upper Egypt, e.g., Bahjūrah and Akhmīm, the Black Death was quite serious.[27] In the year 1389, out of 24,000 *faddans* of productive lands in Luxor, only 1,000 were being cultivated.[28]

In the Palestinian villages, as in the suburbs of Gaza, there was a high death rate among the peasants at the time of plowing, so that many men died in the fields.[29] From Jinīn,[30] no one survived except an old woman who fled from the pandemic.[31] When harvest time came, only a greatly reduced number of laborers was to be found on the land. The amirs and their servants tried to recruit more workers, promising them half the harvest, but found no one to help them collect the crops. From their horses, the landowners personally directed the servants but were unable to accomplish the entire task.[32] As in other epidemics, it can be generally assumed that the amirs employed their soldiers and household servants to cultivate, harvest, and thresh the crops, because of the shortage of peasants.[33] The result of the mortality rate in Egypt was such that "the crops came to maturity on only half the land."[34]

The diminished number of peasants was due to flight from the land, as well as to plague mortality. Everywhere plague occurred, there is evidence of flight from the countryside. Even in the Arabic accounts of Andalusia, the rural laborers are reported to have fled to the cities when plague struck their villages.[35] Leo Africanus, who traveled in North Africa in the early sixteenth century, accepted as a common fact that plague would customarily occur every ten, fifteen, and twenty-five years and that most of the inhabitants would abandon

27 *as-Sulūk*, part 2, vol. 3, p. 784.

28 as-Sakhāwī, *aḍ-Ḍaw' al-lāmi'*, vol. 5, p. 266.

29 *as-Sulūk*, part 2, vol. 3, p. 775; see "La Grande Peste Noire," p. 370, n. 7.

30 *Systematic Notes*, vol. 15, pp. 16, 48; map no. 13.

31 *as-Sulūk*, part 2, vol. 3, p. 774.

32 *Ibid.*, p. 785; Ibn Iyās, vol. 1, p. 191.

33 Rabie, *The Financial System of Egypt*, p. 69.

34 *as-Sulūk*, part 2, vol. 3, p. 779.

35 *Taḥṣīl*, fol. 72a.

the countryside at these intervals.[36] The depopulation of the countryside by death and flight from the Black Death was widely observed. Al-Maqrīzī exaggerates to the point of illogic this phenomenon: "The epidemic spread to the entire country to the extent that almost all the peasants died, and no one could be made to return to the land."[37]

Migration to the urban centers may have resulted from a number of factors, among them the desire to avoid the affliction. The pandemic afforded an opportunity for the peasants to escape from oppressive agrarian conditions and to obtain higher wages in the cities. In addition, the cities offered organized religious services, access to physicians, exorcists, and pharmacists, and large food reserves.[38] The urban grain reserves and the grain trade itself were, however, directly related to plague and plague dissemination because the plague flea, *Xenopsylla cheopis*, breeds most freely and lives longest in the debris of cereals. Grain is the favorite food not only of this species of flea, but also of the domestic rat and of man. The staff of life was perversely the scepter of death during plague epidemics.

Unfortunately, we have no evidence of any formal government action to control the mobility of the peasantry at the time of the Black Death, which would be comparable to European legislation. Generally, the Egyptian peasant was not supposed to leave his village without his overlord's permission, and then only for a specific time. Otherwise, the landowner could bring him back with the help of the government—and was even obliged by the government to do so.[39] The Syrian legal scholar as-Subkī (d. 771/1370), a witness to the Black Death in Damascus, castigated the practice established in Syria, and probably in Egypt, that one was constrained to return, within three years, peasants who had fled their vil-

[36] Quoted in Marchika, *La Peste en Afrique Septentrionale*, p. 14.

[37] *as-Sulūk*, part 2, vol. 3, p. 779.

[38] Ira Lapidus, "The Grain Economy of Mamlūk Egypt," *JESHO*, vol. 12, part 1 (1969), pp. 6-8, especially p. 8, n. 2.

[39] Poliak, *Feudalism*, p. 64.

lages.[40] For this reason, al-Maqrīzī refers to the peasant who worked on an *iqṭā'* as *qinn* ("serf").[41] Nevertheless, there is no indication of the forceful regulation or planned repopulation of the countryside during this unsettled time.[42]

On the contrary, the pattern of rural depopulation continued during the second half of the fourteenth century and the beginning of the fifteenth century.[43] During the recurrences of plague epidemics, villages continued to be deserted in Upper Egypt, as was reported, for instance, in Dhū l-Ḥijjah 808/May 1406.[44] At the beginning of this century, the number of deaths had been so great that forty villages were deserted by their inhabitants, "while the government, insensitive to their suffering, sought only to maintain its receipts by force and terror."[45] As an indication of this depopulation, forty congregational mosques in Upper Egypt reportedly had to be closed.[46] Again in 822/1419, we hear that "the horror of the plague struck the countryside and emptied a number of villages of their inhabitants."[47]

Al-Maqrīzī frequently mentioned the poverty of the Egyptian population in the first half of the fifteenth century, especially in Upper Egypt, where the majority of the inhabitants was not left sufficient revenue to acquire the simple necessities

[40] Darrag, p. 62.

[41] Rabie, *The Financial System of Egypt*, p. 63.

[42] In the earlier pandemic of Justinian, which recurred during the 'Abbāsid Period, Hārūn ar-Rashīd had attempted to prevent the depopulation of the countryside and to maintain its essential agrarian productivity. For in the beginning of his reign an epidemic of plague struck the villages of Palestine, where many fled. The caliph announced that those who would return to the deserted villages and till the land would be exempt from taxation (Belyaev, *Arabs, Islam and the Arab Caliphate*, pp. 229-230).

[43] Gaston Wiet, trans., "Le Traité des famines de Maqrīzī," *JESHO*, vol. 5 (1962), pp. 33, 47, 49.

[44] *as-Sulūk*, part 4, vol. 1, pp. 19-20.

[45] Darrag, p. 62.

[46] Ashtor, *Histoire*, p. 273.

[47] *as-Sulūk*, part 4, vol. 1, p. 487. See below for the other demographic factors affecting the evacuation of villages in the fifteenth century.

of life.[48] The history of the important city of Qūṣ may be representative. The town served as an administrative capital of Upper Egypt during the early Mamlūk Period and as a commercial center for the Red Sea trade to the Far East, Nubia, and the Sudan. Its importance continued until the beginning of the fifteenth century, when it was struck by a severe plague epidemic in 806/1403-1404. In that year, it is stated, 17,000 died in Qūṣ.[49] Thereafter, together with the shift of the Red Sea trade to Ṭūr, Qūṣ sank into oblivion. Upper Egypt suffered a significant decline in population, a result as much, perhaps, of extraordinary Nile flooding and bedouin incursions as of plague.

In Syria, plague contributed to a comparable depopulation where plague epidemics continued throughout the fifteenth century. The European traveler Bertrandon de la Broquière recounted in 1434 that near Ḥamā and Antioch several districts were completely abandoned.[50] Likewise, the Venetian consuls in Syria at the end of the Mamlūk Period mentioned in their consular reports epidemics that devastated the agrarian population.[51]

The Arabic histories are unanimous concerning this decline of population in the countryside following the Black Death, although their estimates of reduced or abandoned villages are widely contradictory.[52] The decline in the rural population

[48] Ashtor, *Histoire*, p. 272.

[49] *al-Khiṭaṭ*, vol. 1, pp. 236-237.

[50] Ashtor, *Histoire*, p. 388.

[51] *Ibid.* During the great plague epidemic of 1643, it is reported that 230 villages in Egypt were depopulated (J. J. Marcel, *Égypte depuis la conquête des Arabes jusqu'à la domination française* [Paris, 1848], p. 216).

[52] Ibn al-Ji'ān, *at-Tuhfah as-sanīyah fī asmā' al-bilād al-Miṣrīyah*, ed. by B. Moritz (Cairo, 1898), pp. 50, 57, 72, 73, 75, 117, 119, 122. (Cf. Omar Toussoun, *Mémoire sur les finances de l'Égypte depuis les Pharaons jusqu'à nos jours* [Cairo, 1924].) In 1375 there were reportedly 2,163 fiscal units (each usually consisting of a large village with surrounding hamlets) but since that time many of these units had ceased to exist and new villages were rarely recorded. Some lands were

and the reduction in agricultural productivity are reflected directly in the cadastral surveys of the Mamlūk Empire, and indirectly in the impoverishment of the Christian monastic communities.

The cadastral material presents serious problems of interpretation. Like Professor Russell in his study of the cadasters, we must assume that the original figures in the land surveys are pre-plague statistics based on the assessment of 1315. The changes in taxation, which are mostly reductions, are assumed to have occurred after the outbreak of the Black Death to about the year 1420.[53] Naturally reluctant to grant exemption from taxation, the government officials appear to have retained evidence of the pre-plague quotas. "The changes are so drastic that only plague, except in certain parts of the valley, seems sufficient as a cause."[54] While twelve villages actually had their assessments raised during this period, the overall effect of plague and the severe fluctuations of the Nile was a decrease in revenue resulting from a diminished population and its agri-

---

abandoned and others submerged by the Nile. This index of agricultural and demographic decline must be viewed in light of the fact that the *dīwān* based its records on information supplied by the estate holders who were naturally unwilling to report increases in revenue but were quick to report decreases. As was learned during the French occupation of Egypt, there was a large number of estates and villages that were not recorded in the official registers at all (Marcel, *Égypte depuis la conquête des Arabes*, p. 197). According to Ibn Taghrī Birdī, the number of territorial units in Egypt had *risen* by 1460 to 2,365 (*Hawādith ad-duhūr*, ed. by Popper, vol. 8, p. 333; see the discussion of this matter by Ashtor, *Histoire*, p. 273). The changes in the number of inhabited places may be considered as a rough index of demographic evolution only if there was a considerable reserve of vacant cultivable land. Otherwise, the increase in population results only in a more intensive cultivation and may eventually cause a diminution of the number of settlements because villages coalesce.

[53] Russell, "Population of Medieval Egypt," pp. 77-80. Russell has used the translation of an emended copy (about 827/1424) of a land survey dating from 777/1375, which was derived from the important cadaster of 715/1315; the translation is by Silvestre de Sacy in his *Relation de l'Égypte par Abd-Allatif*, pp. 581-708.

[54] Russell, "Population of Medieval Egypt," p. 78.

cultural production. Of more than 2,200 villages in Egypt, about forty were totally abandoned; 462 of the total number of villages had their tax assessments reduced. Nearly half of the communities of Atfiḥīyah province, on the east bank of the Nile above Cairo, for example, had their assessments reduced or were completely abandoned. Altogether, about twenty percent of all the Egyptian villages received a lower assessment, and two percent were abandoned. The greatest loss in taxation appears to have been in Atfiḥīyah province, where the taxes declined by 26.5 percent of the pre-plague figure, while Manfaluṭīyah province in Upper Egypt fell by 26.2 percent.[55] The total decline of tax revenue from its pre-plague level to about the year 1420 is estimated at about twelve percent.

The Christian monasteries in the Middle East fell victims to the Black Death, as they did in Europe.[56] A comparison of the pilgrimage account of Poggibonsi in 1347-1349 with that of Leonardo Frescobaldi and his fellow Florentines in 1384 shows a perceptible decline in the number of monks in the monasteries of the Holy Lands. Some monasteries had entirely disappeared, such as St. Gabriel at Nazareth, an unidentified monastery near Hebron, and the Monastery of the Desert of St. John.[57] In Egypt, the records of the famous Christian

[55] *Ibid.*, p. 79.

[56] The impoverishment of the Christian monasteries raises the question of the effects of the Black Death and subsequent plague epidemics on the communities (*ḵhānaqās*) of Muslim *ṣūfīs*, which were, however, located in urban and not in rural regions generally. In later epidemics of plague the mortality at the *ḵhānaqā* in Siryāqūs is specifically mentioned (e.g., *as-Sulūk*, part 4, vol. 2, p. 825). After the rapid development of *ḵhānaqās* in the first half of the fourteenth century in Egypt, the institution apparently deteriorated in the latter half of the fourteenth century and into the fifteenth cenury. Shahira G. Mehrez has outlined the architectural history of the *ḵhānaqā* in Egypt and has suggested the reasons for its decline ("The Ghawriyya in the Urban Context: An Analysis of Its Form and Function," unpubl. M.A. thesis, American University in Cairo, 1972). The entire subject of the *ḵhānaqā* deserves further investigation.

[57] Frescobaldi, Gucci, and Sigoli, *Visit to the Holy Places of Egypt, Sinai, Palestine and Syria*, trans. by T. Bellorini and E. Hoade (Jerusalem, 1948), p. 16.

monasteries at Wādī n-Naṭrūn, in the desert northwest of Cairo, are normal until 1346, when they become conspicuously silent. It is no coincidence that the following year marks the introduction of the Black Death into Egypt. From all indications, the complex of monasteries in Wādī n-Naṭrūn was greatly affected by the Black Death.[58] Particularly, the records for the Monastery of Dayr as-Suriān witnessed a gradual decline in the number of monks from the middle of the fourteenth century, due to plague and, after 1374, to the hardships imposed by hostile bedouin raids. The loss of population caused the abandonment of the Nile irrigation system, on which the life of the monasteries was largely dependent; consequently, severe famines took place in the latter fourteenth century. Al-Maqrīzī, writing in the first half of the fifteenth century, observed the diminished number of monasteries and monks in Wādī n-Naṭrūn. Whereas the desert had harbored about a hundred monasteries in the past, there were only seven remaining in the author's lifetime. The Monastery of Abū Yuhannis al-Qasīr was inhabited by only three monks at this time.[59] By 1413, there was only one monk left at Dayr as-Suriān; this monastery was reinvigorated at the end of the fifteenth century, when it was repopulated by Lebanese and eastern monks.[60]

There is no evidence of large-scale migrations during the Black Death, which befell almost the entire Middle East equally, but the repopulation of the Monastery of Dayr as-Suriān by eastern monks does raise the question of such migrations after later plague epidemics. Volney, a late eighteenth-century traveler in the Middle East, argues that Egypt during the Ottoman Period was saved from severe depopulation by the constant influx of immigrants from other parts of

[58] O.F.A. Meinardus, *Monks and Monasteries of the Egyptian Deserts* (Cairo, 1961), pp. 39, 136, 182, 220-221.

[59] F. Wüstenfeld, *Maqrizi's Geschichte der Copten* (Göttingen, 1845), pp. 109-111.

[60] Jules Leroy, "Un Témoinage inédit sur l'état du monastère des Syriens au Wadi'n Natrūn au début du XVIème siècle," *BIFAO*, vol. 65 (Cairo, 1967), p. 4.

the Ottoman Empire.[61] Immigration did take place during the early Ottoman Period from neighboring countries, especially from North Africa; Maghribī villages were established in Upper Egypt at that time. Similar movements of peoples are suggested also for Syria-Palestine in the same period.[62]

Yet the depopulation of the cultivated lands continued unabated while the mamlūk sultans tried unsuccessfully to reverse this almost inevitable trend.[63] It is reasonable to conclude that during the latter fourteenth and the fifteenth centuries the rural population declined appreciably, partly as a result of plague, and, consequently, that the amounts of cultivated land and production were diminished.

The reduced productivity of the countryside greatly affected the prosperity of the cities, which relied directly on the country for a large part of their income besides their daily sustenance. The cities themselves, as centers of communication, were even more vulnerable to plague. Because of the high density of population, plague spread easily and caused massive mortality. The medieval chroniclers naturally focused on the dramatic consequences of depopulation in the cities where they dwelt and were able to record the immediate and prolonged effects of the epidemics.

C. URBAN DEPOPULATION

The populations of the major cities of Egypt and Syria were diminished by flight and large-scale mortality. This trend was reflected in the physical deterioration of the urban centers.

Many inhabitants certainly fled from the cities despite the religious prohibition against fleeing a plague-stricken region. Flight from the urban centers was not inconsistent with an influx of people into the cities at various stages of a plague epidemic, especially when the disease was not rampant or after it had declined. On the other hand, evacuation of the cities

[61] *Voyage*, p. 143.

[62] Poliak, *Feudalism*, pp. 203-204.

[63] Darrag, pp. 62-65; Russell, "Population of Medieval Egypt," p. 78, Table 4.

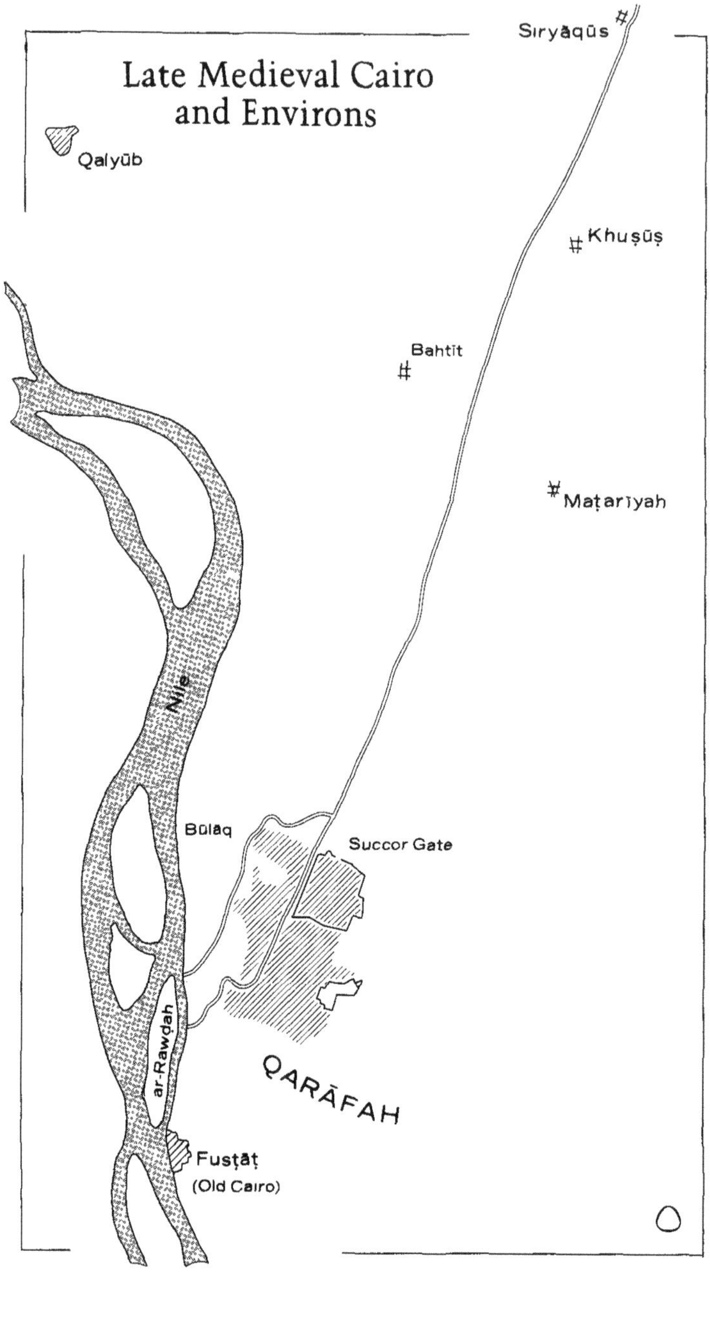

Late Medieval Cairo
and Environs
Qalyūb
Siryāqūs
Khuṣūṣ
Bahtīt
Maṭarīyah
Nile
Būlāq
Succor Gate
ar-Rawḍah
QARĀFAH
Fusṭāṭ
(Old Cairo)

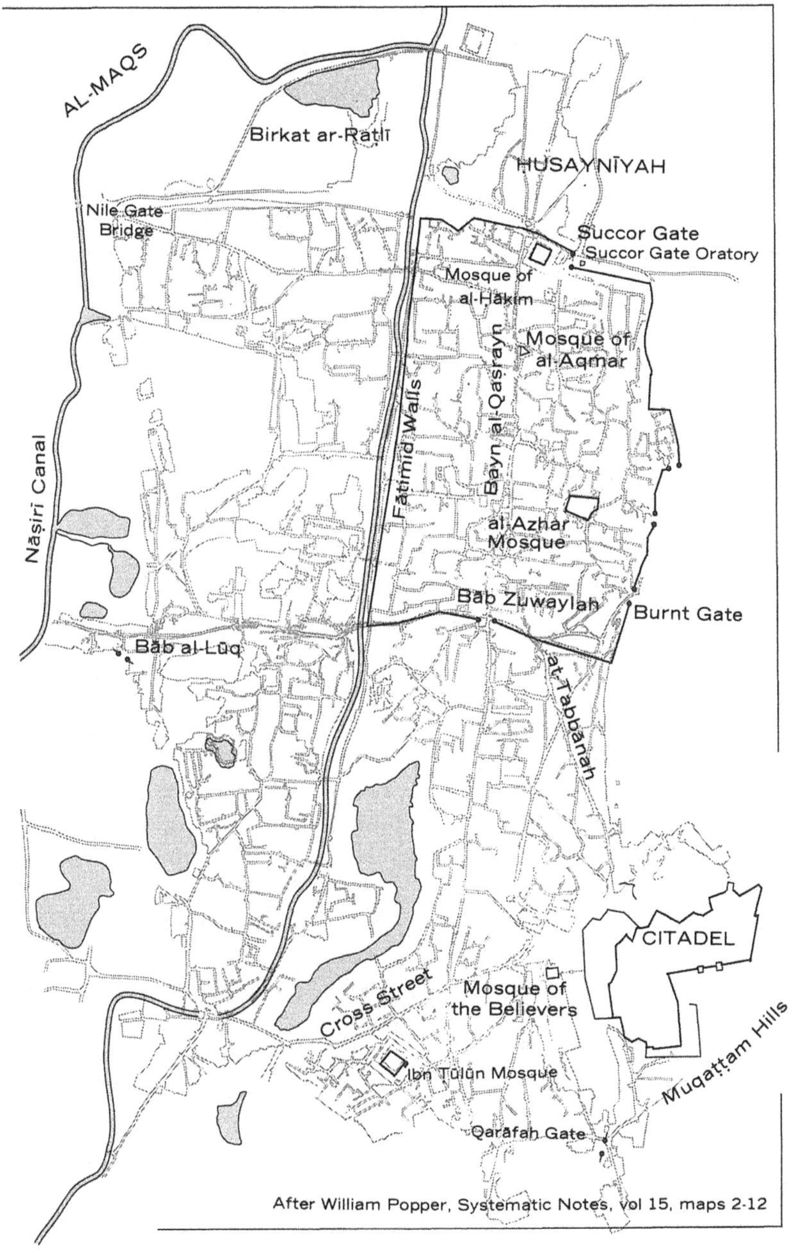

After William Popper, Systematic Notes, vol 15, maps 2-12

during periods when plague was severe may have given contemporary observers a greater impression of plague deaths. A good example of the flight caused by the Black Death is the account of events in Fusṭāṭ.

The Black Death was apparently quite severe in this suburb of Cairo, and it is reported that the destruction was particularly great in the districts of Zuqāq al-Qanādīl and an-Naḥḥāsīn. Because of the high mortality rate, many of the people moved eastward, and the emptied houses were abandoned. The people did not begin to reinhabit the region around the ancient Mosque of ʿAmr ibn al-ʿĀṣ and the east bank of the Nile again until 776/1374-1375. Even after this date, periodic depopulation caused by plague epidemics occurred. For example, in the epidemic of 833/1430 "forty men rode in a ship and went from Old Cairo toward Upper Egypt and all died before they had reached al-Maimūn. And a woman left Old Cairo riding on an ass and intending to go to Cairo; she died while riding, and lay where she was thrown in the road all that day until the corpse began to be fetid; then she was buried without knowledge of who her family were."[1] The continual exodus of population from Fusṭāṭ naturally led to the reduction in the number of its inhabitants and the impoverishment of this suburban region. "The people began to tear down the houses of Fusṭāṭ and to sell its ruins until it became what it is now."[2] The observations of al-Maqrīzī about Fusṭāṭ in the first part of the fifteenth century are supported by the reports of foreign travelers.[3]

Similarly, al-Maqrīzī states that many quarters of Cairo were abandoned and had fallen into ruin by the beginning of the fifteenth century.[4] Flight from Cairo had been common during the Black Death. Many people may have moved to ar-Rawḍah Island in the Nile, believing that the air would be purer there; the migration to this island was observed in

[1] *an-Nujūm*, Popper trans., vol. 18, p. 70.
[2] *al-Khiṭaṭ*, vol. 1, p. 637. [3] Darrag, p. 85.
[4] Quoted in Ashtor, *Histoire*, p. 273.

later plague epidemics.[5] We know that the mamlūk sultan fled the capital with the amirs[6] at the time of the Black Death, recalling the flight of the early Arab rulers of Egypt during the epidemics that followed the Plague of Justinian. The sultan stayed in Siryāqūs with his court from the beginning of Rajab 749/25 September 1348[7] until the end of Ramaḍān/22 December.[8] Later plague epidemics caused sultans to flee Cairo, as in 762/1360-1361 when the sultan escaped to Kūm Birah.[9] When the plague epidemic of 919/1513-1514 occurred in Egypt, some of the amirs in Cairo sent their children—two of the amirs sent some of their mamlūks—to Ṭūr for safety.[10]

Evidence of flight from Syrian towns during the Black Death is found in the story of a peasant in Gaza who had led twenty oxen out to his fields; the oxen died one after another, and the man helplessly watched them collapse. He returned to Gaza and then departed for Cairo. The governor himself abandoned Gaza in order to take refuge in the village of Budda'arsh. Incidentally, flight from the cities gave some an opportunity for larceny, and we get a glimpse of such activity in al-Maqrīzī's account of Gaza. Following the report of the peasant who fled to Cairo, it is related that six robbers entered a house in Gaza in order to burglarize it. They accomplished their crime, but all died shortly thereafter. Al-Maqrīzī frequently mentions the fact that homes, shops, and caravanserais were left unguarded against such depredations.[11]

5 al-Manṣūrī, Dār al-Kutub al-Miṣrīyah MS no. 102 *majāmī' m*, fol. 202b.

6 *as-Sulūk*, part 2, vol. 3, p. 781, clearly states that after the funeral of 'Abdallāh Manufī in Cairo (Ramadān A.H. 748) "the amirs returned to Siryāqūs"; cf. "The Plague and Its Effects," p. 72.

7 *as-Sulūk*, part 2, vol. 3, p. 780.

8 *Ibid.*, p. 781.

9 *al-Khiṭaṭ*, vol. 2, p. 316; see Ramzī, *al-Qāmūs al-jughrāfī*, part 2, vol. 3, p. 63.

10 "The Plague and Its Effects," p. 72.

11 *as-Sulūk*, part 2, vol. 3, p. 775. Concerning the village of "Budda-'arsh," see "La Grande Peste Noire," p. 370, n. 7.

The flight of the governor of Gaza during the Black Death was not an isolated phenomenon. During the severe plague of 897/1491-1492 in Jerusalem, the governor, Khaḍarbak, fled the city and stayed in the orchards in the suburbs. Fear of the disease increased, and the populace rebuked him for fleeing and caused him to return to the city after a short time. Subsequently, his daughter and then his wife died, and finally the governor himself.[12]

Ibn Abī Ḥajalah, who was in the Syrian capital at the time of the Black Death, alludes to a man who harangued a crowd trying to persuade them to leave the city.[13] In Antioch, many of the inhabitants went out from the city when the pandemic struck, as did the Kurds from Qaramān and Caesarea; a number attempted to escape to Rūm (Anatolia), but most died en route. In the case of Antioch, the horses of the dead fugitives returned, and the people who had remained in the city followed the horses back to their dead colleagues. The survivors took what the others had abandoned and came back to the city, only to be overtaken by plague themselves.[14]

We are well informed of the flight of urban populations by not only the historical chronicles but also by the poetic accounts of the Black Death. In some cases, the poetry of the plague observers voices the desirability of flight. For example, the verses of Ibn Nubātah quoted by al-Maqrīzī: "Let us leave Damascus whoever wants to live. I have no desire to remain here. The souls of men have become very cheap; each soul is worth a kernel."[15] Furthermore, the plague treatises attest to

[12] al-'Ulaymī, *al-Uns al-jalīl bi-ta'rīkh al-Quds wal-Khalīl* (Baghdad, 1968), vol. 2, p. 361.

[13] *Daf' an-niqmah*, fol. 80b.

[14] *as-Sulūk*, part 2, vol. 3, pp. 773-774.

[15] *Ibid.*, p. 790. The metaphor of a *kernel* is the most common one in the poetic descriptions of the plague boil because the word *ḥabbah* may mean both plague "pustule" and "seed" or "grain." See also aṣ-Ṣafadī quoted in *ibid.*, p. 789, and al-Mi'mār quoted in *ibid.*, p. 791; aṣ-Safadī, Dār al-Kutub al-Miṣrīyah MS no. 102 *majāmī' m*, fol. 199a; Fadlallāh, *ibid.*, fol. 200a; Nawājī, *ibid.*, fol. 201a; and *Badhl*, fols. 11a, 130a.

flight from plague by their continual discussion of the legality of fleeing from a plague-stricken land. The famous treatise written by Ibn al-Khaṭīb during the Black Death in Andalusia recommends flight from the disease.[16] In addition, flight was advised by the legal scholars as-Subkī and az-Zarkashī in the Middle East.[17] Later writers on plague in the Middle East argue for the advantage and permissibility of fleeing.[18]

Concerning urban mortality, depopulation was estimated in the fourteenth and fifteenth centuries in a number of ways. The deaths of certain individuals in the major cities were recorded in the *dīwān al-mawārīth al-ḥashrīyah*, and these *dīwān* figures were cited by the major chroniclers, particularly for the later plague occurrences contemporary with their own lives.[19] The *dīwān* registered only the deaths of those with taxable legacies. The government would take the entire estate of anyone dying without heirs and the residue of an estate where the heirs were not entitled to the whole inheritance. In some instances, the government would confiscate inheritances even when there were heirs. Cairo and Fusṭāṭ had separate *dīwāns* and included the deaths of Christians and Jews as well as Muslims for both of these areas.[20] The lists were made in duplicate; one for the director of the *dīwān* and the other for his assistant, the *nāẓir ad-dawlah* or auditor. Al-Maqrīzī refers

[16] *Muqni'at*, fol. 43a.

[17] See Appendix 3.

[18] Appendix 3: (1) Idrīs al-Badlīsī; (2) al-Jazā'irī; and (3) al-Yārḥiṣārī.

[19] al-Maqrīzī refers to a *dīwān* for the city of Fez, which excluded from its accounts the deaths of foreigners and the poor; it furnished the total of 36,000 deaths during the plague epidemic of 817-818 A.H. (*as-Sulūk*, part 4, vol. 1, p. 351). This and other references in the Egyptian sources concerning Fez may be explained by the demonstrated connections between the Marinid dynasty of Morocco and the Mamlūk Sultanate (see M. Canard, "Les Relations entre les Mérinides et les Mamelouks au XIVe siècle," *Annales de l'Institut d'Études Orientales*, vol. 5 [Algiers, 1939-1941], pp. 41-81).

[20] Rabie, *The Financial System of Egypt*, pp. 1-2, 7, 127-132, 146-147; *Systematic Notes*, vol. 15, p. 99; B. Michel, "L'Organisation financière de l'Égypte sous les Sultans Mamelouks d'après Qalqachandi," *BIE*, vol. 7 (Cairo, 1925), pp. 136, 139.

to the minute and often severe control of the state over inheritances by this *dīwān* before the Black Death.[21] (The mortality from the *dīwān al-mawārīth* is explicitly stated for the severe famine and pestilence during 694-696/1294-1297 in Cairo.[22])

All the chroniclers writing on Cairo, when referring to the figures of this *dīwān* for plague deaths, exclude those who died "at the hospital (*bīmāristān*) and the corpses (*ṭuraḥā'*) from off the streets."[23] This common expression is conveniently explained by Ibn Taghrī Birdī in his account of plague in 864/1460:

> During those days the plague spread in Cairo; the number of dead whose names came to the bureau [of the controller of escheats] was 35 on Tuesday, 19 Rabī' II . . . This number of deaths on analysis is found to be exclusive of the deaths in the Manṣūrī Hospital and the pious foundation for unclaimed corpses.[24]

The hospital is thus identified as the famous one established by the Sultan al-Manṣūr Sayf ad-Dīn Qalā'ūn (678-689/1279-1290). This hospital included not only wards with a regular medical staff, lecture rooms, and laboratories but also an adjoining library of medical, theological, and legal books. The structure is still functioning today in the old city and is one of the great monuments of mamlūk architecture.[25] The *waqf aṭ-ṭuraḥā'*, or trust for the burial of indigents, is often referred to

[21] Wiet, "Le Traité des famines de Maqrīzī," p. 40; see also Rabie, *The Financial System of Egypt*, pp. 130-132.

[22] *Beiträge zur Geschichte der Mamlūken-sultane*, p. 36; al-Birzālī quoted in Little, *An Introduction to Mamlūk Historiography*, p. 48 (Little shows that the anonymous historian edited by Zetterstéen took this passage from al-Birzālī).

[23] al-Maqrīzī's early use of the phrase during the plague epidemic of 790 A.H. is given in *as-Sulūk*, part 3, vol. 2, p. 578.

[24] *an-Nujūm*, Popper trans., vol. 22, p. 91; see the Arabic text, ed. by Popper, vol. 7, p. 528.

[25] See the description of the hospital in Lane-Poole, *A History of Egypt*, pp. 283-284.

explicitly in the historical accounts.[26] In both cases, the plague victims were poor and were not listed in the *dīwān*.[27] The poor were often the recipients of the personal charity of the sultan and the mamlūk amirs, as in the plague epidemic of 776/1374-1375 in Cairo.[28]

Unfortunately, we have no extant *dīwān* data for the period of the Black Death in Cairo. Al-Maqrīzī mentions very general daily death rates during the Black Death and subsequent epidemics, while his first precise reference to the *dīwān* is made for the epidemic of 790/1388.[29] Ibn Taghrī Birdī does not discuss mortality until the severe plague of 833/1429. Ibn Ḥajar uses the *dīwān* figures from the epidemic of 819/1416-1417, but less exactly than al-Maqrīzī. This does not mean that *dīwān* figures for Cairo did not exist for the Black Death. Ibn Ḥajar states that the number of names registered in the *dīwān al-mautā* decreased as the Black Death waned and that this registration was the normal practice in other times of plague.[30] Likewise, we can be certain that the *dīwān* operated in Damascus during the Black Death. Ibn Kathīr asserts that when the pandemic began to decline in the year 750/1349, "the *dīwān* of inheritance decreased to twenty after it had reached a total of five hundred in the year 749."[31]

We can assume that the people tried to evade taxes and confiscations by the government and were particularly successful during the confusion of a massive epidemic. One treatise

[26] For example, see Ibn Ḥajar, *Inbā' al-ghumr*, vol. 2, p. 260. See also *Muslim Cities*, p. 84.

[27] It is unknown whether this *dīwān* was associated in any way with a tax on coffins; there are no references to funeral taxes in Cairo or their suspension during times of plague. We know that there were taxes on biers, washers, and carriers in Damascus, for the taxes were abolished by the government in that city during the Black Death (*al-Bidāyah*, vol. 14, p. 226; *Daf' an-niqmah*, fol. 75a).

[28] Ibn Ḥajar, *Inbā' al-ghumr*, vol. 1, p. 72.

[29] See n. 23 above. The same reference to *dīwān* mortality figures is found in Ibn al-Furāt, *Ta'rīkh*, vol. 9, pp. 28-29 for the year A.H. 790.

[30] *Badhl*, fol. 124a.

[31] *al-Bidāyah*, vol. 14, p. 250; see also *as-Sulūk*, part 2, vol. 3, p. 779.

writer accepted this evasion as normal during plague epidemics.[32] This also seems to be the point of a passage from al-Maqrīzī:

> On Monday, 4 [3] Jumādā II [833], the number carried out of the gates of Cairo was counted and reached 1,200, aside from the funerals from the Hakkūra, the Ḥusainīya, Būlāq, Cross Street, Old Cairo, the two Qarāfas, and the Desert quarters of Cairo, numbering more than that. At the same time there were registered in the bureau of escheats in Cairo only 390, because some people made coffins for charity, and most of those who carried their dead in these coffins failed to register the names in the bureau.[33]

Furthermore, al-Maqrīzī tells us that during the epidemic of 841/1437-1438 the people prepared their own coffins and that most of the deaths were among children, slaves, and servants.[34]

Support for this statement of the high mortality rate among children and slaves is found in a unique (to my knowledge) summary of *dīwān* mortality figures during the plague epidemic of 822/1419. The great number of deaths among children was a characteristic of the plague recurrences in both the East and the West:

> When I Jumādā began [26 May 1419], the plague abated so that on the first of the month the number of dead listed was seventy-seven. Shaykh Taqī ad-Dīn al-Maqrīzī says: "The number of those who died in Cairo and whose name was entered in the bureau from Ṣafar 20 to the end of I Rabīʿ [March 18 to April 26] was 7,652 souls:[35] 1,065 men, 669 women, 3,969 children, 544 male slaves, 1,369 female slaves, 69 Christians, 32 Jews. That was exclusive of the hospital and exclusive of the Old Cairo bureau, and those whose names did not come to the bureau [in Cairo]; and this does

[32] *Badhl*, fol. 124a.

[33] Quoted in *an-Nujūm*, Popper trans., vol. 18, p. 71. This is copied from the report in *as-Sulūk*, part 4, vol. 2, p. 826.

[34] *as-Sulūk*, part 4, vol. 2, p. 1031.

[35] The total of the figures given is 7,717 and not 7,652.

not fall short of completing 10,000 dead. There died also in the towns of ash-Sharqīya and al-Gharbīya provinces the like number." I say regarding Shaykh Taqī ad-Dīn's words, "this does not fall short of 10,000," that in the plague of 833 there died on one day in Cairo and its suburbs about 10,000 men, and that continued for some days, with between 8,000, 9,000, and 10,000 [deaths daily], as (God Who is exalted willing) will be related in its proper place in the chapter on al-Malik al-Ashraf Barsbay al-Duqmāqī.[36]

This extract from the *dīwān* indicates that the mortality rate had declined from an average of 193 a day from 18 March to 26 April 1419 to 77 on 26 May. As Ibn Taghrī Birdī suggests, the degree of mortality during this epidemic was far below that of the plague epidemic of 833/1429-1430, although it is unlikely that in the latter epidemic the deaths reached 10,000 a day.[37] At the very least, this one excerpt from the *dīwān* demonstrates the effective registration of plague dead and a level of mortality that is not inconsistent with the more severe plague epidemics. Moreover, it shows that the records of the *dīwān* were accessible to the historians and that they examined them.

The list of dead for the plague of 822/1419 must be a greatly abbreviated version of the registry. For example, although it does not specify mamlūks as a distinct class, they must have been recorded separately because of their importance to the state and their sizable legacies. The recording of deaths among the mamlūks was also important for the redistribution of their *iqṭā's*. Thus, in the epidemic of 864/1460, Ibn Taghrī Birdī says, 300 persons were recorded in the *dīwān* for Monday, 15 Jumādā II/8 April, of whom seventy-five were mamlūks, including thirty-five amirs' mamlūks and others; the rest were the sultan's mamlūks.[38]

[36] *an-Nujūm*, Popper trans., vol. 17, p. 66; *as-Sulūk*, part 4, vol. 1, p. 492. Ibn Taghrī Birdī refers to his account of the severe plague epidemic in 833/1429-1430 during the reign of the Sultan Barsbay (825-841/1422-1437), see *an-Nujūm, Popper* trans., vol. 18, pp. 69-76, 181-189.

[37] See below, part E, section 2.

[38] *an-Nujūm*, Popper trans., vol. 22, p. 97.

Regarding the religious minorities in the summary of the *dīwān*, it appears that the government directly supervised inheritances; this practice differed from the independent control of legacies exercised by minority groups in pre-Mamlūk Egypt. An incident in the fifteenth century sheds a good deal of light on this point. In Ramaḍān 841/February-March 1438, when plague was raging in Cairo, the sultan accepted the scheme of a man who suggested the government's taking the inheritances of Jews and Copts, which were not distributed to heirs. The sultan sold to the man the right to carry out this scheme and decreed that the control of all inheritances would be attached *once again* to the public treasury, seemingly referring to the earlier practice. In order to execute this design to the fullest, the controller made the measure retroactive to the first year of the reign of Sultan Barsbay (825/1422). He ruthlessly examined the titles of property and made the minorities pay the tax. The epidemic decimated the population, and a great amount of goods and wealth was found to be without heirs, a fact that rendered his enterprise very profitable. The successor to his office continued the same policy (decree of Rabīʿ II, 842/September 1438).[39]

The chroniclers pay remarkably little attention to the financial burden of the tax on the people or the benefits derived by the government from this source during plague epidemics. The contemporary observers were more interested in the *dīwān* figures as merely indicators of the epidemics' growth and decline. Ibn Taghrī Birdī remarks: "The value of mentioning the statistics (of the bureau) lies in the fact that they indicate the increase and decrease in the plague, so there is some value in mentioning them."[40]

On the basis of these *dīwān* figures, there was an attempt by some to estimate—however unsatisfactorily—total mortality. A chronicler of Damascus recalls that for the plague epidemic of 795/1392-1393:

[39] Darrag, pp. 144-145.
[40] *an-Nujūm*, Popper trans., vol. 22, p. 94.

One of the scribes of the bureau of escheats in Aleppo told me, "I wanted to report accurately how many died in Aleppo and its province; I worked it out and found that from the beginning of the epidemic to its end three hundred and sixty thousand persons died; men, women, children, Jews, and Christians—mostly children. One hundred and fifty thousand died from within the city, and the remainder from outside of the city and its vicinity."[41]

While the scribe makes the valuable observation that children were the primary victims of the epidemic, he must have multiplied the *dīwān* deaths by an unreasonable figure in order to arrive at a total number of deaths. The resulting estimate is far too high for Aleppo's probable population, but the proportional rate of mortality between the city and its suburbs may be correct.

As should be clear, the *dīwāns* for Cairo, Fusṭāṭ, and the other major cities of Egypt and Syria recorded only a fraction of the total urban mortality during a plague epidemic.[42] Other methods were used to ascertain the entire daily death rate. Ibn Taghrī Birdī tried to estimate the aggregate number of deaths by counting the biers that were prayed over in one important oratory in Cairo and roughly multiplying that number by the number of principal oratories in the city.[43] More systematically, the government undertook the counting of deaths in the mosques, for the same historian tells us that in 833/1430: "The

[41] Ibn Ṣaṣrā, *ad-Durrah al-muḍī'ah fī ad-dawlah az-ẓāhiriyyah*, ed. and trans. by William M. Brinner, *A Chronicle of Damascus, 1389-1397* (Berkeley and Los Angeles, 1963), vol. 1, pp. 182-183, vol. 2, p. 137.

[42] See below, part E, n. 45 for the relationship between *dīwān* mortality figures to the number of funerals in the mosques. In addition, the percentage of deaths in the *dīwān* to the number carried out of the gates of the city on Jumādā II, A.H. 833, was 32% (*as-Sulūk*, part 4, vol. 2, p. 826).

[43] *an-Nujūm*, Popper trans., vol. 22, pp. 95-97, gives the number of dead who were prayed over at the major mosques of the city during the plague epidemic of 864/1460. He mentions seventeen oratories whereas al-Maqrīzī numbers only fourteen (*as-Sulūk*, part 4, vol. 2, p. 827).

number of the dead for whom prayers were said in the oratory at Succor Gate on Sunday 10 [9] Jumādā II [5 March], was 505; a large number with inkstands and pens had come to stand there to record this."[44] According to al-Maqrīzī, those who said the prayers over the dead usually recorded the number.[45] During the plague epidemic of 863-864/1459-1460 in Cairo, "Amir Zayn ad-Dīn, the major-domo, sent a number of his men at a designated wage to count all the oratories of Cairo and its environs, and to count the number of those prayed over."[46] Ibn Taghrī Birdī concludes that, as far as he knew, deaths were recorded in this manner only in Cairo and were an approximation of the total number.[47]

Another method employed by the government was to count the number of coffins going out of the city gates. The two methods were probably used concurrently, for Ibn Taghrī Birdī states that during the same month of Jumādā II, 833/February-March 1430, there were 12,300(?) coffins carried out of Cairo's gates in a single day, "as determined by the clerks who made the count by order of some high official or, according to others, by order of the Sultan himself."[48]

These two means of estimating urban deaths by the government during the later plague occurrences are significant because they were used during the Black Death in Cairo and are our only source for estimating mortality. According to al-Maqrīzī, a count was made at the time of the Black Death of the number of people for whom funeral prayers were recited in the oratories of the suburbs to the north and east of the city (outside the enceinte of the Fāṭimid walls). In addition, a count was made within Cairo during Shaʿbān and Ramaḍān/25 October-22 December 1348, when the Black Death was at its worst.[49] Second, Ibn Abī Ḥajalah tells us that he heard from reliable sources that "Majīd ad-Dīn al-Asʿadī, the famous

[44] *an-Nujūm*, Popper trans., vol. 18, p. 71.
[45] *as-Sulūk*, part 4, vol. 2, p. 826.
[46] *an-Nujūm*, Popper trans., vol. 22, pp. 93-94.
[47] *Ibid.*, p. 93, n. 273.
[48] *Ibid.*, vol. 18, p. 72.
[49] *as-Sulūk*, part 2, vol. 3, p. 782.

merchant of the sultan, put in charge of the gates of Cairo in Sha'bān and Ramaḍān a group of his men, and they recorded for him the number of dead who went out from the gates."[50]

The urban mortality rate is observable not only in the high *dīwān* figures, the numbers of funerals, and the counts at the city gates, but also by the sharply decreased commercial activity[51] and the beginning of the deterioration of some of the city quarters. Al-Maqrīzī records, for example, that the previously thriving at-Tabbānah region, between the old city and the Citadel, was deserted and fell into ruin as a result of the Black Death.[52] Within the following fifteen years, plague appeared twice in Cairo; Ibn Abī Ḥajalah claims that many properties around the capital were vacated, and no one dwelt there up to the time of his own account (766/1364).[53] As we have seen, this may very well apply also to Fusṭāṭ.

Despite a brief political and economic recovery under Sultan Barqūq (784-801/1382-1399)—which was witnessed by impressionable foreign travelers unfamiliar with Cairo's earlier greatness[54]—the depopulation of the metropolitan area continued apace into the fifteenth century, paralleling the rural decline in population and cultivation. The effects of the cumu-

[50] *Daf' an-niqmah,* fol. 75a. According to this method of accounting, Ibn Abī Ḥajalah states that 900,000 dead were counted from within the city, and this incredible number is given by al-Maqrīzī (see below, part E, n. 49). It is highly probable that al-Maqrīzī took this figure from Ibn Abī Ḥajalah, as did Ibn Hajar (*Badhl,* fol. 128a). However, Ibn Abī Ḥajalah was in not Cairo but Damascus during the Black Death; he may actually have been told about the accounting of dead in Cairo but given an inflated and more impressive number than the actual total. See also Janet L. Abu-Lughod, *Cairo: 1001 Years of "the City Victorious"* (Princeton, 1971), p. 37, n. 5.

[51] See below, chap. VII, part D.

[52] *al-Khiṭaṭ,* vol. I, p. 361.

[53] *Daf' an-niqmah,* fol. 75a.

[54] See Abu-Lughod, *Cairo,* p. 38 and n. 7. The discrepancies between the native observers of the deterioration of the cities and the foreign visitors is hardly inexplicable considering the relative size and activity of Cairo to contemporary cities in Europe and North Africa (*ibid.,* p. 41). Even the otherwise impressionable Italians, Frescobaldi and Sigoli, attest to the depopulation of the Egyptian countryside, see part B above.

lative decrease in urban population by the early fifteenth century are most clearly seen in the degeneration of the capital. Professor Janet Abu-Lughod has described the conditions of Cairo at this time in the following passage, based primarily on the account of al-Maqrīzī:

> The northern suburb of al-Ḥusaynīyah, which had become relatively deserted after the Black Death, was utterly desolate by 1403. The western suburbs, sorely decimated during the preceding fifty years, were reduced to scattered dwellings and a few orchards. Birkat al-Raṭli, the former resort area to the northwest, was deserted, and even the once-populous industrial district of al-Maqs was in ruins, with only a few markets and mosques still functioning. Ruins bordered the Citadel, and Qāhirah and Fusṭāṭ were once again separated by dusty plains and rubble. In the brief thirty years between the works of Ibn Duqmaq and Maqrīzī [793-823/1390-1420], Fusṭāṭ had undergone a rapid decline, with a devastation of the famous Sūq al-Qanādīl (the covered bazaar so dark and dense it was lit by candles) and the Khiṭ al-Muṣāṣah, and with many buildings destroyed by scavengers. Only the cemetery cities south and east continued to grow, ironically confirming the macabre state of the city. Furthermore, the blight which had hitherto been confined to the suburban ring now spread into the very heart of the central city. Once-bustling markets were abandoned as poverty and depression inhibited commerce. The caravan market had still not recovered from the sequestrations of al-Nāṣir Faraj [801-815/1399-1412], and the luxury markets—fur, candles, gold and silver armor and ornamented bridles for horses—closed for lack of customers; even the prostitutes felt the impact of the depression. Residential quarters suffered a similar fate. The *ḥārāt* [quarters] within the eastern and northern sections of the walled city were deserted at their fringe and decayed into slums near the city's center. It is perhaps significant that almost all of the *ḥārāt* of the city and its environs listed by Maqrīzī were

> located within the longitudinal belt stretching between al-Ḥusaynīyah north of the walled city and the Citadel due south of the walled enclave. It is perhaps also significant that only 31 of the 37 *ḥārāt* identified by Maqrīzī were noted as still in existence. Thus, by the opening decades of the fifteenth century, if we are to be guided by the famous topographer, Cairo had diminished in extent and population, had retrenched toward the portions settled before the expansive era of al-Nāṣir ibn Qalāwūn, and had suffered a severe setback in prosperity and commercial activity.[55]

Later, there was a revival of trade because of the resurgence of the international spice trade in the middle of the fifteenth century, but population and agricultural productivity continued to decline due to successive epidemics of plague, famines, foreign campaigns, and domestic insecurity.[56] The mamlūk élite, who benefited most from this efflorescence of the spice trade, was certainly not immune from the plague epidemics which struck Cairo; they were serious and costly casualties. The deaths of the highly prized mamlūks formed a significant portion of the urban mortality rate, and along with domestic slaves, children, and foreigners, the mamlūks made up a disproportionate share of the total human destruction during the recurrences of plague after the Black Death.

D. A SPECIAL CASE: THE MAMLŪK ARMY

"In almost every epidemic the following formula, or one resembling it, is used: *wafataka al-ṭā'ūn bil-mamālīk wal-aṭfāl wal-'abīd wal-jawārī wal-ghurabā* ('the plague caused death among the mamlūks, children, black slaves, slave-girls and foreigners')."[1] During the successive plague epidemics, there are many references to the death of mamlūks, slaves, children, and foreigners—not all of whom may previously have been

[55] *Ibid.*, pp. 39-40.

[56] *Ibid.*, pp. 40-41, 48-49.

[1] "The Plague and Its Effects," pp. 69-70.

exposed to plague.[2] The modern study of *Pasteurella pestis* has shown that infection is dependent not on age, race, or sex, but entirely on exposure.[3] If the modern form of plague does not differ significantly from its medieval predecessor, it can only be inferred that the frequent references during the Black Death and later epidemics to the high mortality rate among women and children indicate the easy communication of plague in unhealthful conditions of their homes and their closer domestic contact with flea-infested animals and with plague victims.[4] Moreover, it is known that pregnant women are able to transmit their infection to their children, and the cruel death of mothers and their infants during the Black Death attracted particular attention. Al-Maqrīzī states, for example: "It was established during this epidemic [the Black Death] that no infant survived more than a day or two after its birth, and its mother followed it into the grave."[5]

The foreigners and slaves—whether mamlūk or domestic—shared the common plight but were particularly vulnerable to the recurrent plague epidemics because of a lack of immunity to the disease or poor physical health. Slaves were usually brought to Egypt at a young age, generally without immunity

[2] In addition to Ayalon's citations (*ibid.*, p. 70, n. 1), see for the plague of A.H. 775-776: al-Manbijī, *Tasliyat*, p. 3; the plague of A.H. 783: *as-Sulūk*, part 3, vol. 2, p. 441; the plague of A.H. 795: Ibn Sasrā, *ad-Durrah al-muḍī'ah*, vol. 1, p. 183; the plague of A.H. 822: Ibn Hajar, *Inbā' al-ghumr*, vol. 3, pp. 199-200; the plague of A.H. 833: *as-Sulūk*, part 4, vol. 2, pp. 822, 824 *et passim*; the plague of A.H. 841-842: Ibn Ḥajar, *Inbā' al-ghumr*, British Museum Add. MS no. 7321, fols. 332b, 341a, and *as-Sulūk*, part 4, vol. 2, p. 1031 *et passim*, vol. 3, p. 1127; the plague of A.H. 848: Ibn Hajar, *Inbā' al-ghumr*, British Museum Add. MS no. 7321, fol. 365a; the plague of A.H. 881: al-'Ulaymī, *al-Uns al-jalīl*, vol. 2, p. 318; the plague of 987 A.H.: *ibid.*, vol. 2, p. 361; and the plague of A.H. 918-919: al-Badlīsī, Berlin MS no. 6371 (cf. Süheyl Ünver, "Sur l'histoire de la peste en Turquie," p. 479).

[3] Pollitzer, *Plague*, pp. 503-504.

[4] *as-Sulūk*, part 2, vol. 3, pp. 775, 780, 784; *al-Bidāyah*, vol. 14, p. 226; *'Iqd al-jumān*, p. 86; *Muqni'at*, fol. 44a; Ibn Ḥabīb, *Tadhkirat an-nabīh*, British Museum Add. MS no. 7335, fol. 145b.

[5] *as-Sulūk*, part 2, vol. 3, p. 784.

to plague and were consequently susceptible to the disease endemic in the Middle East.[6] The susceptibility of slaves to plague was well known. At the time of the plague epidemic in 841/1437-1438 in Cairo, the slave market was shut because of the large number of slaves who had died of plague. One man had to sell his slave, so he began to hawk him in the streets. But no one responded, regardless of the crowds of people; on the contrary, they fled, fearing the death of the slave by plague.[7] The consistently high mortality rate among the mamlūks, especially, during the Black Death and recurrent plague epidemics deserves special attention because of their pivotal role in Egyptian and Syrian society.

[6] On the unresolved question of immunity to plague, Pollitzer has written: "It is certain that human beings as well as rodents, if surviving a plague attack, are apt to be resistant to the infection. However, owing to the fact that until recently instances of recovery from severe forms of the disease were infrequent in man, little information is available on the solidity and duration of this naturally-produced state of immunity" (Pollitzer, *Plague*, pp. 137-138). Therefore, for reasons that are still not clear, natural human immunity to plague may have existed in the past. Relevant to this subject, Christopher Morris has recently suggested that the mysterious cessation of plague in Europe in the late seventeenth century was due to the fact that "either the rodent or the human population of North-West Europe, including Britain, had by about 1670 begun to 'breed immune.' In other words, only stocks with acquired or inherited immunity were now surviving, the susceptible having died out. The immunity could have been one or both of two different kinds —immunity to plague or immunity to flea-bite. Although second attacks of the disease can and do occur they are not very common and survival from one infection almost certainly confers a considerable degree of resistance. And some people, doubtless, have a natural or inborn immunity. The rodents, certainly, have in some areas been known to 'breed immune.' But, more important, there is reason to believe that some men are much more liable to flea-bite than other men and that this uninviting quality in their blood is often hereditary." ("The Plague in Britain," *The Historical Journal*, vol. 14, no. 1 [1971], pp. 212-213.) Moreover, genetic anthropology may yet prove the greater susceptibility of certain racial groups to plague than others, which would have a bearing on comparative mortality rates during the Black Death.

[7] *as-Sulūk*, part 4, vol. 2, p. 1047.

Professor David Ayalon has shown that the cumulative effect of plague epidemics in Egypt was to reduce the manpower of the mamlūk army and contribute to the steady decline of the army from the late fourteenth century to the Ottoman conquest of Egypt. The records of practically every major plague in Egypt note the high number of deaths among the royal mamlūks (*mamālīk sulṭānīyah*). During the epidemics, the royal mamlūks remained in their barracks in Cairo, regardless of the danger of contagion or infection; their close association could only have encouraged the spread of plague among them. Al-Maqrīzī noted the high mortality in the Citadel during the plague epidemic of 841/1437-1438:

> Death was terrible among the mamlūks inhabiting the barracks; there died in this epidemic about 1,000. And there died of the castrated servants 160 eunuchs; of the slave-girls of the sultan's household more than 160, besides 17 concubines and 17 male and female children.[8]

The mortality was particularly high among the royal mamlūks, compared to the older mamlūks of former sultans and amirs in the later epidemics. The latter groups were able to flee the centers of the epidemics and may previously have been exposed to plague infection and gained a sufficient degree of immunity to withstand its recurrences. We know that the number of the sultan's purchased mamlūks who died in the plague epidemic of 864/1460 was 1,400.[9] On one day during the epidemic in Cairo, Friday, 19 Jumādā II/11 April, 630 of the sultan's mamlūks perished. The historian Ibn Taghrī Birdī, who was stricken by plague at this time, wrote the following verses about plague and the mamlūks:

> To us there came the pestilence, it suddenly was seen imported, did descend on him who eagerly it sought;
> For frequency of sinfulness, of wrong that had appeared, the Lord sent it especially on imports he had bought.[10]

[8] *Ibid.*, p. 834.
[9] *an-Nujūm*, Popper trans., vol. 22, pp. 99-100.
[10] *Ibid.*, p. 98.

In this plague epidemic of 864/1460, it would appear that more than half of the mamlūks whom the sultan had bought died, while the death rate among all the other classes of mamlūks did not reach more than one-third.[11]

The effects of the plague of 833/1429-1430 on the mamlūk army are representative. It provoked the customary communal responses in the cities (see chapter VI). Specifically, the Meccan caravan for the annual pilgrimage, which normally marched through the city before its departure, was delayed until Sha'bān/May; the postponement was caused by the deaths of the mamlūk lancers. The number of people in the procession was also smaller than usual because of the extent of urban mortality and the care extended to the dead.

Ibn Taghrī Birdī tells us that in this year among his father's mamlūks four who had gained prominent government positions died in one day. He also mentions that numerous mamlūks, slaves, and servants died in his own home, aside from members of his family. The mamlūks' estates changed hands rapidly because of the high death rate. Ibn Taghrī Birdī says that "an *iqṭā'* in the standing army was transferred in a few days to nine individuals, each of them dying in turn." Among the governing élite, the sultan's son and brother as well as the Caliph al-Musta'īn were victims of the epidemic.[12]

The mamlūk class as a whole was so severely affected that the sultan was "preoccupied with the death of his mamlūks" and could not be concerned with foreign adventures. "The severest plague was among the Sultan's mamlūks, those living in the Citadel barracks . . . in the morning 450 of them might be sick and in the course of the day more than 50 mamlūks would die."[13] There are no definite figures for the numbers of royal mamlūks or their mortality during this epidemic. However, we know that the corps declined from about 5,500-5,700 in 824/1421 to about 4,000 in 841/1437.[14] Assuming a figure

[11] "The Plague and Its Effects," pp. 71-72.

[12] *an-Nujūm*, Popper trans., vol. 18, pp. 70-74, 184-187.

[13] *Ibid.*, p. 71.

[14] David Ayalon, "Studies on the Structure of the Mamlūk Army," *BSOAS*, vol. 15 (1953), p. 226; Emmanuel Piloti, *L'Égypte au com-*

of about 5,000 mamlūks, a mortality rate of fifty a day—even at the height of the epidemic that lasted four months—would indicate a serious and costly destruction of the military élite. Recurrences of plague not only diminished the manpower of the army, but caused considerable revenue to be spent to replenish its depleted numbers, at a time when the cost of slaves from the Russian steppe was increasing substantially.[15]

Although Professor Ayalon's study concentrates on these later plague epidemics,[16] it is clear that the Black Death appreciably affected the mamlūk army and its organization. The only difference from the later recurrences is that the death rate among the mamlūks was probably not remarkably higher than that of the local inhabitants or disproportionate among the mamlūk classes, who were equally vulnerable to the initial epidemic. The royal mamlūks, particularly, "would not abandon the capital during the Black Death in 1348-1349, for to have done so would have meant relinquishing their power to an opponent mamlūk faction besides losing their feudal estates and other kinds of property which changed hands frequently

mencement du quinzième siècle, ed. by P.-H. Dopp (Cairo, 1950), p. 16; and Darrag, p. 39.

15 Ashtor, *Histoire*, p. 463. One reason that the cost of domestic slaves in Egypt did not increase in the same manner is that they were usually drawn from Africa rather than from southern Russia. In Italy, and the West in general, the cost of domestic slaves from the Balkans and southern Russia did rise considerably from the middle of the fourteenth century and is more comparable to the rise in the cost of mamlūks in Egypt (pp. 501-504).

16 Ayalon fails to note a number of probable plague epidemics in the second half of the fourteenth century ("The Plague and Its Effects," p. 68). The mortality among mamlūks is especially mentioned in the following additional sources. For the plague of A.H. 790-791: Ibn Hajar, *Inbā' al-ghumr*, vol. 1, pp. 350, 353; *as-Sulūk*, part 3, vol. 2, p. 578; al-Jawharī, *Nuzhat an-nufūs*, vol. 1, p. 170; Ibn al-Furāt, *Ta'rīkh*, vol. 9, p. 28. For the plague of A.H. 820: Ibn Hajar, *Inbā' al-ghumr*, vol. 3, p. 139. For the plague of A.H. 833: Ibn Ḥajar, *Inbā' al-ghumr*, vol. 3, p. 437; *as-Sulūk*, part 4, vol. 2, p. 826 *et passim*. For the plague of A.H. 841: *ibid.*, part 4, vol. 2, p. 1037 *et passim*. And for the plague of A.H. 853: Ibn Iyās, vol. 2, p. 32.

during an epidemic when the owners died."[17] The barracks of the sultan's mamlūks in the Citadel were consequently emptied by the pandemic. With respect to the non-mamlūks in the army, al-Maqrīzī tells us that almost all the soldiers drawn from the local population (*ajnād al-ḥalqah*) perished.[18] The corps of drummers of the amirs[19] virtually disappeared; the drum corps of one important amir diminished from fifteen members to three.[20] The estates of the army, as we should expect, were rapidly transferred. Because of numerous deaths, the estates and military property passed from one person to another until artisans, such as tailors, shoemakers, and public criers, assumed military dress and rode on horseback—an unwonted presumption.[21] During the peak of the Black Death, the *iqṭā'* of a non-mamlūk soldier changed hands six times during one week, as other inheritances passed to four or five successive owners.[22] The Black Death, like the severe plague recurrences, vitally affected the army by decreasing the value and revenue of these estates. Al-Maqrīzī asserts that as a result of the Black Death, no landowner received the complete revenue from his estate, and a number received absolutely noth-

[17] Ayalon, "The Muslim City and the Mamlūk Military Aristocracy," *Proceedings of the Israel Academy of Sciences and Humanities*, vol. 2 (Jerusalem, 1967), p. 320.

[18] *as-Sulūk*, part 2, vol. 3, p. 781. As Ayalon has pointed out, this is the only reference to the death of non-mamlūks ("The Plague and Its Effects," p. 71).

[19] The *ṭablakhānah*: amirs of the upper ranks had the privilege of being accompanied by a ceremonial band.

[20] *as-Sulūk*, part 2, vol. 3, p. 784.

[21] *Ibid.*, p. 785. Ayalon remarks: "In another outbreak the number of fiefs that became available was so large, and there was so much confusion and seizure of property, that even the *kuttābiyyah* studying in the military schools, took fiefs before their release and prior to obtaining their horses. In 897 the sultan assembled the entire army, *julbān* and *qarānīs*, and gave each man a horse out of the effects of the deceased Mamlūks. In 919 the sultan distributed among the *khāṣṣakiyyah* 800 helmets, 600 sets of horse armour, and coats of mail, shields, swords, lances, quivers and arrows which had been the property of Mamlūks carried away by the plague." ("The Plague and Its Effects," p. 73.)

[22] *as-Sulūk*, part 2, vol. 3, pp. 780, 782.

ing.[23] This agricultural revenue was essential to the maintenance of the mamlūk establishment.

In another respect, the Black Death affected the waging of wars. In North Africa, as we have seen, it interrupted the battle between the bedouin Arabs and the Marinid king near Kairouwan in 749/1348, and probably was the major cause of the king's defeat.[24] According to al-Maqrīzī, in Andalusia plague provoked the Muslims to attack the weakened Christians until they themselves were equally stricken and forced to retreat to North Africa, where they found that plague had preceded them.[25] Furthermore, as has been previously mentioned, plague broke out in the army of Malik Ashraf, who was besieging Shaykh Ḥasan Buzurg in Baghdad, and he had to withdraw. Plague is also given as the reason for ending the promotion of a crusade among the Christians in Cyprus against the Turks in 1351.[26] In the decade following the pandemic, no major military offensives were undertaken by the Mamlūk Sultanate, a fact that may be indicative of the decline in military strength.[27]

During the rest of the Mamlūk Period, plague disrupted or prevented a number of military expeditions, as well as undermining the effectiveness of the mamlūk army. For example, in 809/1406-1407, the amirs attempted to postpone an expedition to Syria because of plague in Egypt.[28] In two other cases, plague stopped the advance of hostile armies that would have provoked engagements with the mamlūk army. In 833/1429-1430, a plague epidemic in Shāh Rukh's army prevented his

[23] *Ibid.*, p. 785.

[24] Ibn Khaldūn, *at-Taʿrīf*, p. 27.

[25] *as-Sulūk*, part 2, vol. 3, p. 777. This statement appears to contradict the fact that the Muslims in Gibraltar, fighting King Alfonso XI, were stricken first by the Black Death. Either al-Maqrīzī is misinformed about events in Andalusia or he is referring to unidentified Muslim raids against Christians elsewhere in southern Spain.

[26] Hill, *A History of Cyprus*, vol. 1, pp. 301, 307.

[27] Muir, *The Mameluke or Slave Dynasty of Egypt*, pp. 94-97.

[28] *an-Nujūm*, Popper trans., vol. 14, p. 133.

marching into Syria,[29] and in 880/1475-1476, the army of Ḥasan aṭ-Ṭawīl, grandson of Qarā Yalak, was destroyed by plague. The news of this event pleased the mamlūk sultan in Cairo, who had been preparing to send an expedition against him.[30]

In various ways, therefore, plague directly affected the functioning of this special class within medieval Muslim society, and its military operations. Together with the evidence for rural and urban depopulation, the death rate of the mamlūks suggests a dramatic decline in numbers during the Black Death and recurrent plague epidemics. The deaths of the mamlūk corps were a small but vitally important part of the general ruination that afflicted the entire empire.

E. GENERAL MORTALITY OF THE BLACK DEATH

It is tempting but extremely hazardous to estimate the general degree of population decline caused by the Black Death in Egypt and Syria. It is hazardous, first of all, because of the unreliable and inadequate data concerning death rates to be found in the medieval chronicles. The mortality figures for the Black Death and later epidemics of plague are generally exaggerated, fragmentary and contradictory. Most of the contemporary estimates of deaths for plague epidemics in the latter half of the fourteenth and fifteenth centuries are for the major cities, and are of little assistance in estimating the rural depopulation. Moreover, even the urban population for which we do have mortality figures was particularly unstable during an epidemic. Certainly, some fled. On the other hand, the major cities received an influx of population from the countryside which more than offset the reduction by flight; the introduction of additional population before an epidemic would naturally have increased the total number of urban deaths.

[29] Ibn Ḥajar, *Inbā' al-ghumr*, vol. 3, p. 441; *an-Nujūm*, Popper trans., vol. 18, p. 77; *as-Sulūk*, part 4, vol. 2, pp. 836-837.

[30] "The Plague and Its Effects," p. 72.

We are at a further disadvantage in estimating total plague destruction because we do not possess a mathematical formula for determining it, as we have for other communicable diseases. This is because of the complex and highly variable pathology of plague. Apart from deaths resulting from plague, there was continuous natural mortality as well as death from concomitant diseases that may have contributed to population decline, especially during the Black Death.

Second, it is very difficult to estimate the decline in population resulting from the Black Death because of our appalling ignorance of total population figures in the Middle East during the medieval period. A knowledge of the population of Egypt and Syria and their major cities before the Black Death is obviously necessary in order to assess the degree of depopulation caused by the pandemic. There are, however, no extant estimates of regional or urban population in the early fourteenth century, nor has the problem of Middle Eastern population attracted sufficient modern investigation, despite the current interest in historical demography and urban history. The lack of both medieval and modern attention to the study of population, together with the scarcity of information for plague mortality make a reasonable judgment of the demographic effect of the Black Death exceedingly difficult.

With these admissions of ignorance and uncertainty as a caution, I have first brought together what information we have or can deduce about the population of Egypt and Syria and their major cities before the Black Death. Second, I have sought to ascertain the probable magnitude of mortality caused by the Black Death, primarily in Cairo, by comparing it with the relatively well-documented death rate caused by the plague epidemic of 833/1429-1430. Finally, I will consider the approximate mortality rate of the Black Death in the context of total population, in order to make a very tentative estimate of the general scope of population decline.

1. Population History of the Middle East

We have no reliable estimates of Egyptian population until the late eighteenth century, when European travelers took a keen interest in population. For example, Volney, a Frenchman who visited the Middle East between 1783 and 1785, was impressed by the depopulation of Egypt and its capital. He estimated the population of Cairo at a quarter of a million and the entire population of the country at just over two million.[1] Volney's estimates anticipated very accurately the findings of the French expedition in the early nineteenth century. The population of Cairo, excluding Būlāq and Fusṭāṭ, was estimated by Jomard, using various demographic methods,[2] in the classic *Description de l'Égypte*, at 263,700, and the overall population at 2,488,950 (not including the nomadic population of perhaps 130,000).[3] The first census in Egypt in 1821 produced a figure of 2,536,400.[4] Edward Lane estimated the population of Cairo at 240,000 before the plague epidemic of 1835, and a total Egyptian population of less than two million.[5] The population of Cairo in 1847-1848 may have been 253,541, in a total Egyptian population of 4,542,620.[6]

From these general levels of population in the early nineteenth century, it has commonly been assumed that the population of the Arab provinces of the Ottoman Empire declined from the sixteenth to the eighteenth century.[7] This is partly supported by the Ottoman census records that have been pub-

[1] *Voyage*, pp. 134-135. Comparable estimates were made by W. G. Browne, *Travels in Africa, Egypt and Syria from the Years 1792 to 1798* (London, 1799), p. 71.

[2] See the summary of Jomard's methodology in Abu-Lughod, *Cairo*, p. 57.

[3] "Mémoire sur la population comparée de l'Égypte ancienne et moderne," *Description de l'Égypte*, 2nd ed., vol. 9 (Paris, 1829), pp. 118-132.

[4] Russell, "Population of Medieval Egypt," p. 70 and n. 10.

[5] *Manners and Customs*, pp. 23-24.

[6] *Ibid.*, p. 548.

[7] There has been no systematic examination of this assumption, especially for Egypt. Marcel Clerget, *Le Caire* (Cairo, 1934), vol. 1, pp. 240-241, suggests that the population of Cairo declined from the latter half of the fourteenth century and was particularly aggravated in the seventeenth and eighteenth centuries. He estimates the population of Cairo in the middle of the sixteenth century at 430,000, and 245,000 at the end of the eighteenth century.

lished.[8] Specifically, the population of Aleppo declined from 67,344 in 1519 to 56,881 in 1520-1530 and to 45,331 in 1571-1580; Damascus contained 57,326 inhabitants in 1520-1530 and 42,779 in 1595. (These population levels for Aleppo and Damascus in the early Ottoman Period make Professor Russell's recent estimates of 14,000 and 15,000, respectively for the two cities at about 1200, appear greatly mistaken.[9] Such miscalculations lead to justifiable skepticism about Russell's methodology and rejection of his other estimates for Middle Eastern population, particularly for Cairo, which he estimated at 60,000 before the Black Death.[10]) There are no known statistics for Cairo from the Ottoman records.

In lieu of such valuable statistics from the Ottoman censuses for Cairo, the only significant medieval estimate of Cairene population[11] was made by Leo Africanus, who visited Egypt in the early sixteenth century and roughly calculated the population of the city. He states that Cairo, about the year 1526, contained within its walls not more than 8,000 families. The large suburb of Bāb az-Zuwaylah comprised about 12,000 families; Bāb al-Lūq, 3,000; Būlāq, 4,000; Qarāfah, 2,000; al-Fusṭāṭ, 5,000; and ar-Rawḍah Island, 1,500.[12] Multiplying this number by an average family of five to six members, we may place the metropolitan population roughly at between 177,500 and 213,000, with about 40,000-46,000 for the Fāṭimid walled city.

[8] Ö. L. Barkan, "Essai sur les données statistiques des registres de recensement dans l'empire Ottoman aux XVe et XVIe siècles," *JESHO*, vol. 1 (Paris, 1958), pp. 9-36; for Aleppo and Damascus, see pp. 27-28. See also *EI*²: "Daftar-i Khāḳānī" (Ö. L. Barkan).

[9] *Medieval Regions and Their Cities*, pp. 201, 203.

[10] *Ibid.*, p. 208, and "Demographic Comparison of Egyptian and English Cities in the Later Middle Ages," *Texas A. & I. University Studies*, vol. 2 (1969), p. 66.

[11] The estimates of European travelers in the Middle East are fantastic and may be disregarded; see Clerget, *Le Caire*, vol. 1, pp. 138-139.

[12] *The History and Description of Africa*, ed. by Robert Brown (London, 1896), vol. 3, pp. 870-879.

The Ottoman conquest of Egypt in 1517 marks a break in the history of Egypt. "In their first census of Egypt the Ottomans found total revenue reduced from 9.5 million in the fourteenth century to no more than 1.8 million dinars."[13] Presumably, the first figure represents a fiscal level achieved before the Black Death. In any case, if economic productivity is an approximate index to population, the revenue figures at the time of the Ottoman conquest reflect a significant decline in population.

What, then, was the general pattern of Egyptian population before the Ottoman conquest? The population of Egypt appears to have risen appreciably from the twelfth century until the advent of the Black Death, reaching its apogee in the early fourteenth century and declining by various stages thereafter.[14] This general pattern of population increase before the Black Death is based largely on the evidence of cadastral surveys, the most important of which was the survey of an-Nāṣir in 1315.[15] On the basis of the tax returns and the number of *faddans* under cultivation, Professor Russell considers the population

[13] *Muslim Cities*, p. 39.

[14] For works dealing with medieval Egyptian population, see: Clerget, *Le Caire*, vol. 1, pp. 154-172, 238-240; Fernand Braudel, *Le Méditerranée et le monde méditerranéen à l'époque de Philippe II* (Paris, 1949), p. 348; Omar Tousson, *Mémoire sur les finances de l'Égypte*; Jomard, "Mémoire sur le population comparée de l'Égypte," pp. 109-211; M. ad-Darwish, "Analysis of Some Estimates of the Population of Egypt Before the Nineteenth Century," *L'Égypte Contemporaine*, vol. 20 (1929), pp. 273-286; M. ad-Darwish and H. as-S. Azmi, "A Note on the Population of Egypt," *Population*, vol. 2 (1934), pp. 34-56; and Silvestre de Sacy, *Relation de l'Égypte par Abd-Allatif,* Appendix. The only recent study of medieval Egyptian population has been made by Russell: "The Population of Medieval Egypt" (see chap. II, part A, n. 2, and "Effects of Pestilence and Plague, 1315-85," *Comparative Studies in Society and History*, vol. 8, no. 4 [1966], pp. 464-467 [cf. S. L. Thrupp's criticism of this article: "Plague Effects in Medieval Europe," *ibid.*, pp. 474-479]).

[15] There are various conflicting interpretations of population based on the cadasters, particularly for the 1315 survey. See Russell, "Population of Medieval Egypt," pp. 75-82 for bibliographical references.

of Egypt before the Black Death to have been about 4 to 4.2 million.[16] His estimates for urban population are far too low, as I have previously shown to be the case also for Cairo; consequently, the estimate for total population is too small and may be considered a minimum.

The only recent study to propose population figures for Egypt and Cairo is the monograph on the history of Cairo by Professor Abu-Lughod, who suggests without explanation a pre-plague population for Egypt of about eight million and about half a million for Cairo.[17] An estimate of half a million for Cairo is close to the figure of 600,000 for the early fourteenth century proposed by Marcel Clerget in 1934. In spite of the omission of his bases for estimating the population of each quarter of the city, Clerget's suggested figure reinforces one's belief in a population of at least half a million.[18]

There is no easy way to determine more exactly the population of Cairo before the Black Death.[19] One manner of esti-

[16] *Ibid.*, pp. 76-77. On the basis of the estimate of 3,642,159 taxable *faddans*, Russell proceeds to say: "If one may still assume about a person to the feddan and then add ten percent [for urban population] the total for Egypt before the plague was about four million people. This might be raised a little, perhaps to 4.2 millions, if one assumes that the prosperity brought more persons to the cities and raised their percentage." See also Russell, "Demographic Comparison of Egyptian and English Cities in the Later Middle Ages," pp. 64-72, and *Medieval Regions and Their Cities*, pp. 207-213.

[17] *Cairo*, pp. 37, 41, 51, 83, 131. While admitting the economic decline of Egypt in the fifteenth century, the author unaccountably suggests that Cairo's population was still as high as half a million at the time of the Ottoman conquest (p. 57).

[18] *Le Caire*, pp. 239-240.

[19] For example, there are no figures for the importation of wheat into the city by which to calculate urban population, despite the excellent description of the grain trade by Lapidus ("The Grain Economy of Mamlūk Egypt"). Concrete figures for the grain supply would have given us one index to population levels, as it has for the populations of classical Athens and Rome. Other methods may contribute quantitative evidence. There may be important archeological evidence from the American excavation of Fusṭāṭ for urban population in two ways. We know from the chroniclers that many of the residents of Fusṭāṭ left

mating it is by studying the extent of the mamlūk city, including the Fāṭimid city enclosed by walls. Regrettably, no investigations have been made of the extent of the walled cities, the average size of houses, and the average number of persons per family in the Near East during the medieval period, in order to estimate urban density.[20] For the ancient Near East, Professor Robert Adams has attempted to estimate urban population in his intensive study of settlements on the Diyala Plain.[21] He first gives the estimate of 400 persons per hectare made by Professor Henri Frankfort and based on archeological studies of three large and densely populated sites. Frankfort suggests that there were twenty houses per acre with an average area of 200 square meters per house, which would contain six to ten occupants. This amounts to 120 to 200 people per acre; the average of 160 per acre or 400 per hectare was found by Frankfort to be precisely the average density of modern Aleppo and Damascus.

---

their city during the Black Death (see above, part C). The pandemic was very acute in Fusṭāṭ (perhaps because of the granaries located there), and it is reported that the community moved eastward and abandoned the houses. The present American excavation should be able to corroborate these descriptions of abandonment from the mid-fourteenth century and the partial deterioration of the old city from that time, with only piecemeal rebuilding thereafter. Second, the excavation should be able to determine floor plans in order to estimate the average size of homes in Fusṭāṭ and thus the density of human habitation. Another possible method of gaining information for the population of Cairo before the Black Death (when the population was at its height) would be an estimate based on the size of the existing mosques, which should have accommodated most of the adult male population. Another basis of estimation would be the number and size of the baths within the city (see André Raymond, "Signes urbains et étude de la population des grandes villes Arabes a l'époque Ottomane," *Bulletin d'Études Orientales*, vol. 27 [Damascus, 1974], pp. 183-193).

20 Russell has assumed about 250 persons per hectare as the usual density of Islamic cities (*Medieval Regions and Their Cities*, p. 208). The basis for this estimate is not given.

21 *Land Behind Baghdad: A History of Settlement on the Diyala Plains* (Chicago, 1965), pp. 122-124.

Second, Adams cites Professor Yeivin's judgment that Seleucia in the first century A.D. had an average density of 357 persons per hectare. Adams refutes these two estimates on the grounds that they are too high.[22] He considers the estimates of both Frankfort and Yeivin incorrect because of their overestimation of family size and, hence, their measurements of urban density. Adams concurs with Russell that the ancient and medieval family was much smaller; he believes an average of five persons per house to be too high, and considers about 3.5 persons per family as a more accurate average (although he notes that five to seven persons was the norm for families in rural areas at the time of his research). On this basis, Russell suggests 150 persons per hectare for the Near East. For purposes of his own work, Adams has adopted 200 persons per hectare for the ancient settlements.

The only investigation of the population of medieval Muslim cities in this manner has been L. Torres Balbas' study for Muslim Spain.[23] Professor Balbas has gained particularly valuable information about Andalusian cities from reports of these cities when they were conquered by the Christians—which we do not have, of course, for the Middle East. His basis of calculation is primarily the size of the walled enclosures. He reckons the average area of a one-family house to have been 151.61 square meters, which is close to the size of the average American house (1200-1800 sq. ft.). However, on the analysis of three well-documented cities, Balbas raises this figure to 172 square meters for houses inside a walled area. Moreover, he calculates six members per family, hence that number per individual dwelling. The corresponding density per hectare is then approximately 348 persons, which is relatively close to the estimates of Yeivin and Frankfort for the cities of the ancient Near East. Because of the lack of such

[22] *Ibid.*, pp. 24-25. The mean density in Baghdad according to the 1947 census was 137.2 persons per hectare and that of the Khuzestan villages was approximately 223 persons per hectare.

[23] "Extensione y demografia de las Ciudades Hispanomusulmanas," *Studia Islamica*, vol. 3 (1955), pp. 35-59.

research as Balbas' for Middle Eastern cities, we will have to accept uncritically his estimate of urban density—making the unwarranted assumption that the characteristics of the Hispano-Muslim city are comparable to those of the medieval Middle Eastern city, specifically Cairo and Damascus.

In the fourteenth and fifteenth centuries, the principal part of Cairo formed an irregular rectangle measuring approximately two-and-a-quarter by one-and-a-half miles, or about 864 hectares.[24] Within this area, the walled Fāṭimid city covered only about 171 hectares.[25] Because of the significant growth of the mamlūk city as an extension of the Fāṭimid city, primarily to the south, I have assumed a density of settlement similar to the walled area for the entire region in the early fourteenth century. Also, the level of population before the Black Death was greater than at any time during the Middle Ages; consequently, the population density would logically have been at a maximum level and further justifies our using the high degree of persons per hectare suggested by Balbas for the entire region. If we accept 348 inhabitants per hectare as the average density, the Fāṭimid walled area of Cairo would contain about 60,204 persons; the larger region of the mamlūk city gives us a population of about 300,672. (A similar calculation based on Adams' estimate of 200 per hectare for the latter would give 172,800.[26]) These figures do not

[24] *Systematic Notes*, vol. 15, p. 23 (and maps nos. 6-11): "Mameluke Cairo of the fifteenth century A.D. was an irregular rectangle measuring about 2¼ miles from N to S and 1½ miles from E to W. (Actually, the city rectangle lay in a NE direction, so that the SW corner was much nearer the Nile than the NW corner; but N, S, E, and W will be used in the following description.) The N and E limits were defined by walls; the W limit by the Nāṣirī Canal; the S limit, an irregular line, by a series of rubbish mounts, the ruins of earlier constructions. The Citadel projected to the E from the SE corner of the Mameluke City." (The area is computed at 256 hectares per sq. mile.)

[25] *EI*[1]: "Cairo" (C. H. Becker) estimates the walled city under Caliph al-Mustanṣir (427-487/1036-1094) at about 2/3 of a sq. mile or 171 hectares.

[26] These figures may represent the range of population of Cairo before the Black Death; it is possible that it was closer to the former

include the suburbs of Ḥusaynīyah immediately north of the city, the Desert Plain on the east, Qarāfah on the south, Fusṭāṭ to the southwest, and the right bank of the Nile, including Būlāq.

We must, however, add to this estimate a guess at the population of these Cairene suburbs, which is even more imprecise. The suburbs of the mamlūk city were extensive in the early fourteenth century and greatly increase the figure for total urban population.[27] Balbas suggests that the suburban population of the Andalusian cities never exceeded one-half of that of the walled area, although this ratio may have been conditioned by the special circumstances of Muslim cities in Spain in the later Middle Ages.[28] Nevertheless, taking this ratio as a conservative estimate of urban-suburban population according to Balbas, we may raise the figure of 300,672 to 451,008. This rough order of magnitude is slightly lower than the estimates of Professors Abu-Lughod and Clerget, but, considering the significant development of the Cairene suburbs before the Black Death, their judgments are not at all unlikely. As for the total Egyptian population, it may have been between four and eight million, probably closer to the higher figure, due to a far greater urban population and larger family unit than those proposed by Russell.

There is even less certainty about the overall population of the Syrian provinces of the Mamlūk Empire. The only modern historian to deal with the population of Syria in the later Middle Ages is Professor Poliak. According to his reasoning, the mamlūk government levied one soldier from every 250 inhabitants in the districts of Sidon, Beirut, and the Biqāʿ in 1343; the soldiers so enlisted numbered 500, a figure that implies a rough estimate of a total population of 125,000 in these

figure, because of Adams' reliance on Russell's questionable estimate. Comparison with the modern demographic character of the medieval section of Cairo is instructive: see Abu-Lughod, *Cairo*, p. 57 *et passim.*

27 Abu-Lughod, *Cairo*, pp. 27, 31-36.

28 "Extensione y demografia," p. 53.

regions.[29] On this basis, Poliak suggests that the population of the Lebanon (except for Tripoli) would have been about 150,000 on the eve of the Black Death. Poliak proposes that if we apply to the Mamlūk Period the geographical distribution of Syria-Palestine population existing in 1800 (when the population of the Lebanon formed approximately a sixth of the total), the entire population of Syria, Palestine, the Lebanon, and Transjordan prior to the Black Death would have been about 900,000. However, he asserts that the real figure was probably somewhat greater—about 1,200,000—because the transformation of the Lebanon into one of the most densely populated parts of Syria-Palestine took place as late as the seventeenth century.[30]

We have no estimates of Damascene population by either medieval or modern writers except for the Ottoman census figures, which have been mentioned—57,326 in 1520-1530. It is reasonable to assume that the population of Damascus was in excess of this number before the Black Death. Similar to that in Egypt, the period before the Black Death was favorable to population growth, and we can assume a maximum population for the Syrian capital. According to Professor Popper, the city formed an irregular rectangle, "a little more than one mile in extent from E to W, three-fifths of a mile from N to S (including the Citadel)."[31] On the basis of the measurement of 348 persons per hectare for the walled area of a medieval Muslim city, the population of Damascus before the Black Death may have been about 53,453.[32] If we add to this number one-half of the walled population for the extra-

[29] See Ṣāliḥ ibn Yaḥyāh, *Ta'rīkh Bayrūt*, p. 105.

[30] "The Demographic Evolution of the Middle East: Population Trends Since 1348," *Palestine and Middle East*, vol. 10, no. 5 (May, 1938), p. 201.

[31] *Systematic Notes*, vol. 15, p. 37 (and maps nos. 15 and 16).

[32] An area of 153.6 hectares would give this figure. If we take the area of the ancient walls (beginning of the third century A.D.), measuring 1500 by 750 meters, which formed the skeleton of the medieval Muslim city (*EI*²: "Dimashḳ" [N. Elisséeff]), the walled area of 112.5 hectares would give a population of 39,150.

mural population, the total would be roughly 80,180. Again, as with Cairo, the population may have been somewhat higher.

2. The Estimated Mortality of the Plague Epidemic of 833/1429-1430

Turning to the Black Death and the problem of estimating its death rate, we are faced with the difficulty that the reports in the chronicles are particularly scarce and untrustworthy at this time—even for Cairo.[33] Cairene mortality figures were reportedly taken from counts made at the oratories[34] and at

[33] For Muslim society outside of the Middle East, we have estimates only from Andalusia for destruction caused by the Black Death. Ibn Khātimah asserts that the deaths reached a peak of seventy a day in Almería in 749/1348-1349, but says that this was small compared to other cities in both Muslim and Christian lands. He compares this daily mortality rate with reports from trustworthy witnesses; on one day—May 24—1,202 died in Tunis, 700 in Tlemcen, 1,500 in Valencia, and 1,252 in the island of Majorca (*Taḥṣīl*, fol. 57a). The highest estimate of all the Arabic writers for the mortality rate of the Black Death is given by the otherwise most reliable author Ibn al-Khaṭīb, that seven-tenths of mankind perished (*Muqniʿat*, fol. 43b).

[34] The number of oratories where the funerals were counted varies in the historical accounts of the Black Death and later plague epidemics; consequently, it is difficult to estimate urban mortality rates from these counts because of the variable selection of oratories. For example, in the description of the plague epidemic of 864/1460 in Cairo, Ibn Taghrī Birdī mentions the daily number of funerals from different mosques whose number ranges from ten to seventeen (*an-Nujūm*, Popper trans., vol. 22, pp. 91-99). It seems that the rough estimates made by the medieval chroniclers were usually calculated by multiplying the funerals at one of the important oratories by the number of oratories in which funeral services were being held to give the total number of dead of the city. The latter method is indicated in a passage from Ibn Taghrī Birdī's chronicle for the same epidemic of 864/1460 in Cairo: "The statements of the accountants differed because of the preoccupation of everyone with himself and his household; one said that there died on the day 4,000; one said 3,500. The second speaker estimated by the number over whom prayers were said this day in Succor Gate Oratory, and said that each hundred dead in Succor Gate Oratory was at [the rate of] 360 dead [in Cairo]." (*Ibid.*, p. 97; n. 293: "H reads: 'Each 100 was at [the rate of] 1,000 because the number there was

the city gates, but the numbers are highly suspect. The authenticity of the figures for the Black Death is called into question by the lack of first-hand accounts and the failure of the later historians to give the sources for their statements. Almost all the important accounts of the pandemic were written by men, particularly al-Maqrīzī, who did not personally witness the event, although their information may have been gathered from older but lost sources, such as the history of Ibn al-Furāt. Therefore, before proceeding directly to the evaluation of the reports of the mortality rate for the Black Death, we should consider the mortality rate produced by a particularly severe recurrence of plague in the early fifteenth century, which is similar to the Black Death in many respects but relatively well-documented by contemporary historians. Again, the purpose of such a circuitous procedure is to gain some idea of the probable range of plague mortality for Cairo during the Black Death.

The plague epidemic of 833/1429-1430 in Egypt had apparently spread from Syria, where it had raged since Sha'bān 832/May 1429; it had appeared as well in Byzantine Anatolia and in the lands of the Franks. The two important historians, Ibn Taghrī Birdī and al-Maqrīzī, had seen it in Cairo.[35] The former called the epidemic "the Great Extinction" because of its severity, which was almost certainly due to the presence of the pneumonic form—particularly in the winter months.[36] Ibn Taghrī Birdī declares: "In this year occurred the great plague, the like of which we have not known in Egypt and its towns or in the greater part of Syria [for many years]. . . . This

350.' ") The principal oratories that are named and presumably always included in such calculations were: Succor Gate Oratory, Mu'minī Oratory, Farriers' Oratory (Muṣallā al-Bayāṭirah), and al-Azhar Mosque.

[35] *an-Nujūm*, Popper trans., vol. 17, p. 171; vol. 18, pp. 69-76, 181-189; *as-Sulūk*, part 4, vol. 2, pp. 822 ff. See also Ibn Iyās, vol. 2, pp. 18-19; Khalīl aẓ-Ẓāhirī, *Kitāb zubda kashf al-mamālik*, ed. by P. Ravisse (Paris, 1894), p. 112; *Badhl*, fol. 123b; *Mā rawāhu l-wā'ūn*, p. 156; Ibn Hajar, *Inbā' al-ghumr*, vol. 3, pp. 437 ff.; al-Mu'minī, *Kitāb al-futūḥ*, Dār al-Kutub al-Misrīyah MS no. 2399 *ta'rīkh* (photographic copy), vol. 2, p. 296.

[36] *an-Nujūm*, Popper trans., vol. 18, pp. 69, 181.

plague was greater and worse than all those plagues since the general plague that occurred in 749 [the Black Death]. I have not known a plague like this one to occur in Cairo and Old Cairo."[37]

In Rabīʿ II, 833/December 1429-January 1430, the epidemic traveled southward through the Delta to Cairo and then on toward Upper Egypt. The daily death rate in Alexandria was about 100 during this month, while in the provinces of al-Buḥayrah and al-Gharbīyah it was equally severe. Five thousand were reported to have perished in the provincial capital of Maḥallah. Nine thousand were supposed to have died in an-Naḥrārīyah in al-Gharbīyah province, northwest of Ṭanṭā. "Death was so bad in Siryāqūs Monastery that the number reached about 200 every day; and it increased also in al-Manūfīyah and al-Qalyūbīyah [provinces], until 600 would die in a single village."[38] The Christian monastic communities were conspicuous casualties of plague as they had been in the Black Death. Leo Africanus seems to refer to this plague epidemic as destroying the monastery of Saint George in Akhmīm; the monastery was replaced by houses for artisans and merchants.[39] Also as in the case of the Black Death, there are extraordinary accounts of the destruction of animals and crops in the countryside.

In the metropolis of Cairo, the plague epidemic provoked organized religious services in the mosques, popular acts of piety, massive funerals, and communal processions out to the desert plain comparable to those in the earlier pandemic. The entire population of the city suffered also from the rise of prices for shrouds and coffins. Everything the sick required was expensive—for example, sugar, purslane seed, and pears—and few were treated with costly medicines. The general commerce of the city dwindled. As in the Black Death, houses were left vacant and property was abandoned; likewise, there was a disregard for some of the dead and their summary burial in trenches.

[37] *Ibid.*, p. 181. [38] *Ibid.*, pp. 69-70.
[39] *The History and Description of Africa*, vol. 3, pp. 901-902.

Most importantly, we have more information about deaths for this plague epidemic than for any other in the fourteenth and fifteenth centuries, although even this information is very meager. There are three kinds of data besides the medieval guesses at total urban mortality. There are the *dīwān* figures, the number prayed over in the oratories, and the number of coffins counted at the city gates. Regarding the first, the deaths recorded were highly selective, as we have described. Even with these figures, it is still difficult to reconstruct the total urban mortality rate because of the paucity of *dīwān* statistics for the various stages of an individual epidemic. This information is usually given only for periods of greatest human destruction. Furthermore, the use of the *dīwān* figures must be qualified by the failure of many to report deaths to the government bureau. Concerning the mosque funerals, not every plague victim was taken to one of the principal oratories for a funeral service and properly recorded, but the number must have been very close to the total, considering the strict religious observances of Muslim society. The mosque figures have the disadvantage that the number of dead is given from a varying number of oratories by the contemporary historians, so that we cannot assume that a given figure is derived from a fixed number of oratories. I have made, however, a significant distinction (consistent with the data) between the figures given for the principal mosques of the mamlūk city and those from all the mosques of the city, i.e., the mamlūk city and the suburbs. Theoretically, the counts at the city gates would be our best guide to the urban death rate except for the fact that these figures are rare and unreliable; nor does this practice seem to have been employed consistently. It is not clear at which gates the counts were made, but, according to the references in the chronicles, they seem to correspond to the gates of the walled city.[40]

40 For example, Ibn Taghrī Birdī quotes al-Maqrīzī for the plague deaths on Monday, 4 Jumādā II, 833/27 February 1430: "The number carried out of the gates of Cairo was counted and reached 1,200 aside from the funerals from the Hakkūra [NW of the city], the Husainīya,

With these reservations, the following facts seem reasonably clear (see the summary of data, Table 1). The plague epidemic appears to have begun in Cairo about the beginning of Rabīʿ II/the end of December. The Cairo *dīwān* increased its registration of those persons dying with taxable legacies from twelve at the beginning of the month to forty-eight at its end, according to al-Maqrīzī. Further, the total number for the month was 477, indicating a rapid rise in the mortality rate at the end of the month (or a totally erratic pattern throughout). This does not include Fusṭāṭ because this suburb had its own *dīwān*, and it is no surprise to learn from al-Maqrīzī that the reported mortality rate in the Fusṭāṭ *dīwān* was much lower than in the Cairo *dīwān*.[41]

By the end of the following month, 29 Jumādā I/February 23, the number prayed over in Cairo reached 2,100, of whom more than 400 were entered on the pages of the Cairo *dīwān*. In Būlāq specifically, seventy were counted, but only twelve names were placed in the *dīwān*, which indicates that individuals in the Cairene suburbs (again excluding Fusṭāṭ) were included in the Cairo *dīwān* register. It also implies that other methods of accounting were being used; the figure of seventy deaths presumably was reached by counting the number of coffins at the oratories of this suburb. Ibn Ḥajar states that 1,800 died at the end of this month and, if he is correct, he may mean the number carried out of the city gates or recorded in the city mosques.[42]

On 4 Jumādā II/February 28, the number of biers carried out of the gates of Cairo was 1,200; at the same time the *dīwān* recorded 390 deaths. On the seventh of the month, the number

Būlāq, Cross Street [SE of the city], Old Cairo, the two Qarāfas, and the Desert Plain quarters of Cairo." (*an-Nujūm*, Popper trans., vol. 18, p. 71)

[41] On 7 Jumādā II, A.H. 833, the Fusṭāt *dīwān* included only thirty names compared to 350 for Cairo.

[42] If we assume a uniform increase in the mortality rate, which is by no means necessarily true, the *dīwān* figures increased by more than 352 by the end of the month, with an average daily increase of about 12. The total *dīwān* deaths for the month would be about 5,570.

recorded in the Cairo mosques was 1,200, of which only 350 were reported to the *dīwān*, indicating a temporary decline in mortality at the beginning of the month. On 9 Jumādā II/March 5, the figure for those prayed over in the mosques of the city had risen to 1,263; specifically, the funerals at Succor Gate (Bāb an-Naṣr) Oratory, on the northern side of the city, numbered 450. The *dīwān* recorded 400. On the next day, there were 505 coffins recorded at Succor Gate, which according to al-Maqrīzī was only one of fourteen major mosques, but perhaps the most important, for the coffins could then be taken out to one of the large cemeteries nearby. On 11 Jumādā II/March 7, the number recorded in the oratories of Cairo and the suburbs reached 2,246. Before the peak of the epidemic in the middle of Jumādā II, the number at Succor Gate Oratory exceeded 800. The chroniclers state that, on the same day, the number carried out of the city gates amounted to 12,300, which is impossible considering the fairly uniform rise in the mortality rate and its possible range; a more realistic figure would be 10,000 less. At the height of the epidemic, the number of plague victims appears to have reached more than 1,030 on one day at Succor Gate,[43] which is high but not inconsistent with

[43] It is difficult to interpret the following statement that is the only one we possess for the peak in the mortality rate: "In the month of II Jumādā the number over whom prayers were said in the oratory of Succor Gate alone in one day exceeded 800 dead. On the same day the number carried out from the rest of Cairo's gates reached 12,300, as determined by the clerks who made the count by order of some high official, or, according to others, by order of the sultan himself. Then the number over whom prayers were said at the Succor Gate Oratory in the middle third of II Jumādā was 1,030 and some, and the number at the Mu'minī Oratory in the Rumaila approached that number; according to this count [?] there died on this day about 1,500 people." (*an-Nujūm*, Popper trans., vol. 18, p. 72) I have interpreted the figure of more than 1,030 at Succor Gate as being for the one day, 15 Jumādā II. Such a number is possible for the height of the epidemic but far too low for the cumulative mortality over one-third of the month. The latter part of the statement does not make sense; it would appear that Ibn Taghrī Birdī means to say that 15,000 people died that day, which is equally implausible (see *ibid.*, p. 76). If we second-guess Ibn Taghrī Birdī, he seems to have multiplied the figure of 1,030 by fourteen (the number of oratories commonly cited) to reach an estimated 15,000.

the number of funerals at this important oratory. The epidemic declined thereafter until the end of the following month (Rajab/April). There are no figures given for the diminishing death rate, but Ibn Taghrī Birdī seems to imply that the mortality rate declined rapidly after 18 Jumādā II/March 14. The epidemic abated and no longer struck children, mamlūks, foreigners, and servants as usual but, instead, older prominent men.

Can we determine the relationship between the selective *dīwān* record of Cairo and the other sources for mortality data from this plague epidemic and others in the fifteenth century? There is no case where the *dīwān* list, the funerals, and the counts at the city gates are all given for one day. In only one instance is the *dīwān* figure mentioned for the same day as the count of coffins at the city gates—4 Jumādā II/February 28.[44] The *dīwān* register represents about 32.5 percent of the number taken out of the city gates. Only seven instances exist where the *dīwān* list and the number of mosque funerals are mentioned for the same day during the plague epidemics of 833/1429-1430, 841/1437-1438, and 864/1459-1460 in Cairo.[45] The *dīwān* record ranges between twenty and thirty percent of the number of funerals. Within these seven instances, the *dīwān* figure corresponds to approximately twenty percent for all the oratories of the city and thirty percent for the principal oratories. The percentage of the *dīwān* figures is remarkably high and may indicate the efficiency of the bureau of escheats or, more likely, the underestimation of the total number of deaths. The

[44] *as-Sulūk*, part 4, vol. 2, p. 826.

[45] 29 Jumādā I, A.H. 833—19% plus (*as-Sulūk*, part 4, vol. 2, p. 825; *an-Nujūm*, Popper trans., vol. 18, p. 70); 7 Jumādā II, A.H. 833—27% (*as-Sulūk*, part 4, vol. 2, p. 826—Fusṭāṭ: 30%); 9 Jumādā II, A.H. 833—32% (*ibid.*, pp. 826-827); 21 Shawwāl, A.H. 841—27% (*ibid.*, p. 1041); 17 Jumādā I, A.H. 864—28% (*an-Nujūm*, Popper trans., vol. 22, pp. 93-94); 26 Jumādā I, A.H. 864—20% (*ibid.*, vol. 22, p. 94); and 1 Jumādā II, A.H. 864—17% (*ibid.*, p. 95). These estimates should be used with extreme caution because of the meagerness of the data and the inaccuracy of the manner of accounting.

relationship of one to five would give a rough estimate of the *dīwān* mortality figures to total urban depopulation.[46]

On the basis of these very tenuous relationships between *dīwān* mortality rates on the one hand and the funerals and counts at the gates on the other, *dīwān* figures have been estimated to give monthly mortality counts for the plague epidemic of 833/1429-1430, where *dīwān* citations are lacking. Concerning the cessation of the epidemic, we will assume that the mortality rate in the Cairo *dīwān* decreased steadily and consistently in the second half of Jumādā II, by fifty a day from 700 on 16 Jumādā II/March 12 to fifty on 29 Jumādā II/March 25. We will also assume that the mortality rate for Rajab was similar to Rabīʿ II, declining from forty-eight a day to twelve at the end of the month.

According to the very fragmentary figures that the chroniclers supply for daily mortality rates, we can calculate very roughly the *general extent* of the depopulation—*not* the precise mortality. The total figure is based on the following calculations from the estimates of *dīwān* death rates:

	Monthly Dīwān Mortality Rate x 5	=	*Monthly Cairene Mortality Rate*
Rabīʿ II	477		2,385
Jumādā I	5,570		27,850
Jumādā II	11,845		59,225
Rajab	477		2,385
Total	18,369		91,845

This estimate is remarkably close to Ibn Taghrī Birdī's judgment of the mortality figures; he first quotes al-Maqrīzī's

[46] The calculation of the mortality rate according to the *dīwān* figures is given below. These *dīwān* figures do not appear to be excessive to me but are generally consistent with the range of such mortality for the one case where we have an extract from the Cairo *dīwān* during the plague epidemic of 822/1419 (see part C above).

summary for the entire loss of population and then gives his own opinion:

> Al-Maqrīzī says: "This was a year of evils, wars, and seditions; and there was a great plague in Northern and Southern Egypt, in Cairo, Old Cairo, and their environs. The smallest stated number of deaths is a total of 100,000, but the one who merely guesses says that this 100,000 refers to Cairo and Old Cairo alone, aside from the dead in Southern and Northern Egypt, who were equal in number." I say: The statement of the one who places the 100,000 deaths in Cairo and Old Cairo alone is by no means guessing, for the plague lasted more than three months, including its beginning, decline, and cessation.[47]

The calculations according to the *dīwān* figures are very faulty, but they give us an idea of the general scope of mortality as well as substantiating—surprisingly enough—the claims of the medieval chronicler. With this exceptional plague epidemic in mind, therefore, it would not be unreasonable to find during the Black Death in Cairo a daily mortality rate of more than 4,943.[48] Moreover, a total of more than 100,000 is likely for the Black Death, in view of the fact that it lasted for a longer time and attacked a greater population with no possible immunity to plague.

3. Medieval and Modern Estimates of Mortality Caused by the Black Death

Approximately eighty years before the severe plague of 833/1429-1430, the Black Death struck Egypt and caused at least an equal loss of population. After coming to Egypt in the autumn of 1347, the pandemic spread southward throughout

[47] *an-Nujūm*, Popper trans., vol. 18, p. 76.

[48] This figure is based on the fact that the funerals at Succor Gate are about 36% of the funerals of the principal oratories and 21% of all oratories. At the height of the epidemic of A.H. 833, the number at Succor Gate was 1,030 which would give 4,943 for all the oratories of the city and thus close to the total urban mortality figures.

the Delta in 1348. It reached its peak in Cairo during the winter of 1348-1349 and ceased in February 1349.

The plague pandemic probably began in Alexandria, where the death rate rose to 100 and then 200 a day. The highest point may have been reached when on one day 700 coffins were reportedly prayed over in the grand mosque of the city. The Black Death became severe in Cairo from the beginning of Rajab 749/25 September 1348, when the daily figure averaged 300, according to al-Maqrīzī. By the end of the month (October 24), it averaged more than 1,000 a day. The period of greatest mortality was during the following winter: the epidemic intensified in Cairo during Sha'bān/25 October-22 November, and was particularly grave in Ramaḍān/23 November-22 December—to the extent that "it was impossible to count the dead." In Shawwāl/23 December-20 January, a new symptom was observed—blood-spitting—which must refer to highly fatal pneumonic plague. The daily death rate was reportedly 10, 15, and even 20,000 in Cairo and Fusṭāṭ.

Al-Maqrīzī states that, during an indeterminate period of the Black Death, a calculation of plague deaths was made on the basis of the number of funerals at certain oratories of the city. The count was made in the oratories of Succor Gate, Zuwaylah Gate, Burnt Gate (Bāb al-Maḥrūq), below the Citadel (presumably Mu'minī Oratory, where enormous numbers of funerals took place in later epidemics), and the Oratory of the Lion Slayer, opposite the Mosque of Qawsūn (outside of Qarāfah Gate). These oratories were located outside the enceinte of the Fāṭimid walls of the mamlūk city and probably were used for the majority of the dead being taken to the vast cemeteries east of Cairo. At these funeral services, 13,800 dead were counted in two days. This number did not include those who perished in the markets and empty quarters of the metropolis, the region beyond the Nile Gate Bridge (Bāb al-Baḥr) over the Nāṣirī Canal in the northwestern corner of the city leading to Būlāq, the Ḥusaynīyah and Ibn Ṭūlūn quarters, and those who died in their homes and whose burials were delayed. Thus, the count appears generally to have excluded those who were neglected within the city and those dying in the suburbs outside the mamlūk city.

While this detailed account appears reliable, al-Maqrīzī adds that "following another estimation, there were 20,000 deaths in a single day. The count of funerals in Cairo for the months of Sha'bān and Ramaḍān [November and December] was 900,000. Again this did not include the deaths in the regions that were not built up, the quarters of Ḥusaynīyah and Ṣalībah, and other parts of the suburbs; their death rate was double that of the walled city."[49] Ibn Abī Ḥajalah, who lived in Damascus during the calamity, claimed that the deaths in Cairo reached as high as 27,000 a day.[50] Likewise, Ibn Baṭṭūṭah, who was traveling in Syria during the time of the Black Death, gives what may similarly be called "pictorial numbers" in his estimate of maximum daily mortality as 24,000 in Cairo and Fusṭāṭ.[51]

These estimates of maximum daily mortality of 20,000 and more are incredible, given a pre-plague population for metropolitan Cairo of no more than 500,000-600,000 and the long duration of the pandemic. The Black Death in Cairo lasted through the fall and winter, with its greatest destruction in the five months from the end of September 1348 to the beginning of January 1349; we do not even know when the peak

[49] *as-Sulūk*, part 2, vol. 3, pp. 772, 780-782. These statements of Cairene mortality are often repeated in later sources, e.g., Qalqashandī, *Subḥ al-'a'shā*, vol. 13, p. 79, and Ibn Iyās, vol. 1, p. 191.

[50] *Daf' an-niqmah*, fols. 75a, 76a.

[51] *Travels, A.D. 1325-1354*, vol. 1, p. 144. The only European evidence for the mortality in Cairo is the curious report of Giorgio Gucci, who journeyed through Egypt to the Holy Lands in 1384-1385. He relates that during the Black Death in 1348 the mamlūk sultan had written to King Hugh of Cyprus informing him that there were days when over a hundred thousand persons died in Cairo. King Hugh reportedly had these figures written on stone as a memorial in Nicosia and in the principal cities of Cyprus. (Frescobaldi, Gucci, and Sigoli, *Visit to the Holy Places*, pp. 100-101; p. 101, n. 1: "The king is Hugh IV [1324-59] who loved to embellish his palace [Enlart, *L'Art Gothique en Cypre*, Paris, 1899, vol. 2, p. 52] and perhaps put the inscription in some decoration.")

was attained, although it was probably in December. Even if we assume a very rapid decline in the mortality rate from the end of January 1349, the estimate of 900,000 for November-December just within the walled city is fantastic.[52] It is evident that we are dealing with very exaggerated estimates of daily death rates, despite their constant repetition in the chronicles; according to al-Maqrīzī's own figures, the total for urban depopulation is impossible, far greater than the probable population of all of Cairo.

Because of the extreme paucity of reliable data, we have to rely on al-Maqrīzī's one statement of 13,800 funerals at five oratories during two days when the epidemic was presumably at its worst, for some idea of the general level of the death rate. A figure of about 7,000 as the height of the daily number of deaths counted at the five principal oratories of the city is reasonably consistent with the level of maximum daily mortality during the plague of 833/1429-1430. A maximum daily mortality at all the oratories of the city may have been more than 10,000. With this peak of daily mortality, it is possible that the aggregate death rate was in excess of 200,000, given a pattern of mortality similar to that of the epidemics of 833/1429-1430 and 864/1460 (see Tables 1 and 2). This would be about one-third to two-fifths of the total urban population. This rough guess agrees with al-Maqrīzī's statement—probably taken from Ibn Ḥabīb—that the Black Death destroyed one-third of the population of Egypt and Syria.[53]

The question of the rural depopulation of Egypt has been

[52] It would seem that al-Maqrīzī took a figure of 15,000 and simply multiplied it by sixty days to get this number. It is possible that he assumed that this figure represented the daily mortality rate during the period and was the result of doubling the numbers counted at the oratories of the city to give an approximate number for the entire metropolis. A figure of about 7,500 for the funerals at the principal oratories would not have been unreasonable for the severe stages of the epidemic and is close to the 6,900 (half of 13,800) mentioned above.

[53] Quoted in "England to Egypt," p. 120; see also Ashtor, *Histoire*, p. 546: *Durrat al-aslāk*, ed. by A. Meursinge and H. E. Weijers, *Orientalia*, vol. 2 (Amsterdam, 1846), p. 388.

approached in a different manner through the study of the cadastral surveys from before and after the Black Death, but these fiscal surveys have their own inherent difficulties. On the basis of a review of the cadasters for Egypt during the Mamlūk Period, Professor Russell has proposed a twenty to thirty percent loss in total population, or possibly lower percentage from the pre-plague level to about 1420. From a population of about 4.2 million in Egypt in 1348, "the population dropped about fifteen percent by 1378 and another five percent by 1420 where it must have remained at about 3.15-3.36 million until the Turks took over in the sixteenth century."[54]

TABLE 1

THE PLAGUE EPIDEMIC OF 833/1429-1430 IN CAIRO

		Principal Oratories			
Date	*Dīwān*		*Succor Gate*	*All the Oratories*	*City Gates*
1 Rabīʿ II	12				
29 Rabīʿ II	48				
29 Jumādā I	400			2,100	
30 Jumādā I				1,800 (?)	1,800 (?)
4 Jumādā II	390				1,200
7 Jumādā II	350	1,200			
9 Jumādā II	400	1,263	450		
10 Jumādā II			505		
11 Jumādā II				2,246	
? Jumādā II			800		12,300 (?)
15 Jumādā II			1,030		15,000 (?)

Besides the fact that the suggested level of population is too low, there is good reason to believe that the demographic decline was greater than fifteen percent, closer in fact to the medieval chroniclers' estimate of one-third. First of all, there are no grounds for Russell's assumption that the Egyptian population declined significantly between the 1315 cadastral

[54] "Population of Medieval Egypt," p. 80.

TABLE 2

THE PLAGUE EPIDEMIC OF 864/1460 IN CAIRO

Date	*Dīwān*	*Succor Gate Oratory*	*Principal Oratories (17?)*	*Urban Mortality*
17 Jumādā I	170	100	600	
26 Jumādā I	235		1,153	
1 Jumādā II	316		1,910	
3 Jumādā II		350		3,500 (?)
11 Jumādā II	280	570		
14 Jumādā II	300	570	1,416*	4,000 (?)
21 Jumādā II		350	1,154*	
28 Jumādā II		190	434*	
6 Rajab		100		
13 Rajab		25	53*	

* Figures for only three principal oratories: Succor Gate, al-Azhar, and Farriers' Oratory

survey and the outbreak of the Black Death.[55] This assertion is made apparently on the basis of the development of European population before the Black Death. Since there is no evidence that Middle Eastern population declined appreciably in the first half of the fourteenth century but probably was on the increase, the percentage of depopulation resulting from the Black Death would be higher than Russell's estimate. Second, there are a number of misconceptions about plague pathology in Russell's account that result in a lower assessment of the plague mortality rate in Egypt.[56]

Furthermore, it should be emphasized that Russell's cor-

[55] See above, part A.

[56] For example: "Oddly enough a more densely settled area might be expected to have a relatively less decline [*sic*] since there were more persons to the rat." (Russell, "Population of Medieval Egypt," p. 80 and n. 56) This is a completely erroneous assertion. There is certainly no evidence for this statement about the ratio of human to rat population and discounts entirely the importance of infectious pneumonic plague.

relation between the total decrease of about twelve percent in the tax quotas (from before the Black Death to the third quarter of the fifteenth century) and the degree of depopulation is a poor gauge of demographic change and is indeed a minimum. The assessed taxation was certainly highly conservative, and the estimated reduction must be regarded as a very reluctant admission of revenue decline; in addition, as Russell admits, individual peasants may have increased their cultivation, which would distort the equation of tax quotas with population change. An assessment of population based on revenue should be further qualified by the possible rural underemployment, significant monetary inflation, and changes of prices and labor costs.

Thus, the degree of depopulation in Egypt resulting from the Black Death is far from certain. It can only be suggested at this stage of investigation that an Egyptian population of between 4.2 and 8 million may have declined by about one-quarter to one-third.[57] Although Russell is correct in stating that the Egyptian population continued to decline in an irregular manner after the Black Death, there is no reason to assume that the population remained stable or began to increase again in the early fifteenth century, as the European population may have done. On the contrary, the evidence indicates sustained depopulation until the Ottoman conquest of Egypt and Syria and perhaps afterwards.

Turning to Syria during the Black Death, we find that the two historians Ibn Abī Ḥajalah and Ibn Baṭṭūṭah give more credible estimates for the maximum death rate in Damascus, where they were resident, than for Cairo. The former estimated a peak of more than 1,000 and the latter, 2,000 a day.[58] Ibn Kathīr, who was also in Damascus, observed mass funerals at the Umayyad Mosque that reached more than 150 a day, excluding the funerals in the suburbs and those of non-

[57] Poliak accepts the medieval estimate that population in the Middle East declined by one-third and suggests that the population of Egypt declined from about three million to two million ("The Demographic Evolution of the Middle East," p. 201).

[58] See ns. 50 and 51 above.

Muslims. The general mortality rate, according to Ibn Kathīr, rose from 100 a day in Rabīʿ I, 749/June 1348, to more than 200 in Rabīʿ II/July, and 300 in Jumādā I/August.[59] In Rajab/September-October, the number of deaths reached 1,000, and during the month of Shaʿbān/November was excessive, as in Cairo.[60] Similarly, al-Maqrīzī states that the daily total amounted to 1,200 dead during Rajab/September-October.[61]

In the year 750/beginning 22 March 1349, the pandemic began to decline in Damascus. As already mentioned, Ibn Kathīr comments that the *dīwān* of inheritance in the city decreased to twenty after it had reached a level of 500 in the year 749/1348-1349.[62] The figure of 500 is too small for the total *dīwān* list of deaths for the entire year; it may refer to the highest daily mortality rate during the Black Death, compared to an estimated peak of about 915 in the epidemic of 833/1429-1430 in Cairo. The twenty deaths in the *dīwān* may represent the daily mortality rate in Damascus when the epidemic was subsiding at the beginning of 750/March 1349, close to the normal mortality rate in the *dīwān*.

If the death rate rose from 100 a day in Rabīʿ I, 749/June 1348, to over 1,000 a day in Shaʿbān/November, as alleged by Ibn Kathīr, by a simple but highly suspect calculation based on a progressive rise and decline of mortality over at least a five months' period—we do not even know how and when the epidemic diminished—the total would be at least 30,000. The epidemic lasted for another four months, so that this figure is certainly a minimum. Thus, the degree of depopulation based on a population of 80,000 in Damascus may have been about thirty-eight percent.

Despite Ibn Ḥabīb's general estimate that one-third of the population of Egypt and Syria was destroyed by the Black Death, he says that only one-quarter of the population of Damascus perished.[63] According to this figure, the population of the city declined from about 80,000 to 60,000.

[59] *al-Bidāyah*, vol. 14, pp. 226-227.

[60] *Ibid.*, p. 228.

[61] *as-Sulūk*, part 2, vol. 3, p. 779.

[62] See above, part C, n. 31.

[63] *Durrat al-aslāk*, p. 359.

As for the other cities of Syria, a total of 22,000 deaths is given for the city of Gaza in the period from 2 Muḥarram to 4 Ṣafar 749/2 April to 4 May 1348—apparently reported by the governor of the province.[64] A similar report from the governor of Gaza to the government in Damascus claimed that more than 10,000 died in roughly the same period, 10 Muḥarram to 10 Ṣafar/10 April to 10 May.[65] The latter report from a contemporary source is more reliable. Concerning Aleppo, Ibn Ḥabīb remarks that as many as 500 died in one day; he had estimated that 1,000 died daily in Damascus and 20,000 in the entire country of Egypt.[66] Al-'Aynī furnishes the same estimate for Egypt, in addition to the mortality rate of 100 a day in his hometown of 'Ayn Tāb; plague was said to have destroyed about two-thirds of the town's *'ulamā'*.[67] If the population of Syria was 1,200,000, as claimed by Poliak, the medieval estimate of one-third would have reduced the population by 400,000.[68]

Finally, Qalqashandī, an Egyptian historian contemporary with al-Maqrīzī, expresses the resigned consternation of many at the enormous number of deaths. He repeats al-Maqrīzī's more fantastic figures, as others had done for the depopulation of Egypt and Syria, and remarks that it was an extraordinary

64 *as-Sulūk*, part 2, vol. 3, p. 775.

65 *al-Bidāyah*, vol. 14, p. 225. There is a doubt whether these figures refer to the city of Gaza and its suburbs or to the entire province of Gaza, but probably to the former.

66 *Tadhkirat an-nabīh*, British Museum Add. MS no. 7335, fol. 145b.

67 *'Iqd al-jumān*, chapter 25, part 1, p. 85.

68 "The Demographic Evolution of the Middle East," p. 201. Poliak's discussion gives a very brief survey of population from the Black Death to 1914 (pp. 201-205). With regard to the Black Death, Poliak brings some new data into consideration but simply accepts the medieval estimate of the mortality rate as a basis of calculation. He rightly emphasizes the planned depopulation along the Syrian coast by Sultan al-Asraf Khalil in 1291 to prevent any future Crusades from utilizing the region as a military base, but, surprisingly, neglects the demographic effects on Syria of the Mongol invasions (see Ashtor, *Histoire*, pp. 383-384). More surprising and quite erroneous is Poliak's proposal of a gradual demographic *increase* from the Black Death until modern times (see graph, p. 203).

coincidence that the year 749/1348-1349 itself was suppressed in the fiscal records of the government and transferred to the year 750/1349-1350. (This transference was periodically done in order to re-establish the concordance between the solar and lunar calendars.) When the year of the Black Death was transferred to 750/1349-1350, Qalqashandī concludes that: "Everything died, even the year itself!"[69]

All these estimates of population and plague mortality figures in the Middle East are open to serious question; only the statements of death rates when they are clearly attributed to the formal funeral services in specific urban oratories, the *dīwān*, or the counts at the city gates may be reasonably acceptable.[70] We can conclude, however, that the quantity and quality of the mortality data in the medieval Arabic chronicles are insufficient and are unsuitable for modern demographic analysis. A comparable dearth of statistics is found for other facets of medieval Muslim life about which we would like to know a great deal more.[71]

The chroniclers emphasize only periods of severe plague mortality, while we have no idea, for example, of the normal everyday mortality rate in the Cairo *dīwān*. The historians give the dates of the beginning of periods of high mortality rates, but rarely describe the ensuing course of the epidemic—its variations, peak, and decline—to enable us to pinpoint its evolution.[72] The *dīwān* figures are reasonably accurate but, as

[69] *Subh al-'a'shā*, vol. 13, p. 79.

[70] For example, such ambiguous statements as al-Maqrīzī's that the daily mortality rate at the beginning of Rajab 749/25 September 1348, was 300 in Cairo is problematic, for it is unclear what this figure actually refers to—the *dīwān* figure for Cairo, the number of funerals in the oratories of the city, the number taken out of the gates, or someone's guess.

[71] For example, see the conclusions of Montavez P. Martinez, *La oscilación del precio de trigo en el Cairo durante el primer régimen mameluco (1252-1382)*, unpubl. diss., Madrid, 1964 (summary published by the Faculty of Philosophy and Letters, Madrid, 1964).

[72] In attempting to estimate total mortality, this is crucial since it is incorrect to assume—as I have in part done—a constant increase and decrease during an epidemic. The actual evolution of a plague epidemic is highly irregular; for example, Ibn Taghrī Birdī wrote about the

has been repeatedly stressed, these figures are quite scarce and reflect only very roughly the total urban death rate. This urban bias of the historical information itself makes it almost impossible to generalize about the depopulation of the entire country. Barring the unlikely discovery of complete *dīwān* records for this period, quantitative and comparative data will have to be sought through a critical re-examination of the cadastral surveys and indirectly through the study of biographical dictionaries.[73] For general population estimates of

---

plague epidemic of 864/1460 in Cairo: "One of the characteristics of this plague was that it would diminish slightly from the day before, then would increase greatly on the morrow until it reached its limit on the pattern [of movement] and subsided." (*an-Nujūm*, Popper trans., vol. 22, p. 93)

[73] A study of the *tabaqāt* literature for fourteenth- and fifteenth-century Egypt and Syria may furnish comparative data for years when plague was known to occur. For the Black Death, a survey of deaths in the fourteenth-century biographical dictionaries would suggest the relative degree of mortality that is otherwise impossible to obtain because of the lack of precise mortality figures. If the *ṭabaqāt* mortality rate is correlated to the recurrences of plague, the general proportion of deaths should be related to the determined plague years even if plague is not mentioned as the cause of death in the biographies. The comparative death rate would also be an indication of the plagues' severity within the specific group of the dictionary and would aid in distinguishing between pneumonic and bubonic plague epidemics. (The two most important collections of biographies that should be studied in this way are: Ibn Ḥajar, *ad-Durar al-ḵāminah* [Hyderabad, A.H. 1348-1350] and his student, as-Sakhāwī, *aḍ-Ḍaw' al-lāmi'* [Cairo, A.H. 1353-1355], which are devoted to the eighth and ninth centuries A.H. respectively. Such investigation should also include Ibn Taghrī Birdī's *al-Manhal aṣ-ṣāfī wal-mustawfī ba'da al-wāfī* [one volume published, Cairo, 1956] and Ibn Rāfi', *Kitāb al-wafayāt* [unpublished] for Syria during the period of the Black Death; see E. Ashtor, "Some Unpublished Sources for the Bahrī Period," *Scripta Hierosolymitana*, ed. by U. Heyd, vol. 9 [Jerusalem, 1961], pp. 24-27. Equally, the *ṭabaqāt* literature for fourteenth-century Andalusia may yield significant demographic data; the most conspicuous work is by Ibn al-Khaṭīb, *al-Ihātah bi-mā tayassara min ta'rīḵh Gharnāṭah* [*GAL*, vol. 2, p. 262, n. 3; the extant portion is published in an abridged version by M. 'Abdallāh Enan, Cairo, 1955].)

the Middle East, methods applied to the study of medieval European population and new techniques peculiar to the circumstances of Muslim society must be developed and employed. Of particular importance is the evidence produced by archeological excavations of Islamic sites for questions of urban density.

What may be said with some assurance is that, on the basis of the fragmentary mortality figures for the disaster and comparison with the comparable plague epidemics of 833/1429-1430 and 864/1460, the Black Death substantially reduced the Middle Eastern population. The description of the economic and social repercussions of the Black Death will also reinforce this conclusion. However, the initial depopulation caused by the Black Death, despite all of its dramatic qualities, is far less significant for the history of the later Mamlūk Empire than the cumulative loss, as exemplified by the deterioration of the mamlūk army. Middle Eastern population was unable to recover successfully from the holocaust of the Black Death because of a number of adverse factors. By the early fifteenth century, the aggregate decline may have been more than one-third of the entire population from its pre-plague level, with no discernible recovery thereafter. It is necessary to turn, therefore, to an examination of the recurrence of plague and the other unfavorable conditions for population recovery to substantiate the claim that plague contributed to a sustained decrease in population.

F. THE PERIODICITY AND NATURE OF PLAGUE RECURRENCES

Plague recurred during the 174 *hijrah* years between the outbreak of the Black Death in the Middle East in 748/1347 and the conquest of Egypt and Syria by the Ottoman Empire in 922/1517. In Egypt and Syria, plague is cited for fifty-eight years (including the Black Death) of this period. Without regard to the intensity or nature of the plague epidemics, a number of pertinent observations may first be made about the plague recurrences, given a reasonable margin of error in the determination of the reappearances because of a lack of complete historical-medical evidence.

The repetition of plague epidemics in Egypt after the Black Death follows very closely the pattern of plague outbreaks subsequent to the Plague of Justinian.[1] In the latter case, the reappearances of plague occurred in cycles of between nine and twelve years from 540 to 770, comprising fifteen cycles. Taking the evidence only for Egypt in the 174 *hijrah* years after the Black Death, there is a possible total of twenty-eight outbreaks of plague. This excludes the epidemics in the rest of the Middle East (which may, however, be related to an epidemic in Egypt) because the evidence is more fragmentary than for Egypt and only inflates the number of possible plague years. The recurrences in Egypt appear in a somewhat cyclical pattern on the average of about every five and a half years, with a median of five years. The intervals are generally shorter than during the aftermath of the Plague of Justinian or the Black Death in Europe. The medical reasons for these cycles are far from clear. The explanation must lie in the complex relationship of men to rats and fleas. The loss of immunity and the replacement of human, rat, and flea population densities as well as the unpredictable re-introduction of the disease from outside the country may account for the pattern. In any case, the frequent recurrence of plague in Egypt suggests an endemic focus of plague in the later Middle Ages and the periodic destruction of its population.

Of greater demographic and historical importance than the mere cyclical appearances of plague is the nature of the plague recurrences themselves. For Europe, it is generally accepted that the Black Death in all three of its forms caused a dramatic demographic decline. This severe depopulation was followed by further demographic decline resulting from the periodic reappearances of plague epidemics into the fifteenth century. However, recent historical study of the plague recurrences in Europe has critically questioned the nature of these recurrent

[1] Biraben and Le Goff, "La Peste," pp. 1492-1493.

epidemics and asked whether they had the significant demographic importance that had earlier been attributed to them.[2] Professor J.M.W. Bean has examined the later plague appearances and has refuted the hypothesis that *continued* outbreaks of plague caused *continued* demographic decline, as suggested by other scholars.[3] His criticism is based on the ex-

[2] The recent study by Shrewsbury (*A History of Bubonic Plague*) is largely an example of extreme revisionism of earlier works on the Black Death and plague recurrences, particularly G. Creighton's *A History of Epidemics in Britain* (Cambridge, 1894). Shrewsbury's work rightly insists that epidemics of *other* diseases were important factors in the demographic and medical history of Great Britain. However, while the study is devoted primarily to the better documented epidemics of the sixteenth and seventeenth centuries, a major objective of the author is to refute the demographic importance of the Black Death and to deny the existence of recurrent plague epidemics through the fifteenth century. As for the Black Death, Shrewsbury argues that it destroyed, at most, 20% of the population (p. 123). He does not consider the epidemics of the second half of the fourteenth century as outbreaks of bubonic plague at all. This is surely mistaken. Without a lengthy review of Shrewsbury's criteria and the historical evidence, it may be said that he (a professor of bacteriology) has generally applied our modern medical knowledge of plague too rigorously to the medieval evidence. Despite the self-imposed limitations placed on the study, the most serious fault of the study is the exclusion of pneumonic plague from consideration. A discussion of pneumonic plague is imperative in any historical account of plague. The important question, therefore, remains unanswered: Did pneumonic plague occur in Britain after the Black Death or was it excluded because this study was narrowly confined to bubonic plague? (I concur fully with Christopher Morris' criticism in his review of Shrewsbury's work in *The Historical Journal*, vol. 14, no. 1 [1971], pp. 205-215.)

[3] "Plague, Population and Economic Decline in England in the Late Middle Ages," *The Economic History Review*, 2nd series, vol. 15 (1962-1963), pp. 423-437. The disputed hypothesis for continued demographic decline in England due to plague may be found in John Saltmarsh, "Plague and Economic Decline in England in the Later Middle Ages," *Cambridge Historical Journal*, vol. 7 (1941), pp. 23-41. Saltmarsh attributes to the plague recurrences (until 1665) the demographic decline of England and the economic consequences of a reduced population, i.e., declining rents, marginal lands falling out of cultivation, higher prices for manufactured articles, etc. (See also R. Mols, *Introduction à la démographie historique des villes d'Europe du*

amination of the nature and form of these plague epidemics, of their mortality figures, and of their chronology in England in the fourteenth and fifteenth centuries.

The gist of Bean's argument is that the recurrence of plague in Europe rarely included pneumonic plague after the Black Death, and thus allowed for a rapid replacement of population. Similarly, the leading medical historian of plague has written that "primary infectious pneumonic plague played an insignificant part in the spread of plague in Europe after the decline of the Black Death except, perhaps, in a few Russian epidemics."[4] Bubonic plague, it will be recalled, is medically the least contagious of epidemic diseases, while primary pneu-

---

XIVe au XVIIIe siècle [Louvain, 1954-1956], vol. 2, pp. 437, 483.) Saltmarsh's thesis is accepted by Russell in his many works on medieval population; see, for example, his *Medieval Cities and Their Regions*, p. 246. The thesis of declining European population has also been related to the economic "depression" of early Renaissance Europe; see H. A. Miskimin, *The Economy of Early Renaissance Europe, 1300-1460* (Englewood Cliffs, N.J., 1969). The argument may be briefly summarized in the following proposition: (1) demographic decline causes economic decline (and conversely, demographic increase causes economic prosperity); (2) there was a marked economic decline from the mid-fourteenth century to the mid-fifteenth century in Europe; therefore, (3) the period of economic decline following the Black Death resulted from a sustained demographic decline. The second premise has not been proven conclusively, and the conclusion is the subject of considerable controversy. (See Robert Lopez and H. A. Miskimin, "The Economic Depression of the Renaissance," *The Economic History Review*, 2nd series, vol. 14 [1962], pp. 297-407, and the strong rebuttal by C. M. Cipolla in *The Economic History Review*, 2nd series, vol. 16 [1964], pp. 408-426. For a clear statement of this controversy, see D. Herlihy, "Population, Plague and Social Change in Rural Pistoria, 1201-1430," *The Economic History Review*, 2nd series, vol. 18 [1968], pp. 225-227.) If the decline of population is the basic cause of economic decline in Europe, greater emphasis should be placed on other demographic factors besides plague. In the face of these two major controversies—demographic and economic—of late medieval Europe, we should be especially careful of facile comparisons and conclusions.

[4] Hirst, p. 34; see also Wu Lien-Teh, *A Treatise on Pneumonic Plague*, p. 7; and Sticker, *Abhandlungen*, vol. 1, p. 20.

monic plague is probably the most infectious epidemic disease and is almost always fatal.[5]

Bean has concluded that the instances of pneumonic plague after the Black Death were indeed rare.[6] This is supported by the observation that the European plague reappearances, particularly in England, were gradually limited in geographical scope, which would be indicative of contagious as opposed to infectious pneumonic epidemics. Altogether, the lack of persuasive evidence for pneumonic plague after the Black Death in Europe should lead to a much lower estimate of plague mortality for these recurrences, or the investigation of other concomitant demographic causes of the reduction of population if there was a sustained population decline in the late fourteenth and the fifteenth centuries.[7]

The same criteria used by Bean may be applied to the material for the plague recurrences in Egypt and Syria during the same period. In the Middle East, we are faced with a remarkable difference in the nature of the plague epidemics. The historical evidence shows that pneumonic plague recurred regularly after the Black Death and consequently implies a significant demographic effect. Using the methods of examination applied to plague in Europe, the Arabic sources clearly describe the spitting of blood, the appearance of plague in the winter months, and the general or "national" character of these epidemics.

As for the comparative mortality rates of successive plague epidemics in the Middle East, the precise but very limited

[5] Hirst, p. 29.

[6] "Plague, Population and Economic Decline," p. 426.

[7] Modern studies of late medieval European population suggest an "overpopulation" in the thirteenth century followed by a steady demographic decline before the Black Death. The Black Death and later plague epidemics as well as other demographic factors are considered only to have accelerated the decline and not to have been an absolute "Malthusian check" to population growth. This view leads correctly to the more careful examination of a declining birth rate of the population itself, caused by deteriorating economic and social conditions. (See Herlihy, "Population, Plague and Social Change in Rural Pistoria," pp. 234-244.)

mortality figures given by the contemporary historians, particularly for Cairo in the fifteenth century, are very poor indices of severity and do not allow us to draw any firm conclusions. As I have already mentioned, the *dīwān* figures are very fragmentary, and the comparison of relative severity is not satisfactory, because the *dīwān* accounts are usually quoted only for the more severe plague epidemics, which included the pneumonic form of plague, and generally not for the milder epidemics of plague. Where limited comparison of severity can be made between what are believed to have been non-pneumonic and pneumonic plague epidemics in the early fifteenth century, the evidence is consistent except for the year 819/1416. In this year, the *dīwān* figures are as high as those of 833/1429-1430 or 864/1459-1460 (where there is strong evidence of pneumonic plague). The plague epidemic of 819/1416 began in the spring, and the brief historical description of al-Maqrīzī does not mention the distinctive symptoms of pneumonic plague. Secondary pneumonic plague may have occurred, in which rapid death takes place without any signs of coughing or expectoration,[8] or the epidemic may have been accompanied by other communicable diseases. In general, the statistical data for measuring relative severity are far too scanty —there are only thirty-six statements of daily mortality for the fifty-eight plague years—to either substantiate or challenge the historical conclusions based on the other criteria for pneumonic plague.

There is a possible approach to plague mortality that may prove to be very profitable. The evidence of archeological excavations, particularly of Muslim cemeteries, may be used to corroborate the historical accounts, not only by adding quantitative data but by indicating the manner of burials, the age and sex ratios of the victims, and the possible effect on urban settlement. There is a strong probability that such material may soon be available. A Polish expedition has excavated the Arab necropolis situated above a classical site at Kūm ad-Dikkah, in the center of modern Alexandria. A large Muslim

[8] Pollitzer, *Plague*, pp. 445-446.

cemetery overlies the entire acropolis of the Roman theater (perhaps a council hall) and baths.[9] Only during the Muslim period did the site serve as a burial ground. After the Arab conquest of Egypt, the population of Alexandria apparently declined considerably, and during the Middle Ages the cemetery was on the outskirts of the city. There is some confusion in the preliminary reports about the stratigraphy and dating of the cemetery, but generally there appear to be two layers of the necropolis; the lower dates from about the end of the ninth century.[10] Between the upper and lower necropolises was a layer of rubble.[11] The upper layer served as a cemetery, according to stratigraphical data, in the eleventh century and continued in use during the Mamlūk Period.[12]

Mass burials were conspicuous in the upper necropolis. The tombs contained no funeral equipment; burials were mixed and incomplete; and most skeletons were poorly preserved. In the majority of the tombs, various animal bones were found,

[9] T. Dzierżykray-Rogalski and E. Promińska, "Studies of Human Bones from Sector M-IX of the Moslem Nécroples at Kom el-Dikka, Alexandria (Egypt)," *Études et Travaux*, no. 2, vol. 6 (1968), pp. 174-175.

[10] *Ibid.*, p. 176. See also Leszek Dąbrowski, "Two Arab Nécroples Discovered at Kom el Dikka, Alexandria," *Études et Travaux*, no. 2, vol. 3 (1966), pp. 176-178; for tomb inscriptions and dating, see W. Kubiak, "Stèles Funéraires Arabes de Kōm el-Dick," *Bulletin de la Société Archéologique d'Alexandrie*, no. 42 (Cairo, 1967), pp. 17-26 (p. 17, n. 2 gives a useful bibliography of evidence for the use of the site as a burial ground in the Middle Ages).

[11] T. Dzierżykray-Rogalski, "An Anatomical and Anthropological Analysis of Human Skeletal Remains from the Arab Nécroples at Kom el-Dikka, Alexandria (Egypt)," *Études et Travaux*, no. 2, vol. 3 (1966), pp. 202-203.

[12] Dzierżykray-Rogalski and Promińska, "Studies on Human Bones from Sector M-IX," p. 176; T. Dzierżykray-Rogalski, "Human Bones from Trench F and G of the Moslem Nécroples at Kom al-Dikka, Alexandria (Egypt)," *Études et Travaux*, no. 2, vol. 9 (1968), pp. 229-242. For the disputed dating, see Kubiak, "Les Fouilles Polonaises à Kōm el-Dick en 1963 et 1964," *Bulletin de la Société Archéologique d'Alexandrie*, no. 42 (Cairo, 1967), pp. 47-80, particularly p. 70; Dzierżykray-Rogalski, "An Anatomical and Anthropological Analysis," p. 204.

and the tombs were very poorly constructed. Mortality among females was highest during the period of maximum fertility (thirty to forty years), and mortality among children aged one to six years was exceptionally high. Naturally, there would be no evidence of the plague symptoms, but there is no evidence of any other cause of death, and the manner of burial is consistent with hastily constructed plague cemeteries. Thus, if this were a plague cemetery, it supports the literary evidence that plague had a marked demographic effect by limiting fertility, as well as destroying children.

Despite the lack of quantitative data to make it possible satisfactorily to gauge the levels of severity for successive plague epidemics, on the basis of Bean's other criteria we can establish that the pneumonic type of plague occurred in Egypt at the following times: 748-750/1347-1349 (the Black Death), 776/1374-1375, 781-782/1379-1381, 806/1403-1404, 813-814/1410-1411, 833/1429-1430, 841/1437, 852-853/1448-1449, and 864/1459-1460.[13] From the Black Death to 864/1459-1460, when the historical sources decrease sharply in number and quality, pneumonic plague occurred in fourteen years out of 116 *hijrah* years on the average of every 13.75 years.

The average of intervals is deceiving, since the most outstanding characteristic of the recurrent pneumonic plague epidemics is the gradual leveling in the duration of alternating long and short intervals. From the Black Death to 864/1459-1460, the intervals are: 25-5-24-7-19-8-11-11. The frequency and intensity of such epidemics within each generation would have effectively prevented the population from successively replacing its numbers, and might indicate either no growth or an absolute demographic decline.

An absolute decline is highly probable, due to the fact that the endemic disease struck primarily young women and chil-

[13] In some cases, these epidemics naturally included Syria and Palestine. Parenthetically, a pneumonic plague epidemic probably occurred in Tabrīz in the winter of 893/1488: "Suddenly in the beginning of the winter the cloud of the plague (*ṭāʿūn*), for the second time, covered the hills and plains of Tabrīz." (Minorsky, *Persia in* A.D. *1478-1490*, p. 87)

dren, thus greatly limiting fertility and replacement. In Europe, where young women and children formed a disproportionate element among the plague victims, the same phenomenon is noted by chroniclers and physicians.[14] Yet Bean and others have criticized the assumption that frequent plague outbreaks would result in population decline, by comparing the epidemics to recent and more fully documented experiences of epidemic diseases in areas similar to medieval England, such as among the peasant population of India. The latter shows that severe death rates from epidemics are followed by rapid rises in the birth rate, which enables the population to recover its pre-epidemic level. Short-run demographic decline may decrease the number of dependents on survivors and, along with a rise in living standards, permit marriage at an earlier age.[15] The comparison makes us alert to the resilience of population and its ability to recover under favorable conditions. But it does not describe the demographic situation in the Middle East, where recurrent pneumonic plagues were an overriding factor.

The study of plague epidemics in England by Bean does make us highly skeptical of a prolonged demographic decline in Europe. On the other hand, the same criteria for the plague recurrences in the Middle East strengthen the case for repeated and substantial reductions in population after the Black Death. This decline was aided by other unfavorable demographic factors that retarded population recovery.

G. OTHER FACTORS LIMITING POPULATION GROWTH

Other factors, such as other epidemic diseases and famines resulting from the severe fluctuations of the Nile, contributed substantially to the demographic decline in Egypt in the later Middle Ages. Damaging Nile variations were exceptionally

[14] Bean, "Plague, Population and Economic Decline," p. 431.

[15] *Ibid.*, pp. 431-432. Although this may be true of rural India, it is doubtful whether it is actually applicable to medieval England where, as Bean has shown, plague epidemics became an increasingly urban phenomenon.

frequent during the century following the Black Death. Destructive flooding occurred in 761-762/1360, 778/1376, 784/1382, 797-798/1395, and 812/1409, with an above-average water level from 722/1322 to 824/1421. On the other hand, low water levels provoked famines in 776/1374-1375, 796-799/1394-1396, and particularly 806/1403-1404.[1] Malnutrition may have been the natural consequence of these conditions for many and predisposed them to plague. Famine and flooding may also be associated with the recurrence of plague by causing the movement of infected rats to centers of human settlement in search of food.[2] Furthermore, the neglect of the irrigation system added to the decrease in cultivated land and encouraged rural population to move away from the land, particularly in the fifteenth century.[3]

[1] See Russell, "The Population of Medieval Egypt," p. 79 (based on *as-Sulūk* and Popper, "The Cairo Nilometer, Studies in Ibn Taghrī Birdī's Chronicles of Egypt," *University of California Publications in Semitic Philology*, vol. 12 [1951]). Unfortunately, there is no study of famines in Egypt during the Middle Ages that might show the nature and reasons for severe food crises. Such a study would benefit from the comparative data for Europe during the same period, where there was a similar succession of famines, resulting perhaps from previous overpopulation (see Miskimin, *The Economy of Early Renaissance Europe*, pp. 25-27). However, these data have also not been the subject of any thorough investigation. (For a list of the fourteenth-century famines in England and France, see Helen Robbins, "A Comparison of the Effects of the Black Death on the Economic Organization of France and England," *Journal of Political Economy*, vol. 36 [1928], pp. 447-479.) Even though the famines in the two areas may not be related to similar problems of population density, they would be comparable in climatic conditions and in their social responses to crises, as with plague epidemics: religious rituals and interpretations, migrations, prices and wages, etc.

[2] A number of pilgrims to Mt. Sinai relate a miracle about the Monastery of Saint Mary, where the monks were forced to abandon the monastery because of the lack of food and a subsequent invasion of rats; the monks were miraculously supplied with provisions (Niccolò da Poggibonsi, *A Voyage Beyond*, pp. 109-110). See also Ibn Iyās' description of the rats' attack on the grain reserves in Egypt during the famine of A.H. 917 (*Badā'i' az-zuhūr*, Mostafa rev. ed., *Bibliotheca Islamica*, vol. 5d [Cairo, 1960], p. 217).

[3] Labib, *Handelsgeschichte*, p. 419; "England to Egypt," pp. 115-116; Darrag, pp. 63-66; Ashtor, *Histoire*, p. 268; Xavier de Planhol, *Les*

Professor Russell has suggested that the pattern of rural depopulation was directly related to Egypt's foreign trade, particularly in grain. According to this hypothesis, the inability of the peasantry to sell their surplus grain at a profit in the free market would lead to the impoverishment of the *fellaḥīn* and their migration from the countryside. The younger men who stayed on the land would be forced to remain unmarried for a longer time. Since the medieval birth rate and death rate were generally quite close, any postponement of marriage by a significant number would cause a decline of the total population.[4]

The peasants' sale of surplus grain may indeed have been important, and the reduction of this source of income by increased taxation, low agricultural prices, or poor agrarian conditions may have had an appreciable effect on rural population by encouraging migration and limiting marriage. However, this does not appear to be related at all to foreign trade, as Russell suggests. The foreign commerce of the Mamlūk Empire with Europe was largely a transfer trade, which had only a very marginal effect on the internal economy.[5] Neither were there significant grain exports from the Middle East during the Ayyūbid and Mamlūk Periods.[6] The expansion of European trade with the Middle East following the Black Death was immensely important to the development of European cities and their populations, but it can be argued that the greatly increased volume of European trade with the Mamlūk Empire after the Black Death was more indicative of the economic weakness and population decline in the Middle East than the reverse. Overall, the pattern of Mediterranean population from the early Christian era can scarcely be said to support the theory that "Egyptian population moved with its foreign commerce."

Fondements Géographique de l'Histoire de l'Islam (Paris, 1968), pp. 85, 88.

[4] "Population of Medieval Egypt," pp. 80-82.

[5] *Muslim Cities*, pp. 24-25.

[6] See Labib, *Handelsgeschichte*, p. 323, and Lapidus, "The Grain Economy of Mamlūk Egypt."

Another, more serious, cause of demographic decline in the Middle East was the practice of birth control, which may have been more common in the later Middle Ages than before. Together with the recurrences of pneumonic plague, birth control may have greatly retarded the customarily rapid replacement of population. A number of manuscripts dealing with the circumstances and use of birth control date from the Mamlūk Period. It may be assumed that the worsening economic conditions of this period were legitimate grounds for the widespread recommendation and employment of birth control, since one of its legal justifications is the inability of a family to support additional children.[7] Moreover, at the time of plague epidemics, the Muslims' serious concern for ritual purity in case of sudden death may have limited sexual intercourse and, consequently, the birth rate.

We have learned that the birth rate of a community is highly sensitive to social, economic, and political conditions. The political instability of the mamlūk regime, along with constant warfare and personal avarice from the late fourteenth century, could hardly have been conducive to population growth. A good description of the combination of these circumstances, which we can relate to demographic decline, may be taken from Ibn Taghrī Birdī's chronicle of Egypt from the year 806/1403-1404:

> During this year there was a vast extent of uninundated land in Egypt, and extreme scarcity resulted, followed by the plague. And this year was the beginning of a series of events and trials in which most of Egypt and its provinces were ruined, not only because of the failure of the inundation but also because of the lack of harmony in the government and

[7] The subject of Muslim birth control has been the topic of Basim F. Musallam's dissertation at Harvard University: "Sex and Society in Islam: The Sanction and Medieval Techniques of Birth Control." Further consideration of the topic, in a paper entitled "Birth Control and Middle Eastern History: Evidence and Hypotheses," was presented by Professor Musallam to the Princeton Conference on the Economic History of the Near East, June 16-20, 1974.

> the frequent change of officials in the provinces, as well as other causes.[8]

All these factors outlined by the Egyptian historian, and not plague alone, may account for the prolonged decline of the total population in Egypt and Syria at the time of mamlūk hegemony.

The substantial decline in population could not help but influence the social and economic life of Egypt and Syria. The Black Death and the recurrent plague epidemics had both immediate and protracted consequences. The numerous facets of the periodic disasters are not easily separable, nor is it always easy to distinguish between what may properly be considered direct and indirect consequences of depopulation. Yet the careful marshaling of the plague epidemics' social and economic effects give credibility to the historical event.

[8] *an-Nujūm*, Popper trans., vol. 14, p. 80. Ashtor places primary emphasis for the depopulation of cultivated land on the oppression and insecurity under the later mamlūk regime (*Histoire*, p. 273). See the description of Egypt in the early fifteenth century by Lane-Poole, *A History of Egypt in the Middle Ages*, pp. 327-328.

VI

URBAN COMMUNAL BEHAVIOR DURING THE BLACK DEATH

The metropolis of Cairo was naturally the focus of the chroniclers' attention and, in varying degrees, is representative of most of the other urban centers of the Mamlūk Empire. The chroniclers are quick to relate the morbid aspects of the massive urban death rate. The historians leave little doubt of the severity of the Black Death in Cairo. Speaking of the abandonment of property around the capital, Ibn Abī Ḥajalah claimed that all the previous diseases compared to the Black Death were as "drops in the sea or a point on a circle."[1] Their descriptions of the calamity are supplemented by more pungent depictions of the Black Death, for an unusually large amount of poetry was written during the pandemic.[2] There is an im-

[1] *Daf' an-niqmah*, fol. 75a.

[2] The poetic accounts of the Black Death are relatively abundant (see Appendix 3), and most of the historical records contain a number of quoted verses. The *Risālat an-naba' 'an al-waba'* by Ibn al-Wardī is a good example of the frequent use of literary conceits and metaphors employed in describing plague. Some of the common metaphors and similes for plague and their sources are the following: (1) a cup of poison (aṣ-Safadī quoted in *as-Sulūk*, part 2, vol. 3, p. 789; *Durrat al-aslāk*, p. 358; *Daf' an-niqmah*, fol. 77a); (2) an invading army or a warrior (as-Subkī, Dār al-Kutub al-Miṣrīyah MS no. 102 *majāmī' m*, fol. 198a; Ibn al-Haymī, *ibid.*, fol. 200a; *Durrat al-aslāk*, p. 358; *Daf' an-niqmah*, fol. 81a); (3) an arrow or sword (*Muqni'at*, fol. 42b; *Durrat al-aslāk*, p. 358; *as-Sulūk*, part 2, vol. 3, p. 790; al-Manṣūrī, Dār al-Kutub al-Miṣrīyah MS no. 102 *majāmī' m*, fol. 201a; as-Subkī quoted in *Badhl*, fol. 13a); (4) a predatory animal (aṣ-Safadī quoted in *as-Sulūk*, part 2, vol. 3, p. 789; al-Manṣūrī, Dār al-Kutub al-Miṣrīyah MS no. 102 *majāmī' m*, fol. 202a; as-Subkī quoted in *Badhl*, fol. 130a); (5) a bolt of lightning or fire (aṣ-Safadī quoted in *as-Sulūk*, part 2, vol. 3, p. 790, and Dār al-Kutub al-Miṣrīyah MS no. 102 *majāmī' m*, fol. 199b; as-Subkī, *ibid.*, fol. 198b; *Daf' an-niqmah*, fol. 77a). Besides the pestilential

mediacy in these poetic accounts because the authors speak generally in the first-person about their experiences and interject a rare personal apprehension of the disaster. The accounts may be contrived in style and over-colored in detail, but the basic elements of their ordeal are confirmed by the historians.

To call attention to the excessive mortality rate, the Arabic authors make extraordinary claims about the numbers of dead in the cities and note the scarcity of coffins and shrouds, preachers and gravediggers. Funeral processions passed constantly through the narrow streets. The normally active avenues of everyday life and trade became the conduits of plague dead. Although biers and benches for carrying the corpses were manufactured gratuitously in Cairo, there was not an adequate supply. Bodies were transported on simple wooden planks, ladders, doors, window shutters, and even in baskets. In some cases, a single bier or plank would be used to carry two or three bodies;[3] the same observation is made of the plague dead by Boccaccio in his description of the Black Death in Florence. In Damascus, Ibn Abī Ḥajalah observed camels transporting the dead to their graves.[4] For some inhabitants of Cairo, the final indignity was a summary burial in open trenches, where thirty or more were deposited.[5] If the Black Death in Cairo was like the plague of 800/1397-1398, the dead were carried from the city on camels and thrown into the Nile or into trenches.[6]

In Alexandria the dead were likewise carried on stretchers and planks during the Black Death.[7] In Damascus, there were

---

wind, the snake is particularly associated with plague (*as-Sulūk*, part 4, vol. 1, p. 490; Ibn Hajar, *Inbāʾ al-ghumr*, vol. 3. pp. 199-200; *Dafʿ an-niqmah*, fols. 83b-84a). See Kriss, *Volksglaube*, vol. 2, p. 15 for the magical significance of the snake. The relationship of snakes to jinn and thus to plague may have a Qur'ānic basis, for *sūrah* 72 associates the jinn with serpents.

[3] *as-Sulūk*, part 2, vol. 3, pp. 772-773.

[4] *Dafʿ an-niqmah*, fol. 80b.

[5] *as-Sulūk*, part 2, vol. 3, pp. 772-773.

[6] al-Jawharī, *Nuzhat an-nufūs*, vol. 1, p. 472.

[7] *as-Sulūk*, part 2, vol. 3, p. 777.

delays in removing the dead; at the same time the costs of burial greatly increased, making a particular burden for the poor.[8] People ceased asking permission from the administration to bury the bodies; some of the corpses were even abandoned in the gardens and on the streets.[9] The governor ordered the abolition of the fees on biers, washers, and carriers of the dead in Damascus (16 Rabīʿ II, 749/14 July 1348) to facilitate proper burials. Many coffins were prepared in the suburbs, so that the shortage was relieved outside of the city.[10] The same scarcity and high costs impeded the removal of bodies in Cairo, where, at the height of plague in Shawwāl 749/December 1348-January 1349, bodies and rubbish were heaped in the streets and markets.[11]

In Bilbais, as in most of the towns of the Nile Delta, bodies filled the mosques, hostelries, and shops; the roads stank with the smell of cadavers.[12] Likewise, the cadavers in Qaṭyā were scattered under the palm trees and before the shops.[13] Ibn Abī Ḥajalah describes in his macabre account of the Black Death, "these dead who are laid out on the highway like an ambush for others."[14]

Provision for the poor and chronically unemployed was common in Egypt during the Mamlūk Period; there were pious endowments for the care and burial of the destitute, like those we have already described for plague epidemics. In addition to private alms-giving, the sultan made lavish distributions in times of distress. When the number of vagrants became extremely large during the Black Death, partly, perhaps, because of rural immigration, the sultan distributed the indigent among the wealthy amirs to make provisions for them.[15] We are told specifically that the amirs Shaykhū and Mughulṭāy, the grand constable, directed the washing, shroud-

[8] *Ibid.*, p. 783.

[9] *Ibid.*, p. 779.

[10] *al-Bidāyah*, vol. 14, p. 226; *Dafʿ an-niqmah*, fol. 75b.

[11] *as-Sulūk*, part 2, vol. 3, p. 181.

[12] *Ibid.*, pp. 778-779.

[13] *Ibid.*, p. 775.

[14] *Dafʿ an-niqmah*, fol. 83b.

[15] *ʿIqd al-jumān*, p. 86; *as-Sulūk*, part 2, vol. 3, pp. 778, 781; *Badhl*, fols. 112a-112b.

ing, and burial of the common people in Cairo.[16] In later plagues, the amirs also took some responsibility for burying the destitute.[17]

Begging in the streets, in fact, became almost a profession at such times of hardship, and able-bodied men with gainful employment preferred to join the infirm. An Egyptian historian relates an occasion in Ramaḍān 841/March 1438, when plague was severe in Cairo. The sultan Barsbay had large sums distributed in the streets, where his official was attacked by those eager to partake of the gift. The sultan summoned the head of the vagabonds (*sulṭān al-ḥarāfīsh*) and the shaykh of the beggars' guild (*shaykh aṭ-ṭawā'if*) and compelled them to have the able-bodied return to their trades and send any of them found begging afterward to work on the city's construction sites.[18]

During the Black Death in Cairo, crews were appointed to carry out the burials, and pious men were permanently stationed at various places of worship in the city and in neighboring Fusṭāṭ to recite the requisite funeral prayers.[19] Many men left their normal occupations to profit from these funerals. Some turned to reciting the funeral prayers at the head of processions, others took up the treatment of the ill or washing and carrying the dead, but all received substantial salaries. For example, a Qur'ān reader made ten *dirhems* for each reading. It was said that such a reader would hardly have arrived at an oratory before disappearing in order to officiate at another funeral. A carrier demanded six *dirhems*, and the gravedigger fifty *dirhems* for a grave.[20] However, the majority of the people of Cairo could not afford these high prices.[21]

[16] *as-Sulūk*, part 2, vol. 3, p. 783.

[17] For 776 A.H., see Ibn Hajar, *Inbā' al-ghumr*, vol. 1, p. 72; for 806 A.H., see *ibid.*, vol. 2, p. 260; and for 819 A.H., see *as-Sulūk*, part 4, vol. 1, p. 351.

[18] *an-Nujūm*, Popper trans., vol. 18, pp. 148-149; see also *Muslim Cities*, pp. 55, 83-85, 177-183.

[19] *as-Sulūk*, part 2, vol. 3, p. 781.

[20] Cf. *Risālat an-naba'*, pp. 186-187, for Aleppo.

[21] *as-Sulūk*, part 2, vol. 3, pp. 782-783.

The same high prices and scarcity clearly existed during later plague epidemics, such as the severe epidemic in Cairo during 833/1429-1430. The chronicler Ibn Taghrī Birdī tells the story of one of his slave girls who died of plague in his home. The servants were not able to secure a bier for her, but a number of the old women took charge of washing the body and shrouding her in her best clothing. It was necessary for Ibn Taghrī Birdī also to go to the funerals of two important amirs that day. As he stood at the door of his house while the dead girl was being carried out, a funeral procession for another woman passed by the door. Ibn Taghrī Birdī took the coffin down by force and placed the slave girl beside the dead woman on her bier. Then the two were transported away on the shoulders of the men. The girl's mother and some of the servants went along with her until they were near the tombs, where they took her from the bier and buried her.[22]

The funeral processions to the cemeteries and to the mosques filled the streets of Cairo during the Black Death.[23] They were so numerous that they could not pass in the roadways without disturbing one another.[24] The poet Ibrāhīm al-Mi'mār wrote: "The approaching funeral processions frighten us, and we are delighted when they have passed by—with the alarm of a gazelle when it sees a jackal and then returns to ease when the jackal is gone."[25] The processions of coffins through the streets looked to observers like camel caravans; the biers were carried in such numbers from the Mosque of the Believers[26] to the

[22] *an-Nujūm*, Popper trans., vol. 18, p. 72. For comparable descriptions during the plague of A.H. 833: see *ibid.*, pp. 70, 73 and *as-Sulūk*, part 4, vol. 2, p. 826.

[23] See the descriptions of traditional Muslim funerals by M. Galal, "Essai d'observations sur les rites funéraires en Égypte actuelle," *REI* (1937), books II and III, pp. 131-299 and plates i-xviii; Louis Massignon, "La Cité des Morts au Caire (Qarāfa—Darb al-Aḥmar)," *Opera Minora*, vol. 3, pp. 233-285, plates i-x; and Lane, *Manners and Customs*, pp. 515-533.

[24] *as-Sulūk*, part 2, vol. 3, p. 782.

[25] Quoted in Ibn Iyās, vol. 1, p. 192.

[26] *Systematic Notes*, vol. 15, p. 26, map no. 8.

gate of Qarāfah cemetery that the portal looked like a great white vulture hovering over the dead.[27] Added to this activity were the hysterical weeping and lamentations of the mourners —a traditional part of Muslim funerals.[28] Lamentations were everywhere, and no one could pass before a house without being upset by the plaintive cries coming from within.[29] At the same time that the names of the dead were probably being announced through the streets, many of the survivors accompanied the processions out to the cemeteries to visit the graves, because of the common belief that the souls of the deceased resided in the tombs.[30]

The enormous cemeteries of Cairo, which extend from Succor Gate (Bāb an-Naṣr) to the Qubbat an-Naṣr in length and as far as the Muqaṭṭam Hills to the east of the city, were rapidly filled. In addition, the cemeteries situated between Ḥusaynīyah and Raydānīyah (north of the city) and outside Burnt Gate (Bāb al-Maḥrūq) and Qarāfah Gate were too small for the great numbers of dead.[31] Families resorted to laying their dead on the earth because of the impossibility of burying them.[32]

Ibn Taghrī Birdī relates a graphic account of an unusual burial during the plague epidemic of 833/1429-1430 in Cairo, which may have been a frequent occurrence at the time of the Black Death:

> The child of an individual in our service named Shams ad-Dīn adh-Dhahabī died, and we went out with him to the oratory. The boy was less than seven years old, and when we set him down to pray over him among the dead, a large

[27] Ibn Ḥajar, *Inbā' al-ghumr*, vol. 3, p. 438, for 833 A.H.; for the same year, see *as-Sulūk*, part 4, vol. 2, p. 827.

[28] Galal, "Essai d'observations sur les rites funéraires," pp. 172-174.

[29] *as-Sulūk*, part 2, vol. 3, p. 782. For a description of the mourning after the funeral, see Galal, "Essai d'observations sur les rites funéraires," pp. 184-187.

[30] See Galal, "Essai d'observations sur les rites funéraires," pp. 193-200.

[31] For the location of these areas, see *Systematic Notes*, vol. 15, map nos. 5, 8, and 9.

[32] *as-Sulūk*, part 2, vol. 3, p. 783.

number of others were brought, until their numbers went beyond counting. Then prayer was said over them all, and we went to take up the dead body but found that someone else had taken him and left us another one of about the same age. His family took him up but did not become aware of it; I, however, perceived this and told a number of others; but we did not inform his parents of it and said: Perhaps the one who took him will give him the best interment; there is no profit in talking about it—there would only be an increase in grief. But when the boy had been buried and the proprietors of the funeral office took up the bier they cried out and said, "This is not our bier; this is an old one and its furnishings also are worn out." I advised them to be silent, and then one of the mamlūks threatened to beat them; then they took it and went away.[33]

As Ibn Taghrī Birdī indicates, mass funeral services took place during plague epidemics at the principal mosques of Cairo. Al-Maqrīzī tells us that on one Friday during the Black Death after the public prayer in the great Mosque of al-Ḥākim, the funeral prayers were recited over a double line of coffins that reached from the *maqṣurah* or prayer enclosure to the main entrance. The *imām* or prayer leader stood at the threshold of the entrance door, and the people were obliged to stand behind him on the outside of the building.[34]

In Syria, the father of the historian al-ʿAynī was an *imām* in the garden quarter of ʿAyn Ṭāb (modern Gaziantep) during the Black Death. He later told his son that during the winter he used to go out with the funeral processions to the mosque in order to pray for them, but finally he stayed in the mosque of ʿAyn Ṭāb and waited for the biers to be brought to him. Sometimes he would pray over fifty biers or more at one

[33] *an-Nujūm*, Popper trans., vol. 18, pp. 71-72. Two plague treatises written about the plague of A.H. 764 are devoted almost entirely to the proper manner of burial and the consolation of the bereaved: Ibn Abī Hajalah, *Jiwār al-akhyār fī dār al-qarār*, and al-Manbijī, *Tasliyat ahl al-maṣā'ib fī maut al-awlād wal-aqārib* (Cairo, A.H. 1347).

[34] *as-Sulūk*, part 2, vol. 3, p. 782.

time.[35] In the capital city of Damascus, there was popular dismay and fright at the mass funerals.[36] The number of dead mounted at the Umayyad Mosque as the pandemic increased;[37] at one time (8 Rajab 749/2 October 1348), there was not enough room inside the mosque for the rows of biers, so that it was necessary to place some outside the Gate of as-Sirr. The preacher and the leaders went out to them and read the prayers over all the coffins there.[38] Ibn Abī Ḥajalah witnessed these prayers over the dead at the Umayyad Mosque; on Friday, the 7th of Sha'bān 749/31 October 1348, the dead numbered 263. "The people saw in this a dreadful thing, and there was a great clamor in the mosque."[39] Ibn Ḥajar reports this event from Ibn Abī Ḥajalah in his own plague treatise and states that a reliable person told him that he had seen a similar commotion in the Mosque of 'Amr ibn al-'Āṣ in Fusṭāṭ.[40]

As in the incident of the child's burial recorded by Ibn Taghrī Birdī during the epidemic of 833/1429-1430, confusion among the numerous biers in a mosque may have provoked such a commotion. However, at the time of another violent plague epidemic in Cairo in 841/1437-1438, both Ibn Taghrī Birdī and al-Maqrīzī witnessed extraordinary confusion in al-Azhar Mosque for another reason:

> Friday, Shawwāl 9 [8]. A strange thing happened: The people had rumored that men were all to die on Friday, and the resurrection would come. Most of the populace feared this, and when the time for prayer arrived on this Friday, and the men went to prayers, I too [Ibn Taghrī Birdī], rode to Azhar Mosque, as men were crowding to the baths so

[35] *'Iqd al-jumān*, p. 86.

[36] *al-Bidāyah*, vol. 14, p. 227 (10 Jumādā I, 749 A.H.).

[37] *Ibid.*. pp. 227-228.

[38] *Ibid.* For instances of mass funerals during later plague epidemics in Cairo, see *as-Sulūk*, part 4, vol. 1, p. 349 for A.H. 819; *an-Nujūm*, Popper trans., vol. 18, pp. 71, 73, and Ibn Hajar, *Inbā' al-ghumr*, vol. 3, pp. 437-439, for A.H. 833; and al-'Ulaymī, *al-Uns al-jalīl*, vol. 2, p. 286 for plague in Jerusalem in 873 A.H.

[39] *Daf' an-niqmah*, fol. 76a.

[40] *Badhl*, fol. 128b.

that they might die in a state of complete purity. I arrived at the Mosque and took a seat in it. The muezzins chanted the call to prayer, then the preacher came out as usual, mounted the pulpit, preached, and explained traditions to the people; when he had finished his first address he sat down to rest before the second sermon. He sat a long time, and people were worried, until he arose and began the second preaching, but before he had finished his address he sat down a second time and leaned against the side of the pulpit a long time, like one who had fainted. As a result the crowd, because of the previous report that men were all to die on Friday, was agitated; they believed the rumor was confirmed, and that death had made the preacher the first victim. While men were in this condition someone called out, "The preacher is dead." The Mosque was thrown into confusion, people cried out in fear, wept with one another, and went up to the pulpit; there was much crowding against the preacher until he recovered, rose to his feet, came down from the pulpit, and entered the prayer niche; he recited the prayer inaudibly, and abbreviated it until he had completed two bows. A number of biers then arrived, and the men prayed over them, led by one of their number. Then while they were praying for the dead the crowd cried out that the Friday service was not valid, since the preacher who had prayed after his ritual purity, secured through ablution, had been interrupted when he fainted. Then one of the men came forward, stood up, and recited the noon-prayer, four bows. After the one who recited the four bow prayer had finished, a number of others stood up and at their order the muezzin chanted the call to prayer in front of the pulpit; a man mounted the pulpit, recited two sermons according to custom, and came down to lead in prayer; but they prevented him from advancing to the niche, and brought the prayer leader of the regular five daily prayers, took him forward, and he led them in the Friday service a second time. But when he had finished leading the men in prayer others rose

> and cried out that this second Friday service also was not valid, and they performed the prayer service with another man leading them in the noon-prayer of four bows. So on this day in Azhar Mosque the address from the pulpit was given twice and the noon-prayer twice also. I arose, immediately, and behold! men were auguring the sultan's end because of the performance of two pulpit addresses in one place in one day.[41]

This description vividly illustrates the Muslims' obsession with ritual purity, including complete personal ablutions, in case of sudden death. During the severe plague epidemic of 1835 in Cairo, the English traveler Arthur Kinglake noted this popular response: "It is said that when a Mussulman finds himself attacked by the plague he goes and takes a bath. . . ."[42] The account of the disorder in al-Azhar Mosque in the fifteenth century also demonstrates the Muslims' piety in the face of calamity by the rigorous performance of correct religious rituals if possible. In general, the events in al-Azhar Mosque should be associated with the belief in the coming of the Last Judgment, which is a central teaching of Islam; they should not be interpreted, despite a certain element of mob hysteria, as part of any millennial expectations like those found in Europe during the Black Death.

Ibn Taghrī Birdī furnishes us with another glimpse into his personal life during the severe plague of 833/1429-1430 in Cairo; it may be fairly typical of the educated urban-class response during these horrors. He and his friends would return home from the Friday prayer and mass funerals and would take account of how many were present to compare with the number on the following Friday. Each man had resigned himself to death, having made his will and repented. Each of the young men carried a string of prayer beads in his

[41] *an-Nujūm*, Popper trans., vol. 18, pp. 149-150; *as-Sulūk*, part 4, vol. 2, pp. 1038-1040.

[42] *Eothen* (Lincoln, Nebraska, 1970 reprint), p. 246.

hand and did little besides attending the prayers for the dead, performing the five daily prayers, weeping, directing his thoughts to God, and showing his humility.[43]

Needless to say, in such a parlous state, family rejoicings and weddings no longer took place in Cairo. No one was reported to have held a feast during the entire duration of the Black Death, and no one heard the melodious voices of women, even though the government had lightened the tax on singers by a third. The call to prayer was omitted at a number of mosques, and even the most popular mosques had only one muezzin who had survived. Many of the mosques and shrines were closed because of their greatly diminished congregations and officials.[44] When the traditional ceremonies were carried out at the Umayyad Mosque in Damascus on the night of the 27th of Rajab—the night commemorating Muḥammad's miraculous ascension to heaven (*mi'rāj*)—the people did not attend as usual because many had died, and the survivors were busy with the ill and their dead.[45]

Aside from the mass funerals and their processions, an important aspect of urban activity during plague epidemics was the communal supplication for the lifting of the scourge. During the greatest severity of the Black Death, orders were given in Cairo to assemble in the mosques and to recite recommended prayers in unison.[46] On Friday, 6 Ramaḍān 749/28 November 1348, the people were invited to group themselves behind the caliphal banners and the carriers of the Qur'ān close to the Qubbat an-Naṣr, for a pious procession.[47] Other ceremonies took place in various mosques of Cairo and Fusṭāṭ. One procession was organized to the Oratory of Khawlān,

[43] *an-Nujūm.* Popper trans., vol. 18, p. 72.

[44] *as-Sulūk*, part 2, vol. 3, pp. 783-784.

[45] *al-Bidāyah*, vol. 14, p. 228.

[46] A number of these prayers were suggested in the plague treatises, e.g., *Badhl*, fols. 101b-119b; al-Ḥijāzī, *Juz' fī ṭ-ṭā'ūn*, fols. 154a-155a; and *Kitāb at-tibb*, fols. 141a-142a.

[47] On Sunday, 8 Ramaḍān/30 November, the amir Shaykhū, the wazir Manjak, and a number of other amirs dressed proudly in gold attended the ceremonies at Qubbat an-Naṣr (*as-Sulūk*, part 2, vol. 3, p. 781).

near al-Qarāfah cemetery. The reading of the *Ṣaḥīḥ* of al-Bukhārī[48] was performed without interruption for several days at the Mosque of al-Azhar and in other mosques, in the midst of large praying crowds.

Along with the reading of the Qur'ān, the recitation of the *Ṣaḥīḥ* of al-Bukhārī—the most famous collection of the traditions of the Prophet and the companions—was a customary practice during the Black Death and later occurrences of plague. The reading of al-Bukhārī was always an important feature of worship during the Mamlūk Period, whether at time of rejoicing (e.g., the succession of a sultan)[49] or at times of distress (e.g., when the Nile failed to rise).[50] During the difficult time of rebellion in Cairo in 791/1389, the *Ṣaḥīḥ* was read as a practical guide to conduct for the Muslims.[53] Surely at the time of plague, the chapters in the *Ṣaḥīḥ* which dealt specifically with plague were read aloud,[52] as well as related *ḥadīths*. Furthermore, the traditions regarding plague were expounded in sermons, as in the account of the extraordinary events at al-Azhar Mosque in 841/1437-1438. The oral presentation of these traditions must have informed the people of the three major tenets regarding plague, which we have discussed. In later plagues, the sultan frequently distributed money and appointed men to read al-Bukhārī and the Qur'ān in the principal mosques of the city for the people, and in the Citadel for the sultan himself.[53]

[48] *EI*²: "al-Bukhārī" (J. Robson).

[49] *an-Nujūm*, Popper trans., vol. 13, pp. 112-113.

[50] *Ibid.*, vol. 19, pp. 137-138.

[51] al-Jawharī, *Nuzhat an-nufūs*. vol. 1, p. 199.

[52] See A. J. Weinsinck, *Concordance et indices de la tradition musulmane* (Leiden, 1936), vol. 22, pp. 3-4 for *hadīths* relating to *ṭā'ūn*. See particularly, al-Bukhārī, *Kitāb al-jāmi' as-ṣaḥīḥ*, vol. 2, p. 209; vol. 4, pp. 59-60.

[53] For 790 A.H.: Ibn al-Furāt, *Ta'rīkh*, vol. 9, p. 28; al-Jawharī, *Nuzhat an-nufūs*, vol. 1, p. 170; *as-Sulūk*, part 3, vol. 2, p. 577; Ibn Ḥajar, *Inbā' al-ghumr*, vol. 1, pp. 353-354. For A.H. 833: *an-Nujūm*, Popper trans., vol. 18, p. 73; *as-Sulūk*, part 4, vol. 2, pp. 828-829; Ibn Ḥajar, *Inbā' al-ghumr*, vol. 3, p. 438. For A.H. 841: *as-Sulūk*, part 3, vol. 2, p. 577; *an-Nujūm*, Popper trans., vol. 18, p. 146.

A good example of the awareness of these traditions was the conflict of opinion among the religious classes as to whether supplication for raising the pestilence, and especially the religious processions of the community out to the desert, were canonical, since plague was supposed to be a mercy and a martyrdom for the faithful.[54] Nevertheless, fasting and ceremonial processions out to the desert were a conspicuous sign of distress during the Black Death and subsequent epidemics; the supplication followed the traditional form of the prayer for rain because plague was legally considered to be analogous to drought.[55] "At the most pathetic moment of the pandemic in Cairo, some of the *'ulamā'* counseled the population to unite for prayer to raise the pestilence. The people went *en masse* to the desert adjoining the city to perform the rituals similar to those for rain."[56]

When the plague epidemics of 822/1419 and 833/1429-1430 occurred in Cairo, such fasting and prayer took place outside the city.[57] The excellent description of this ceremony during the plague of 822/1419 by Ibn Taghrī Birdī deserves to be quoted *in extenso*:

> On Thursday, the 8th of Rabī' II [4 May 1419], it was proclaimed to the people by the market inspector that they were to fast for three days. On the last day, Thursday the

[54] This conflict is well illustrated by the criticism of Imām Aḥmad (Shahr ibn Ḥawshab) concerning the elaborate ceremony in the desert during the plague of A.H. 822 in Cairo (quoted below). He cites the *hadīth* of the plague of 'Amwās; their pious forefathers accepted plague as a mercy and summons (*da'wah*) from God while the Muslims of his own day sought to escape from it—"wa qad 'akasa ahl zamāninā al-amr, faṣārū yas'alūn allāh rafa'ahu 'anhum" (*as-Sulūk*, part 4, vol. 1, pp. 489-490).

[55] See the prayer for rain in 854/1450 in *an-Nujūm*, Popper trans., vol. 19, pp. 137-138.

[56] Ibn Iyās, vol. 1, p. 192; see also *Badhl*, fol. 110a.

[57] For A.H. 822: *an-Nujūm*, Popper trans., vol. 17, pp. 64-66; Ibn Hajar, *Inbā' al-ghumr*, vol. 3, pp. 198-199; *as-Sulūk*, part 4, vol. 1, pp. 487-490. For A.H. 833: *an-Nujūm*, Popper trans., vol. 18, p. 69; Ibn Ḥajar, *Inbā' al-ghumr*, vol. 3, p. 439; *as-Sulūk*, part 4, vol. 2, pp. 822-823.

15th, they were to go out with the sultan [al-Mu'ayyad Shaykh] and to beseech God in the desert to lift up the plague. . . . Many of the people fasted on Tuesday, Wednesday, and Thursday, and many of the merchants ceased to sell foods during the fast of the day, as is the custom in the beginning of the month of Ramaḍān. And on Thursday the 15th it was announced to the people to go out to the desert on the following day. The *'ulamā'*, the *fuqahā'*, the *mashāyikh al-khawānik*, the *ṣūfīs*, and the common people went out. The wazīr as-Ṣāḥib Badr ad-Dīn ibn Naṣrallāh and Amir at-Tāj al-Ustādār accompanied them to the tomb of al-Malik aẓ-Ẓāhir Barqūq. They set up cooking facilities in the southern courtyard of the tomb, and they brought sheep and goats. They spent the night there preparing foods and bread. After the sultan had performed the morning prayer, he rode out to them. He came down from the Citadel dressed in wool, and on his shoulders he wore a woolen shawl hanging down in back as in the custom among *ṣūfīs*.[58] On his head was a small turban twisted in the style of the celibate;[59] the end of the turban fell between his beard and his left shoulder. He displayed humility and contrition. His horse was covered in plain fabric—there was no gold or silver. The people drew near to the tomb with him in groups; the Shaykh al-Islām, the chief *qāḍī*, Jalāl ad-Dīn al-Bulqīnī set out from his house walking among a large crowd. The majority of the *'a'yān* (notables) set out from their houses either on foot or riding until the sultan came to the desert near the shrine of Bāb an-Naṣr. They carried flags and copies of the Qur'ān. And when "God is Almighty" was proclaimed, there were ringing shouts. The sultan dismounted from his horse and before him and to his right and

[58] This is one instance of the association of the mamlūk sultans with *ṣūfī* practices similar to the later practice of the Ottoman sultans. Unfortunately, there is no systematic study of ṣūfism during the Mamlūk Period in Egypt and its relation to the mamlūk army, despite the great amount of circumstantial evidence that Cairo was the center of *ṣūfī* organization and learning at this time.

[59] *'uzbahan.*

left were the *qāḍīs*, the men of learning, and the caliph. An innumerable crowd followed him. He spread out his hands and prayed to God, and he cried and lamented. The large crowd saw him and witnessed it for a long time. Then the procession appeared at the courtyard of the tomb of aẓ-Ẓāhir, and the people surrounded him as he ate what had been prepared. He made a sacrifice there to God of 150 fat rams at the cost of five *dīnārs* apiece. Then the sultan sacrificed ten fat cows, two *jāmūs* and two camels. He wept and his tears were stopped by the fullness of his whiskers. He left the sacrifices, as they were, and he returned to the Citadel. The sultan authorized the wazīr at-Tāj to divide the food properly among the principal mosques, the *khawānik*, the shrine of Imām ash-Shāfi'ī, and the tomb of al-Layth ibn Sa'd, the shrine of as-Sayyidah Nafīsah, and a number of *zāwiyahs*. It was distributed to them equally. He divided it among a number of people in the courtyard, and they portioned the food among the poor. Pure bread was distributed to them which numbered 28,000 *raghīf* [flat loaves of bread] which the poor received from the wazīr. He sent to every prison 500 *raghīf* and a number of large cauldrons filled with a great amount of food. The Shaykh al-Islām read the Qur'ān among a large number of people and supplicated God where the sultan had stopped. And Shaykh al-Ḥadīth an-Nabawī Shihāb ad-Dīn Aḥmad ibn Ḥajar from the *ṣūfīs* of the monastery of Baybars[60] and others did likewise until the heat of the day increased and they departed.[61]

[60] See *Systematic Notes*, vol. 15, p. 30 and map no. 9.

[61] *an-Nujūm*, Popper trans., vol. 17, pp. 64-66. Based primarily on *as-Sulūk*, part 4, vol. 1, pp. 487-489 (Bodleian Or. MS no. 458, fols. 141a-142b); see the other descriptions in the sources cited in Appendix 1 for the year A.H. 822. Although this activity included sacrifices, there are no reports of sacrifices comparable to the pre-Islamic rites as described by J. Chelhod in his *Le Sacrifice chez les Arabes* (Paris, 1955), p. 123. Donaldson notes the sacrifice of a black lamb and a specific prayer when plague or cholera appears in Iranian communities (*The Wild Rue*, p. 88).

Supplications and processions comparable to those in Cairo took place in Damascus during the Black Death. On Friday, 7 Rabīʿ I, 749/5 June 1348, the *Ṣaḥīḥ* of al-Bukhārī was read after the public prayer; the ceremony continued with a recitation of a section of the Qur'ān and public supplication.[62] At the evening prayer on Friday, 6 Rabīʿ II, the preacher recited the *Qunūt*[63] in the course of the prayers and begged God to lift the epidemic.[64] As the plague epidemic worsened, a proclamation was made in Damascus on Monday, 23 Rabīʿ II, inviting the population to fast for three days and to go out on the fourth day (Friday) to the Mosque of the Foot (*Qadam*)[65] in order to pray to God for the removal of the disease. Most of the Damascenes fasted, and several spent the night in the Umayyad Mosque, performing acts of faith as in the ritual during the holy month of Ramaḍān, and reading al-Bukhārī. In the morning of Friday the twenty-seventh, the inhabitants came out from all sides of the city, including Jews, Christians, Samaritans, old men and women, infants, the poor, amirs, notables, and magistrates. They marched before the morning prayer from the Umayyad Mosque to the Mosque of the Foot and did not cease chanting the prayers throughout the day.[66]

Previously, a man had come from the mountains of Asia Minor to visit the grand judge of Damascus, as-Subkī, and informed him that when plague had occurred in Asia Minor, he had seen the Prophet in a vision. The man had complained to Muḥammad about the calamity that had struck his people, and the Prophet declared to him: "Read the *sūrah* of Noah[67] 3,363 times[68] and ask God to raise from you your affliction." This was announced in Damascus, and the people assembled

[62] *al-Bidāyah*, vol. 14, p. 225; *Dafʿ an-niqmah*, fol. 75a.

[63] Qur'ān 2:110. See EI^1: "Ḳunūt" (A. J. Wensinck).

[64] *al-Bidāyah*, vol. 14, p. 226.

[65] See "La Grande Peste Noire," p. 383, n. 38.

[66] *al-Bidāyah*, vol. 14, p. 226; for the same event, see also *Dafʿ an-niqmah*, fols. 75a-75b, and *as-Sulūk*, part 2, vol. 3, p. 780.

[67] Qur'ān 71.

[68] 3,360 times according to *as-Sulūk*, part 2, vol. 3, p. 779.

in the mosques to carry out these instructions from the ninth of Rabīʿ I.[69] For a week the Damascenes performed this ritual—praying and slaughtering great numbers of cattle and sheep whose meat was distributed among the poor,[70] as described in the passage from Ibn Taghrī Birdī concerning the plague epidemic of 822/1419.

Similarly, a letter from the governor of Aleppo arrived in Cairo informing them that a pious man, perhaps the same individual from Asia Minor, had seen the Prophet in a dream. The pious man had also complained to the Prophet about plague. The Prophet communicated a prayer to recite, and a number of copies of this prayer were made and sent to Ḥamā, Tripoli, and Damascus, as well as Cairo.[71]

Other examples of religious visions during the Black Death are found in the plague treatises. As-Subkī wrote to his son that a good man had seen the Prophet in a dream in the Umayyad Mosque. The people questioned him about it, and he related to them a special prayer.[72] Apparitions were often reported during the recurrent plague epidemics; for example, during the plague in Egypt in 833/1429-1430, the sultan Barsbay ordered, according to a dream that he had had, that all the preachers, muezzins, teachers, and storytellers should end their supplications with the Qur'ānic verse: "Our Lord, lift from us the punishment; we are believers."[73]

At the time of the Black Death, the tombs of the prophet Mattā and Ḥanẓalah ibn Khuwaylid (brother of Khadījah)

[69] *al-Bidāyah*, vol. 14, p. 226; *Badhl*, fol. 128a.

[70] *as-Sulūk*, part 2, vol. 3, pp. 779-780.

[71] *Ibid.*, p. 780. the prayer is almost identical to the one given above, chap. IV, part C.

[72] Quoted in *Badhl*, fols. 110a-110b.

[73] Qur'ān 44:11. *Badhl*, fol. 109b. Other visions are reported, such as that of a man from Mahallah who was said to have seen the Prophet during the plague epidemic of A.H. 764 (*Kitāb at-tibb*, fol. 142a; *Badhl*, fol. 110b); see also the report of the plague of A.H. 795 in Aleppo (Ibn Saṣrāh, *ad-Durrah al-muḍī'ah*, vol. 1, p. 183); for the plague of A.H. 833 (Ibn Hajar, *Inbā' al-ghumr*, vol. 3, p. 439); and for the plague of A.H. 897 (Ibn Iyās, *Badā'i' az-zuhūr*, Mostafa rev. ed., vol. 5c, pp. 286-287).

were reportedly revealed to the people of Manbij (in northern Syria). Streams of light also shone from the shrines of Shaykh 'Aqīl al-Manbijī and the Shaykh Yanbub outside of the city, and the light from them came over the city. Light came from the tomb of Shaykh 'Alī and his shrine on the north side of the city. The lights passed from one to another; they came together and lasted for four nights until the lights blinded the people of Manbij. The judge of the city observed this phenomenon, gathered witnesses, and then reported it to the provincial capital of Aleppo.[74] Observations of such supernatural phenomena may have been common in the countryside during plague epidemics; judging by modern experience, belief in and veneration of local saints are very prominent during periods of crisis. In this regard, the Black Death and the plague reappearances may have been stimuli or, at least, favorable conditions for the spread of popular Muslim mysticism in the later Middle Ages. Misery and mysticism are often closely related to one another.

In the immediate aftermath of the Black Death, there is no evidence of a fundamental disruption of the functioning of the government in the major urban centers in Egypt and Syria, perhaps because of a simpler and more resilient bureaucratic apparatus than that of present-day governments and the enforcement of normative Muslim behavior on the community. The urban survivors responded to the plague pandemic by trying to protect the living and by caring for the dead and dying. Popular anxiety and fear were allayed by magical and religious practices, which included special services and ceremonial processions. Large-scale funeral services in the mosques, burials, and visitations to the vast cemeteries outside Cairo dominated the life of the city. The European response to the Black Death included the abandonment of religious rites and services for the dead; in the Middle East, on the contrary, there appears to have been a rigorous exercise of traditional Muslim religious practices during the crisis. There was, admittedly, a degree of social disorganization caused by the

[74] Ibn al-Wardī, *Tatimmat al-mukhtaṣar*, vol. 2, pp. 353-354.

scarcity and high prices of certain commodities and the temporary flight of some from plague-stricken communities. More lasting changes, however, took place in income and status relationships because of the underlying economic effects of the Black Death.

VII

THE ECONOMIC CONSEQUENCES OF THE BLACK DEATH

The economic life of Egypt was seriously disrupted by the Black Death and the successive epidemics of plague.[1] The demands of the plague-stricken naturally inflated the prices of certain commodities and services, with the obvious consequences of scarcity and high prices for shrouds,[2] coffins, and pharmaceuticals, as well as the high cost of labor. The substantial modifications in prices and salaries were symptomatic of a sustained dislocation of commerce and labor caused by depopulation.

There is a necessary caveat to the description of prices during the Black Death. It cannot be assumed in an evaluation of the economic consequences of the pandemic that the value of money remained constant. Al-Maqrīzī, who was sensitive to the effects of epidemic diseases on prices, salaries, and exchange rates,[3] states that in Cairo the gold *dīnār* declined in value relative to the silver *dirhem* during the Black Death; one *dīnār* was worth fifteen *dirhems*, while its normal value was

[1] S. Labib, "Egyptian Commercial Policy in the Middle East," *Studies in the Economic History of the Middle East*, ed. by Michael Cook, p. 77; "England to Egypt," pp. 119-123. Cf. the effects of the Black Death in Europe: Langer, "The Black Death," p. 121, where the author postulates that the Black Death was the main cause of economic change in late medieval Europe, and M. Postan, "Some Economic Evidence of Declining Population in the Later Middle Ages," *Economic History Review*, 2nd series, vol. 2 (1950), pp. 222-246.

[2] For the active trade in cotton cloth and shrouds in Damascus during the Black Death, see *Daf' an-niqmah*, fol. 80b.

[3] See *Ighāthah*, pp. 14-17, 36-38 (Wiet trans., "Le Traité des famines de Maqrīzī," pp. 15-17, 37-40).

twenty *dirhems*.[4] During the decade after the Black Death, the ratio of one to twenty was re-established.[5] The normal exchange rate of coined *dirhems* remained twenty units to the standard gold unit up to 760/1358-1359.[6] The observed change in the

[4] *as-Sulūk*, part 2, vol. 3, p. 786: "The prices of all goods declined until *al-fiddah an-nuqrah*, which was called in Egypt *al-fiḍḍah al-hajar*, sold for ten to nine of the *dirhem Kāmilī*. The *dīnār* remained at fifteen *dirhems* after it had been twenty." The first part of this passage is problematic because we do not know the normal exchange rate of this silver coinage or the precise meaning of these terms. As for the terminology, the *nuqrah* was a flan of silver alloy; it was made from an unmeasured globule of silver that was heated and struck in the dies. Because it was not weighed or adjusted, size and weight were of course variable. (The casting of the *nuqrah* is well described in Ibn Ba'rah's manual on minting; see Paul Balog, "History of the Dirhem in Egypt," *Revue Numismatique*, 6th series, vol. 3 [1961], pp. 123-124, and *The Coinage of the Mamlūk Sultans of Egypt and Syria* [New York, 1964], pp. 54-55. See also *nuqrah* in M. H. Sauvaire, "Matériaux pour servir à l'histoire de la numismatique et de la métrologie musulmanes," *JA*, 7th series, vol. 19 [Paris, 1882], pp. 61-64, 151; *Systematic Notes*, vol. 16, pp. 42-43, 51.) The *dirhem nuqrah* was minted at the very beginning of the Mamlūk Period, carrying on an Ayyūbid practice; however, it does not seem to have been minted after the third quarter of the thirteenth century (Balog, *Coinage of the Mamlūk Sultans of Egypt and Syria*, nos. 2a, 2b, 2c, 5). Yet the term is commonly used during the entire Mamlūk Period (Ashtor, *Histoire*, pp. 276, 452; Balog, "History of the Dirhem in Egypt," p. 136; Sauvaire, "Matériaux," pp. 63-64). The word apparently had many meanings, which is the cause of confusion. As for the designation of *hajar*, I have found no other historical reference to *ḥajar* relating to silver coinage in Mamlūk Egypt and Syria. (Cf. the reference to *al-ḥajar* in E. W. Lane, *Arabic-English Lexicon* [New York, 1955], p. 518, based on the fifteenth-century dictionary of al-Fayrūzābādī.) If *ḥajar* is meant in the sense of *tibr* as a piece of unstruck metal, *al-fiḍḍah an-nuqrah* (and not the *dirhem nuqrah*) mentioned by al-Maqrīzī may mean that an ingot of unminted silver, containing two-thirds silver and one-third copper (see *Systematic Notes*, vol. 16, p. 51), sold at the ratio of ten to nine for a theoretical value of minted silver coins containing the same amounts of silver and copper, i.e., the *dirhems Kāmilī*, or simply that *al-fiḍḍah an-nuqrah* was a silver coinage that contained a little more than one-third copper (Ashtor, *Les Métaux précieux*, p. 40).

[5] Ashtor, *Histoire*, p. 276.

[6] *Systematic Notes*, vol. 16, p. 52; Balog, "History of the Dirhem in Egypt," p. 134.

value of the *dīnār* at the time of the Black Death would seem to indicate that silver increased in value and/or that gold decreased in value. Thus, the plague epidemic appears to have directly affected the specie in circulation. The movement in the exchange rates of the two metals may have resulted from the very high costs of medicines, scarce commodities, and labor, which would have tended to draw out family gold reserves during the emergency. The terror of plague may have discouraged saving, so that survivors' inheritances of additional wealth may have added to the quantity of circulated specie and depressed the value of gold. Conversely, silver was used especially for magical talismans and amulets, which may have temporarily inflated its value. In general, the exchange rate was very sensitive to an increase or decrease in the supply of specie.[7]

A. PRICES

Although economic historians have not always been careful to distinguish among various types of agricultural and manufactured products, such a distinction has been made in the review of prices below. The effects of the Black Death on the following commodities will be traced briefly: medicines, essential foodstuffs, essential manufactured products, and luxury goods.

1. Medical Commodities

As in later plague epidemics, business generally stagnated and markets were closed during the Black Death, except for those commodities directly related to prevention of the disease,

[7] An incident slightly before the Black Death illustrates how the increase in the volume of coinage appreciably affected the silver-gold ratio. In 741-742/1340-1342 the ratio was twenty to one; it was violently upset in 742/1342 after the looting of the palace of the mamlūk amir Qawsūn, when so much gold was put into circulation that the ratio fell to eleven to one. The earlier ratio was restored later in the same year. (*al-Khiṭaṭ*, vol. 2, p. 73; *an-Nujūm*, Cairo ed., vol. 10, p. 45; see also Balog, "History of the Dirhem in Egypt," p. 134, and Ashtor, *Histoire*, p. 276.)

treatment of the plague victims,[8] and burial of the dead. Naturally, the prices of medicines show a dramatic rise. Many of the recommended articles, such as aloes, amber, sandal, camphor, and incense were an important part of international trade.[9] The letters to the Venetian merchant Pignol Zucchello from his partner, Vannino, in Alexandria from August to December 1347, give exceedingly high prices for such spices and other goods.[10] The Venetian paid very high prices, particularly for incense, camphor, and cardamom.[11] Even for sugar, Vannino had to pay 23-27 *dīnārs* for a *qinṭār*, while the normal price was usually 6.4 *dīnārs*.[12] Although plague—or any other cause for the steep rise in prices—is, unfortunately, not mentioned specifically, we may infer that the high level of prices resulted from the exigencies of the Black Death.[13]

In the later plagues of 790/1388 and 806/1403-1404 in Cairo, the chroniclers mention the high price of articles that were thought to be beneficial for the plague-stricken.[14] In the latter epidemic, one *qadaḥ* of pumpkin seed (*lubbat al-qar'*) reached

[8] *an-Nujūm*, Popper trans., vol. 18, p. 71; *as-Sulūk*, part 4, vol. 2, p. 819 *et passim*.

[9] See Heyd, *Histoire du Commerce*, vol. 2, p. 563 *et passim*, for a thorough description of each commodity in this long-distance trade.

[10] *Lettere di Mercanti a Pignol Zucchello (1336-1350)*, (Venice, 1957), pp. 86-112.

[11] See Ashtor, *Histoire*, pp. 335, 337. The explanation by Ashtor of the oscillation in the price of spices, characterized by a rise in the fifth decade of the fourteenth century, is insufficient. He interprets the rise in prices as a result of the great demand for Indian commodities, supported by the economic prosperity during the reigns of an-Nāṣir and his immediate successors, or by a general rise in the cost of living, which was of short duration (p. 339). The obvious explanation is the strong demand for spices to purify the air or for medicinal purposes during the Black Death.

[12] *Lettere di Mercanti a Pignol Zucchello*, nos. 44, 45, 56, 57; see Ashtor, *Histoire*, p. 317.

[13] One letter does discuss the Black Death in 1349: *Lettere di Mercanti a Pignol Zucchello*, pp. x, 120-123.

[14] A.H. 790: Ibn Ḥajar, *Inbā' al-ghumr*, vol. 1, pp. 350, 353; *as-Sulūk*, part 3, vol. 2, p. 577; al-Jawharī, *Nuzhat an-nufūs*, vol. 1, p. 170. A.H. 806: Ibn Ḥajar, *Inbā' al-ghumr*, vol. 2, p. 260.

100 *dirhems*, and a *waybah* of garden purslane seed sold for between one and two *dirhems*.[15] Other goods that were demanded during the plague epidemic became expensive, such as white sugar, watermelons, Syrian pears, and molasses. Prepared medical remedies increased eightfold in price. Two years later, in another plague, the prices of medications in Cairo rose sharply again:

> . . . the garden purslane to 80 *dirhems* for every *qadaḥ*. The weight of a *dirhem* of the product was sold for a *dirhem* of money. A *qinṭār* of *shīrkhushk* reached 30,000 after it had been 1,400 and a *qinṭār* of citron 15,000 after being 400. A doctor prescribed a remedy for the illness; in it was *sanāmakī*, *shīrkhushk*, citron, rosewater, and sugar. It was sold for 120 *dirhems*. The seeds of pumpkin reached 120 *dirhems*. . . . Three pomegranates sold for 60 *dirhems* and a *raṭl* of pears sold for 20 *dirhems*, and prices became high in Gaza too . . . watermelons sold in Cairo for 160 *dirhems* while its normal price was only one *dirhem*. And a *raṭl* of the milk of quince was 130 *dirhems* because of the numerous demands of the dying.[16]

We can assume that these varied commodities associated with plague prevention and treatment in later plague epidemics were also demanded during the Black Death and commanded unusually high prices.

2. Essential Foodstuffs

Unlike that of famine, the *immediate* effect of plague on essential agricultural goods and normal domestic commodities was a general decrease or stabilization of prices because of the decrease in the general demand and constant supply (assured by urban reserves). This seems to be the sense of al-Maqrīzī's

[15] Ibn Ḥajar, *Inbā' al-ghumr*, vol. 2, p. 260.

[16] *as-Sulūk*, part 4, vol. 1, pp. 5-6; *an-Nujūm*, Popper trans., vol. 14, p. 128. During the severe plague of A.H. 833 in Cairo, it is reported that people were unable to buy the medicines for the ill or cloth to shroud the dead (*as-Sulūk*, part 4, vol. 2, pp. 826-827). See Ashtor, *Histoire*, pp. 322-323 for the general history of fruit prices.

summary statement that goods declined in price during the Black Death.[17] Despite the epidemic, the price of wheat did not exceed fifteen *dirhems* for an *irdabb*,[18] which was the normal price of wheat during the early Mamlūk Period.[19] An Egyptian historian asserts that much later, when plague appeared in the spring of 864/1459-1460, the prices were extremely high, so that the people were caught between three evils: plague, inflation, and the tyranny of the mamlūks. What is of particular interest in this remark is that it was very peculiar that plague and inflation of food prices should occur together at one time.[20]

While the immediate consequence of a plague epidemic on agricultural prices would thus be negligible, the eventual effect would be a sharp rise in prices after the following poor harvest and the depletion of urban reserves. Added to this would be the increased cost of transportation.[21] The protracted period of the Black Death in Egypt—approximately ten months in Lower Egypt—definitely witnessed this decline in supply and rise in prices. This is probably the situation Ibn Iyās describes as a "famine" during 749/1349, accompanied by an extreme rise in the cost of wheat; one *waybah* (one-sixth of an *irdabb*) sold for 200 *dirhems*.[22] Similarly, in Tunis there is evidence of famine conditions resulting from the long period of the Black Death; great quantities of wheat were dispatched from Sicily to Tunis in March-April, 1350.[23]

In the long run, the prices of primary agricultural commodities adjusted to the new levels of supply and demand. Both Professors Udovitch and Ashtor have argued that the

[17] *as-Sulūk*, part 2, vol. 3, p. 786.

[18] *Ibid.*

[19] See *Systematic Notes*, vol. 16, p. 63, and Ashtor, *Histoire*, p. 293.

[20] *an-Nujūm*, Popper trans., vol. 22, p. 95.

[21] See the account of Ibn al-Furāt cited below, part D.

[22] Ibn Iyās, vol. 1, p. 191; *'Iqd al-jumān*, p. 86 reports that every *waybah* of barley cost 104 silver *dirhems*. Cf. *as-Sulūk*, part 2, vol. 3, p. 772.

[23] Brunschvig, *La Berbérie Orientale sous les Hafsides*, vol. 1, p. 171.

price of cereals remained comparatively low and stable after the Black Death, as a result of depopulation.[24] For if the Egyptian population had remained constant while the agricultural production decreased, there would be evidence of sustained inflation of agricultural goods and/or mass starvation. "Since we have no evidence that either of these occurred, nor of any continued massive grain imports, we must conclude that demographic factors were at the root of Egypt's agricultural decline, and that smaller harvests were being produced by, and were feeding substantially fewer people."[25] This argument implies that there was a negligible underemployment and unemployment in the agricultural sector before the Black Death. In any case, there can be little doubt that overall production in Egypt diminished after the Black Death.[26] Moreover, the same phenomenon of cereal prices is to be found in contemporary Europe.[27]

3. Essential Manufactured Products

The short- and long-term effects of the Black Death on essential manufactured products were a substantial rise in prices due to the increased cost of labor. During the pandemic, the dearth of laborers drove up the prices of processed foodstuffs, such as bread and sugar. The cost of having an *irdabb* of wheat ground in Cairo was 15 *dirhems*.[28] Ibn Kathīr and Ibn Baṭṭūṭah observed this effect of the inflated cost of labor during the Black Death; they specifically noticed the sharp rise in the price of bread in Damascus during Sha'bān-Ramaḍān 748/November 1347-January 1348.[29] In the plague

[24] "England to Egypt," p. 118; Ashtor, "Prix et salaires à l'époque Mamlouke," *REI* (1949), p. 51.

[25] "England to Egypt," p. 118.

[26] Ashtor, "Prix et salaires à l'époque Mamlouke," p. 50.

[27] Ashtor, *Histoire*, p. 548.

[28] *as-Sulūk*, part 2, vol. 3, p. 786; see "La Grande Peste Noire," p. 380, n. 32.

[29] *al-Bidāyah*, vol. 14, p. 224; Ibn Baṭṭūṭah, *Voyages*, ed. by Defrémery and Sanquinetti, vol. 4, p. 317.

of 806/1403-1404, meat also increased in price, expressly because of the cost of slaughtering; a small calf sold for 2,000 *dirhems fulūs*.[30]

Together with the cost of bread and slaughtered meat, that of sugar must have risen considerably during the Black Death, not only because of the cost of labor but also because of the demand for sugar, which was used in various plague remedies. A common remedy and refreshment for plague victims, particularly among the poor, was simply sugar-sweetened drinks with various additives. The high price paid by the Venetian merchant, Vannino, for sugar in Alexandria at the time of the Black Death may be due to this increased demand. From the end of the fourteenth century the price of sugar rose greatly, without any improvement in its production or quality, because of the shortage of labor caused by the Black Death and plague recurrences in the second half of the century. During the epidemics of the fifteenth century, the government monopoly of sugar in Egypt and Syria added to its cost and thereby only increased further the burden on the poor.[31] After the plague of 833/1429-1430, the sultan gave 1,000 *dīnārs*, resulting from the sale of sugar, to the grand mosque of Damascus in order to soothe his conscience.[32]

An exception to this general rise in prices of essential manufactured products was a short-term decline in prices for nonperishable manufactured commodities. People inherited such goods as clothing, cooking utensils, furniture, etc., or would have been able to buy them at very low prices. It was observed that in the deserted streets of Cairo, the abandoned furniture in the empty houses could not be sold. Some people simply appropriated for themselves the furniture and movables of

[30] Ibn Hajar, *Inbā' al-ghumr*, vol. 2, p. 260.

[31] Heyd, *Histoire du Commerce*, vol. 2, pp. 683-684; Darrag, p. 149 for the high prices of sugar in Cairo during the plague epidemic of 833/1430.

[32] Darrag, p. 150; similarly, the sultan made an enormous profit during the famine and plague of 841/1438 in Cairo from his monopolies (pp. 152-153).

others without scruple. Al-Maqrīzī states that very few lived long enough to profit by these acquisitions, and those who survived had no need of them. Because of the scarcity of customers and the abundance of goods, the prices of linens and similar objects declined to one-fifth of their real value, or less. This decline in demand explains the report that the crafts virtually disappeared during the Black Death. Most businesses ceased because many of the artisans could make more money by transporting and burying the dead. Others devoted themselves to selling at auction the movable property and clothes of the plague victims. A proclamation was issued in Cairo that the artisans should resume their trades; some recalcitrants were even beaten.[33]

In the long run, the costs of these non-perishable products rose drastically. Professor Ashtor rightly emphasizes that the increase in prices of industrial products, such as clothing, was much greater than the increase in the prices of processed agricultural products.[34] This would be only natural because of the greater amount of skilled labor required for the former. The sharp rise in the cost of cloth in general—cotton, wool, and linen—directly affected the living standard of the Muslim middle class, since cloth goods were the most important forms of bourgeois wealth and display.[35]

4. Luxury Goods

There would appear to have been a short-run drop in the demand for customary luxuries, and hence a decline in prices. For instance, during the Black Death in Cairo, books of religious science were hawked by weight and were sold at trifling prices.[36] However, the cost of industrial commodities after the pandemic was considerably higher than before it. We know, for example, that the price of an astrolabe doubled in price following the Black Death.[37] This dramatic rise in price was

[33] *as-Sulūk*, part 2, vol. 3, pp. 783, 786.
[34] *Histoire*, p. 344.
[35] *Muslim Cities*, p. 31.
[36] *as-Sulūk*, part 2, vol. 3, p. 786.
[37] Ashtor, *Histoire*, pp. 353-354.

due to the increased cost of skilled labor and/or the increased demand. In the long run, it is possible that the survivors of the plague epidemics, benefiting from their newly acquired affluence, indulged themselves in more luxurious commodities. This pattern of prices is similar and related to the prices for non-perishable, essential manufactured goods, for the circumstances may have made essential many commodities that had previously been considered luxurious.

Historians of post-plague Europe have emphasized the increased demand for luxury goods; according to this argument, a larger number of wealthy individuals of the towns were able to buy expensive commodities as the total population declined.[38] The combination of temporary affluence and the fear of imminent death may have generated a general European taste for lavish Italianate fashions and stimulated luxury crafts. Moreover, the life style of European society may have been strongly affected by the younger generation; the demographic contraction undoubtedly gave greater opportunity to the young, allowing for greater physical and social mobility.[39] Apart from purely economic matters, such considerations about the nature of European society raise broader questions about Muslim social life that can, at present, only be posed: What were the effects of the Black Death and recurrent plagues on the internal structure of the Middle Eastern family, the relationships between its members, and consequently on the nature of its culture?

In any case, there is no marked change that can be discerned in the fashions of the Egyptians or Syrians in the later fourteenth century, reflecting a change in economic and psychological attitudes. Certainly there was no expansion of the luxury textile industry. On the contrary, the Black Death vitally affected the famous cloth factory (*dār aṭ-ṭirāz*) in Alexandria

[38] Miskimin, *The Economy of Early Renaissance Europe*, pp. 91-92, 135-136; A. H. de O. Marques, *Daily Life in Portugal in the Later Middle Ages* (Madison, 1971), p. 38.

[39] David Herlihy, "The Generation in Medieval History," *Viator: Medieval and Renaissance Studies*, vol. 5 (1974), pp. 347-364.

by the destruction of its highly skilled workers.[40] Thereafter the textile industry in Egypt deteriorated rapidly; the number of weavers in Alexandria is reported to have fallen from about 12,000-14,000 in 1394 to 800 in 1434.[41] This decline by the fourth decade of the fifteenth century was observed by both Ibn Taghrī Birdī and the Cypriot merchant Piloti.[42] The reduction of the textile industries in the Middle East resulted from important social and economic changes. Professor Ashtor has shown that after the Mongol conquests the supply of raw materials from Iraq and Persia, particularly dyes, became very scarce. The decline was also due to technological stagnation. The European textiles imported into the Middle East were cheaper, because of technological innovations, and were made of better quality wool. The native textile industry failed to make these innovations. The great *ṭirāz* factories of the government were the only ones who had the resources to adapt to the new competition of foreign textiles, but the royal ateliers in Alexandria and Cairo were closed in the early fifteenth century. The private manufacturers lacked sufficient patronage and risked government confiscation.[43] Added to these poor conditions for investment, the Black Death and the subsequent plague epidemics destroyed the skilled laborers and drove up the price of labor.[44]

In the same manner that high quality, low-cost European textiles were introduced into the Middle East to the detriment of local industry, European paper and sugar and Chinese ceramics flooded Middle Eastern markets and for the same

[40] *Risālat an-nabaʾ*, p. 185; see M. A. Marzouk, "The Tirāz Institution in Medieval Egypt," *Studies in Islamic Art and Architecture in Honor of Professor K.A.C. Creswell* (Cairo, 1965), pp. 157-162, particularly p. 161; and *EI*[1]: "ṭirāz" (A. Grohmann).

[41] Darrag, pp. 70-71; Labib, *Handelsgeschichte*, p. 420; Ashtor, *Histoire*, p. 270.

[42] Ashtor, *Histoire*, p. 270; Darrag, pp. 68-73.

[43] Darrag, pp. 69-71.

[44] Ashtor, "Levantine Sugar Industry in the Later Middle Ages—A Sample of Technological Decline," pp. 27-30 (paper presented at the Princeton Conference on the Economic History of the Near East, June 16-20, 1974).

reasons: they were better and cheaper. The native industries—suffering from oppressive mamlūk control and capriciousness, lack of technological innovation, and the periodic destruction of workers by plague—encountered a greatly limited market from the late fourteenth century. Sultan Barsbay, in the early fifteenth century, was unsuccessful in stopping the dumping of these foreign commodities on the Egyptian market.[45] Concurrently, the mamlūk sultans tried to restore the country's finances; they were unable, however, to improve the country's currency and to stem the collapse of Egypt's economic position.[46]

Related to the decline in the quantity of Middle Eastern luxury production is the question of the effect of plague epidemics on the quality of Islamic art. Once the question is posed, it is enticing to suggest that the destruction of skilled artisans may have contributed to artistic decline from the middle of the fourteenth century. Such a decline during the later Mamlūk Period is, in fact, generally accepted by Islamic art historians. For example, Professor Oleg Grabar, in a recent discussion of the dating of the illustrations of the *Maqāmāt* of al-Ḥarīrī, states that the illustrations' "upward limit is the second half of the fourteenth century when there occurred a general decline in artistic creativity within the Arab world."[47] Moreover, a change may be hypothesized not only in the quality but also in the subject matter of artistic expression, comparable to the change in Sienese and Florentine art after the Black Death, which has been studied intensively.[48] Although we do not

[45] Ashtor, *Histoire*, p. 270.

[46] Balog, *The Coinage of the Mamlūk Sultans of Egypt and Syria*, p. 9.

[47] Oleg Grabar, "The Illustrated Maqāmāt of the Thirteenth Century: The Bourgeoisie and the Arts," *The Islamic City*, ed. by A. Hourani and S. M. Stern (Oxford, 1970), p. 209. See also Eric Schroeder, "Aḥmed Musa and Shams ad-Dīn: A Review of Fourteenth-Century Painting," *Ars Islamica*, vol. 6 (1969), pp. 114-116, and Richard Ettinghausen, *Arab Painting* (Geneva, 1962), pp. 179-187.

[48] Meiss, *Painting in Florence and Siena after the Black Death*; see also Crawfurd, *Plague and Pestilence*, pp. 111-132; and Ziegler, p. 276.

have the abundance of visual evidence for the influence of the Black Death in Muslim society that we do in European art, there is a marked change in subject matter and emotional content. For example, in Persian miniature illuminations from this time, we can observe a perceptible morbidity and an increased emphasis on non-objective representation.[49]

In general, the long-term economic effects of the Black Death and successive plague epidemics produced what Professor Ashtor has called a "price revolution," which occurred at the beginning of the Circassian Period (783/1382).[50] As Professor Udovitch has demonstrated, the discrepancy between the modest rise in the prices of essential agricultural goods and the severe rise in those of industrial goods and processed foodstuffs (such as bread[51] and sugar) resulted from the increased cost of urban labor, and this disparity was accentuated, perhaps, by an increased demand for manufactured commodities. The latter may be attributed to an increase in *per capita* wealth of some plague survivors who benefited from inheritance and the renewed prosperity of the international spice trade.

> These two factors apparently combined to generate an increased demand for goods and services, while the inelastic nature of the demand for agricultural products limited the transfer of the greater per capita wealth and revenues to the

[49] For example, the miniature paintings of the period include numerous scenes of death, funerals, and a panoply of jinn and divs, as in the Demotte *Shāh Namah*; see Doris Brian, "A Reconstruction of the Miniature Cycle in the Demotte Shāh Namah," *Ars Islamica*, vol. 6 (1969), pp. 96-112. Brian's suggested reconstruction involves the controversial dating of the Demotte manuscript. However, if the paintings are after the mid-fourteenth century, it is reasonable that the Mongol court at Tabrīz would have suffered from plague, for we have evidence that Azarbayjan was repeatedly stricken by plague (see chap. ii, part B, n. 35 and chap. v, part F, n. 13). See also Marshall G. S. Hodgson, "Islām and Image," *History of Religions*, vol. 3 (1964), pp. 246-247 and n. 10 by Oleg Grabar.

[50] "L'Évolution des prix dans le Proche-Orient," p. 16.

[51] Ashtor, *Histoire*, p. 457 (graph of bread prices).

agricultural sector thus diverting a large portion of income toward urban products.[52]

The unprecedented and uneven movement of prices was thus directly related to demographic decline.

B. LABOR

Both the processed foodstuffs and the manufactured commodities of all types were directly conditioned by the changes in the price of labor. The immediate effect of the Black Death on labor was the opposite of its effect on agricultural prices and is comparable to that of the European plague: a rapid increase in the cost of labor services resulting from depopulation.

With regard to the highly specialized services of doctors, it is natural to assume that they were in great demand and that physicians' fees increased markedly during the pandemic, considering the danger as well as the need. Plague must have been very profitable for doctors and druggists, bloodletters and magicians. According to the poet Ibrāhīm al-Mi'mar, the herb-seller did not fear plague but rapidly grew prosperous from it.[53] Al-Maqrīzī must be exaggerating when he says that no one in Cairo during the Black Death had time to consult doctors.[54] At the same time, Ibn al-Wardī, who witnessed the Black Death, was surprised by how many men in Aleppo abandoned religious guidance and trusted in doctors.[55] Unfortunately, we have practically no information about the medical profession during the Black Death, but the number of physicians must have declined substantially because of their exposure to the disease. Regarding medical practice in general, Ibn Khaldūn appears to confirm this situation in the second half of the fourteenth century: "In contemporary Muslim

[52] "England to Egypt," pp. 121-122.

[53] Quoted in *as-Sulūk*, part 2, vol. 3, p. 791.

[54] *Ibid.*, p. 781.

[55] *Risālat an-naba'*, p. 186.

cities, the craft of medicine seems to have deteriorated because the population has decreased and shrunk."[56]

Despite an influx of people into Cairo from the countryside, shortages of unskilled labor are conspicuous in the historical accounts. Al-Maqrīzī states that the monthly salary of a groom reached 80 *dirhems*, whereas it had formerly been 30 *dirhems*. Because of the loss of men and horses, a goatskin of water reached the price of 8 *dirhems*.[57] The cost of transporting water to a house in Cairo appears to have risen to more than 10 *dirhems*.[58] Laborers were offered one and a half *dirhems* and three loaves of bread a day in 749/1348 for work on a dam being built on the Nile.[59] A comparison with the pay provided in the endowment deeds for menial labor in 823/1420 and 875/1470 would indicate a high level of payment for such unskilled workmen during the Black Death.

Increased building activity would help to explain the substantial rise of labor costs in the cities after the Black Death, a period that witnessed an increased number of endowments for religious, educational, and philanthropic purposes. The construction of schools, mosques, and tombs may have resulted directly from bequests of the plague victims and from the generosity of survivors who had inherited wealth. The decline of land values may also have encouraged the donation of unprofitable lands for charitable purposes. Since the government's death duties and confiscation of properties belonging to plague victims added greatly to its revenue, the funds may have been used for new monuments and other structures.[60]

[56] *The Muqaddimah*, vol. 3, p. 149.

[57] Comparative price in 1346: 2 *dirhems* (formerly one-half *dirhem*) (as-Suyūṭī, *Husn al-muhāḍarah*, vol. 2, p. 214; cf. *al-Khitat*, vol. 2, p. 167, which gives the price as 2 *dirhems* [formerly three-quarters *dirhems*]). In 1348-1349: 12 *dirhems* (Ibn Iyās, vol. 1, p. 191); during the winter of 1373, the price was 5 *dirhems* (*ibid.*, p. 229).

[58] *'Iqd al-jumān*, chap. 24, p. 86.

[59] *al-Khitaṭ*, vol. 2, p. 168; cf. *Systematic Notes*, vol. 16, p. 117.

[60] Rabie, *The Financial System of Egypt*, p. 136. We have no figures for the revenue received by the Egyptian government from death

In fact, there were an unusually large number of monumental buildings constructed in the sixth decade of the fourteenth century. Although such an assertion is difficult to substantiate because of the lack of documentation, it is possible to suggest in one instance that the remarkable Mosque of Sultan al-Ḥasan,[61] the most impressive monument of the Mamlūk Period in Cairo, was financed largely from the additional revenue accruing to the government.

The artisan class as a whole prospered.[62] Al-Maqrīzī's description of the various classes in early fifteenth-century Egypt indicates clearly the well-being of this class, in an otherwise bleak picture of the economy. His remarks are proof of the continued shortage of urban workers and their increased wages due to the recurrent plague epidemics. He comments on this class in the following manner: "As for the sixth category, these are the artisans, wage workers, porters, servants, grooms, weavers, laborers, and their like. Their wages multiplied many times over; however, not many remain, since most of them died. A worker of this type is not to be found except after strenuous searching."[63] Thus, the long-term effects of the pandemic parallel the short-term in regard to the relative position of the urban laboring classes and the propertied classes, by drastically shifting relative returns and incomes in favor of the former.

After comparing the prices and salaries of the countries of the Mediterranean littoral, Professor Ashtor concludes that the Mediterranean formed an economic unity during the Mamlūk Period.[64] The salaries of Egyptian urban laborers conformed to

---

duties during the Black Death or subsequent plague epidemics. However, it was prodigious under the Ottoman administration of Egypt in the seventeenth century; see Toussoun, *Mémoire sur les finances de l'Égypte*, p. 62.

[61] See *Muslim Cities*, Appendices A, B, and C. For some reason, the Mosque of al-Hasan is omitted from Appendix A.

[62] See Ibn Khaldūn, *The Muqaddimah*, vol. 2, p. 277, for a discussion of the reasons for the prosperity of urban craftsmen and labor.

[63] *Ighāthah*, p. 75. Quoted in "England to Egypt," p. 122.

[64] *Histoire*, p. 511.

the general increase in pay resulting from the Black Death in other countries. The real urban wages of the Egyptian, in terms of buying power of essential commodities, was higher after the Black Death than in all of the other Mediterranean countries.[65]

In the countryside, higher wages may have been obtained by agrarian laborers in the short term. However, because of the attempts of the mamlūk regime to maintain and even increase agricultural revenues through heavier taxation, probable underemployment and unemployment (which may explain the absence of governmental legislation to control peasant mobility that we find in Europe), unfavorable natural conditions for cultivation in the period following the Black Death, and decreased demand, the Egyptian peasant did not benefit as did his urban colleague. The disparity in benefits between the countryside and the cities would partly explain the high standard of living that was made possible for the urban laborer and the constant attraction of the rural population to the cities. The general decline of rural population does not seem to have aided the long-term improvement of agrarian technology or the re-allocation of resources, specifically by the upgrading of holdings, in line with the changing supply of land and labor, as in Europe. Thus, the impoverishment of the rural population, together with the decrease in agrarian production, led to a very considerable decline in the incomes of the Egyptian landowners.

C. LAND

The disruption caused by the Black Death accelerated the decline of the *iqṭāʿ* system, which was the basis of land distribution and the source of agricultural revenue. The *iqṭāʿ* in

[65] *Ibid.* The explanation of this phenomenon, if correct, may be manifold. It may indicate a greater demographic decline in Egypt, a greater imbalance in the urban-rural economies in Egypt, or the comparatively lower cost of essential commodities in Egyptian towns, which could have increased the buying power of urban salaries.

Egypt and Syria was not equivalent to the *fief* in western European feudalism, although they were both essential elements of their respective sociopolitical forms of government.[66] Rather, they were for the most part opposites. The *iqṭā'* from one point of view, was an instrument of governmental centralization, whereas the *fief* was necessitated by governmental weakness and regional particularism. The *iqṭā'* organization was carefully supervised and administered by the state (*dīwān al-jaysh*), which carried out a number of important cadastral surveys during the Mamlūk Period to facilitate the equitable and efficient distribution of grants and to eradicate the hereditary character of the grant. In 715/1315, the most important land survey before the Black Death was made; its total effect was to concentrate control of the revenue resources of the army in the hands of the sultan and to stabilize the Egyptian economy.

Under the mamlūk regime, the *iqṭā'* was a limited and revocable assignment of revenue, unlike the hereditary *fief*. Although it was non-hereditary, the recipients constantly struggled to convey to their descendants at least a portion of their estates. The transference of wealth to a mamlūk's family was made possible by the existence of a particular category of estates granted as pensions and turned into allodial estates, or by setting aside land or money as a *waqf* (pious endowment) devoted to some social or religious purpose, which may have been a common occurrence during the plague epidemics. In the latter case, the descendant was made an hereditary manager of the *waqf* with a regular stipend.

The landed estates were assigned according to the rank of the military officer; the estate had a predetermined income that would be sufficient for the expenditures of that rank. The grant entailed no manorial jurisdiction or subinfeudation; the assignment could be only a fraction of a single village or region and could be made up of distant components. Moreover, the

[66] See the thorough discussion of this topic for the period immediately preceding the Black Death by Rabie, *The Financial System of Egypt*, pp. 26-72.

grantee did not usually live on his land, for the mamlūks greatly preferred to live in Cairo, at the center of power, politics, and wealth. The *iqṭa's* of the amirs were administered by their officials; at the time of harvest, each amir sent his estate officials to measure the crops. The crops or their equivalent in money were taken to the amir's storehouse or treasury in Cairo.

The *iqṭā'* was not necessarily a landed estate; it could be a share of the income from a tax, customs duty, or excise levied by the central government, or special taxes levied by the grantee on areas belonging to the state. The royal mamlūks stationed in the Citadel of Cairo were paid according to their "class" in the garrison schools. Their pay consisted of a monthly stipend, food and clothing allowances, horses and camels and their provisioning, and extraordinary gifts before a military campaign or religious festival.

At the time of the Black Death, *iqṭā's* were sold freely by the mamlūks and militia for cash. In 746/1345, the selling and exchange of land grants had been officially organized (*dīwān al-badal*).[67] This bureau was abolished and then re-established by the amir Manjak, wazir in 749/1348, to accommodate the rapid transfer of properties during the Black Death. Similarly, during the plague in 833/1429-1430 the Egyptian chronicler Ibn Taghrī Birdī observed the transfer of a single estate to as many as five soldiers.[68]

During the turbulent times of the later fifteenth century, the unruly royal mamlūks sought to acquire *iqṭā's* outright. Ibn Taghrī Birdī gives us a vivid description of this confusing state of affairs at the time of a plague epidemic in Cairo in 864/1460:

> When they [the royal mamlūks] had finished taking the goods of men, there appeared among them during the plague the practice of taking the *iqṭā's* of the soldiers of the standing army. Whenever they saw a man at a druggist's shop they would seize him and say to him, "Perhaps the sick man has

[67] *Systematic Notes*, vol. 16, p. 115.
[68] *an-Nujūm*, Popper trans., vol. 18, pp. 70-71.

an *iqṭāʿ*?" If he had an *iqṭāʿ*, the man would tell about it, but if the sick man had no *iqṭāʿ*, he would have a long affair with the mamlūk, unless one of the notables would release him from him. Then after this, it occurred to them that they should take the *iqṭāʿ* of any emir's son (or descendant) or any veteran trooper of whom they heard that he had an *iqṭāʿ*; if it was true they would hope for his sickness, and if he were sick they would look for his death. By this practice the *iqṭāʿs* of most of the men, living and dead, were vacated; and they even did this with [the *iqṭāʿs* of] one another. So both the Sultan and the men engaged in a pressing business, for the purchased mamlūks began to crowd upon him to get the *iqṭāʿs* of the men; and as soon as he was finished with the mamlūks, everyone whose *iqṭāʿ* had been vacated while he was still alive would lodge a complaint; then he could do nothing but return it to him. Thus an *iqṭāʿ* would be vacated today and returned to its [original] possessor tomorrow, and on one day a number of patents could be written, both of annulment and restoration. The men continued to be in these circumstances from the beginning to the end of the season.[69]

These practices may have taken place during the Black Death and would explain the reports of the rapid transfer of estates. The transfer of properties occurred not only during the emergency of the pandemic but continued in the years following the Black Death, principally because of the mamlūks', as well as others', desire to augment their landholdings and revenue at the expense of the non-mamlūk corps. In 753/1353, "the operations of buying the grants by merchants and artisans became so frequent that one group of individuals, almost 300, became brokers of this property and made a profession of visiting the *jundīs* (soldiers) and pressuring them to cede or exchange their *iqṭāʿs*, charging a commission of ten percent."[70] The government was unable to prevent the ex-

[69] *Ibid.*, vol. 22, pp. 95-96.

[70] Gaudefroy-Demombynes, *La Syrie à l'époque des Mamelouks*, p. xlv; see also Poliak, *Feudalism*, pp. 29-30.

change and ceding of such properties. In addition to the land-grabs attempted by the mamlūks during plague epidemics, the continued process of land transfers may indicate the tendency of small landowners to relinquish unprofitable land investments (as well as rights to taxation) for alternative investments in trade or simply for consumption.

The same may be said for urban real estate, which was subject to lower revenue from rents. Professor Ashtor attributes this decline in rents directly to a decreased demand caused by depopulation.[71] Ibn Ḥajar, who lived during the century following the Black Death, may be representative of the investor as well as the scholar of this period. He believed that trading was the most profitable enterprise and consistently refused to build or buy buildings as his son urged him to do. He said that all the great merchants whom he knew did not have a high regard for those who invested in real estate for rental purposes.[72]

The aggregate decline in revenue derived from the *iqṭā's* vitally affected the fixed incomes of religious foundations and the mamlūk ruling class, whose most important single source of income was agricultural profits from their estates. As would be expected in the first group, the salaries of the members of the religious classes drawn from endowments did not rise equally with urban salaries, but were comparatively lower in the Circassian Period (783-922/1382-1517).[73]

The drastically reduced revenue of the mamlūk establishment from its estates accounts for the attempts of the mamlūk regime to supplement its incomes by heavier taxation on rural areas and urban commerce.[74] The inescapable impoverishment of the countryside led the government to increase the rights of the mamlūks to supplementary sources of revenue, i.e., their monthly pecuniary pay (*jāmakiyah*), payment in kind (*rawā-*

[71] *Histoire*, p. 360.

[72] Kawash, "Ibn Ḥajar al-'Asqalānī," pp. 236-237 based on the biography of Ibn Ḥajar by as-Sakhāwī, *Jawāhir*, Paris MS no. 2105, fol. 253a. Cf. Ibn Khaldūn, *The Muqaddimah*, vol. 2, pp. 283-285.

[73] Ashtor, *Histoire*, pp. 376-378. [74] *Muslim Cities*, p. 36.

tib), and extraordinary grants (*nafaqah*),[75] and to non-agricultural taxation. The government intervened in the urban economy, in the form of confiscations, forced purchases, and finally government monopolies in the fifteenth century, in order to meet its expenditures, but its actions contributed to a descending spiral of urban economic life.[76] Thus, the government's attempts to raise the pay of the army produced economic deterioration, and the failure of these expedients accelerated political instability.

It is interesting to note in this regard that during the plague of 833/1429-1430 in Cairo the sultan called together the *'ulamā'* for their opinions concerning the reasons for plague and what should be prescribed for the community. When the *'ulamā'* returned with their opinions, the Shāfi'ī judge stated that in this year three economic hardships had been imposed by the sultan: pressure on the merchants to sell spices to the sultan (otherwise they were forbidden to trade in it); pressure on the merchants to give up the trade in *naṭrūn* (for cloth dying); and the monopoly on sugar cane, so that it was sown only on the sultan's lands. Nothing came of this explanation for the plague epidemic, although it reflects the long-term economic consequences of sustained population decline. In response, the sultan merely ordered the judges and amirs to instruct the people to be penitent and to increase their pious deeds.[77]

The general economic and political tumult that characterized the second half of the fourteenth century in Egypt was, in part, the result of the struggle to readjust revenue to previous, pre-plague levels. In both Europe and the Middle East, there was a comparable search by landowners for profitable agrarian production. The burden of lower agricultural revenue was shifted by the mamlūks to the peasantry in the form of higher government taxes, higher interest rates on grain, and extraordinary payments. The perpetual agrarian revolts of the later Mamlūk Period may be interpreted as a second phase of a cycle which had begun with the enrichment of the peasants by higher temporary wages and inheritance, with consequent rising ex-

[75] Ashtor, *Histoire*, pp. 379-381. [76] "England to Egypt," p. 123.

[77] Ibn Ḥajar, *Inbā' al-ghumr*, vol. 3, pp. 438-439.

pectations. But later these expectations were confronted by the desire of the landowners to re-establish pre-plague incomes.[78] Moreover, it would seem that the mamlūk political-military insurrections themselves arose not at the time of dramatic demographic decline, but during the long process of unsuccessful recovery in the latter half of the fourteenth century, when men tried to maintain their personal positions and interests.[79]

D. COMMERCE

Commerce underwent a marked decline, judging by the tax returns and the contemporary observations of urban commercial activity.[80] After the height of the Black Death in January 1349, Cairo had become an abandoned city, and few people were seen in the streets. Even the most animated commercial street in the old city of Cairo, Shārī' Bayn al-Qaṣrayn, was deserted.[81] We are fortunate that a description of this important avenue of Cairene life during the Black Death has been preserved from the lost segment of the history of Ibn al-Furāt, a witness to the pandemic in Cairo. The account is contained in the plague treatise of Ibn Ḥajar, who states:

> I read in his own handwriting the history of Shaykh Nāṣir ad-Dīn ibn al-Furāt that he performed the Friday prayer in 749 [A.H.] on the terrace [*saṭḥ*] of the Mosque of al-Ḥākim. He observed the biers which were arranged in three rows from the front of the mosque to the door of al-Khirā'if; the third row was slightly decreased. He said: "The deaths had increased until it had emptied the streets. I had walked at night between the two palaces,[82] between sunset prayer and evening prayer, from the square of the Ḥarīrīyīn [silk manu-

78 Poliak, "Les Révoltes populaires," pp. 251-273.

79 Cf. A. R. Bridbury, "The Black Death," *The Economic History Review*, 2nd series, vol. 26, no. 4 (1973), pp. 577-592.

80 "England to Egypt," pp. 116-117.

81 See *Systematic Notes*, vol. 15, p. 29, map no. 9.

82 This refers to the two Fāṭimid palaces within the old city; thus, the origin of the name of the main thoroughfare: *Bayn al-Qasrayn*.

facturers] to the Sūq ad-Dajāj [fowl market] close to the Mosque of al-Aqmar. I only saw lamps burning in a few of the shops along the street. I didn't find merchandise because of the scarcity of people who bring the merchandise to the shops. The cost of one pomegranate reached half a *dīnār*. Flour from an *irdabb* of wheat reached the price of a *florin*. The horror of this is too long to recount, but this is indicative of the calamity."[83]

The scarcity and high prices were thus clearly due to the lack of labor to bring merchandise to market and sell it or, in the case of flour, to process it. Al-Maqrīzī states that the Black Death was particularly acute among the shopkeepers in Cairo and Fusṭāṭ, after the women and children. The markets were logically the areas of greatest danger because of the high density of human and rat populations, the constant influx of individuals and commodities, and the apparently common practice of selling the discarded clothing of plague victims. Many of the merchants fled the danger; in Bilbais, the markets were deserted because no one would stay there, and the rare vendor who still existed moved out of the city and installed himself in the suburban orchards. The markets of Alexandria were likewise closed, along with the government tax bureau that collected taxes of a fifth on the merchandise of natives and foreigners.[84]

The foreign merchants, who probably introduced the Black Death to Alexandria and to other Levantine ports, were also victims of plague. Al-Maqrīzī mentions specifically, in his ac-

[83] *Badhl*, fols. 130a-130b. The section of the *History* of Ibn al-Furāt for the years A.H. 690 to 788 is apparently lost. Therefore, this portion has been omitted from the published text (vol. 8: 683-689 A.H.; vol. 9: 789-799 A.H.). According to C. K. Zurayk, there is a possibility that the three manuscript volumes in Brussa (Hussein Čelebi Collection; see *GAL*, vol. 2, p. 50) may cover a part of this period (communication of January 7, 1970). If this important work could be located, it might show that Ibn al-Furāt was a major source for later historians, particularly al-Maqrīzī.

[84] *as-Sulūk*, part 2, vol. 3, pp. 777-780.

count of the Black Death in Alexandria, a ship of European merchants which anchored in the port. The merchants told of having seen a drifting ship off Tripoli. They followed it and found that everyone on board had died of plague. Leaving the death ship, they sailed on to Alexandria, during the trip losing two-thirds of their number.[85]

Because of the death of such foreign merchants and the devastation of the pandemic in Europe, it is natural that foreign merchandise became rare in the Near Eastern markets for a time.[86] In Alexandria, the caravanserais had to close because of the scarcity of clients, which must have included the European merchants and their cargoes.[87] During the later plague epidemics in Egypt and Syria, the death of European merchants was noted by the Arabic chroniclers. For example, in Alexandria and Damietta during the epidemic of 919/1513, all the Venetian, Catalan, and Ragusan merchants died of plague.[88] At the time of the plagues in 903/1497-1498 and 919/1513-1514 in Damascus, the European merchants immediately fled to Cyprus for safety.[89]

Regarding this European trade, the reduction of Middle Eastern population and other unfavorable economic conditions reduced productive power in agriculture and handicrafts, diminishing its exporting capacity and, to a corresponding extent, its capacity to import.[90] The shrinkage of agricultural goods "must lead to a decline in the surplus available for export or other uses, unless it is accompanied by an improvement in

[85] *Ibid.* See also his other description of a merchant ship coming to the port of Alexandria (*ibid.*, p. 776).

[86] Ibn Iyās, vol. 1, p. 191.

[87] *as-Sulūk*, part 2, vol. 3, p. 777.

[88] Marino Sanuto, *I Diarii di Marino Sanuto* (Venice, 1879-1903), vol. 16, col. 649.

[89] For 903 A.H.: Girolamo Priuli, *I Diarii*, ed. by L. A. Muratori, *Rerum Italicarum Scriptores*, tome 24, part 3, vol. 1 (Lapi, 1912-1921), p. 71; Sanuto, *I Diarii*, vol. 1, col. 856. For A.H. 919: Sanuto, *I Diarii*, vol. 18, col. 155.

[90] Charles Issawi, "The Decline of Middle Eastern Trade, 1100-1850," *Islam and the Trade of Asia*, ed. by D. S. Richards (Oxford, 1970), p. 266.

technology or greater use of capital (which obviously did not take place in the Middle East) or unless the marginal product of labor is lower than the consumption of the worker and his dependents, which is very unlikely to have been true of that period."[91] The high cost of urban labor caused by sustained depopulation, the technological stagnation of industrial production, the very unfavorable fiscal policy of the mamlūk regime, and a decreasing demand by Europeans for Middle Eastern manufactured goods placed Egypt and Syria in an increasingly weak economic position vis-à-vis Europe.

The overall trend of wages and prices, industry and trade in the Middle East is explicable largely by the declining population in the second half of the fourteenth and the fifteenth centuries.[92] Under normal circumstances, Malthusian forces would be expected to operate to increase population once again, with concomitant changes in prices and wages. However, the corrective forces were inhibited partly by continual plague outbreaks, which limited recovery and reduced incentives to bear children and raise families. In sum, the complex economic problem of the later Mamlūk Period remains largely a population problem.

[91] *Ibid.*, p. 249.

[92] Cf. Postan, "Some Economic Evidence of Declining Population," pp. 221-246.

VIII

CONCLUSIONS

> Neither the sun nor death can be
> looked at with a steady eye.
> —La Rochefoucauld

If the full meaning of the Black Death and the recurrent plague epidemics in the Middle East could be easily expressed in concluding remarks, it should scarcely have been necessary to recount at length the story of plague and its impact on medieval Muslim society. However, the existence and nature of the pandemic and subsequent plague reappearances in the Middle East had to be determined as clearly as possible. Equally important has been the attempt to estimate plague mortality and to suggest the diffuse consequences of depopulation for most aspects of Muslim life in the latter half of the fourteenth and fifteenth centuries.

By the last decade of the fourteenth century, the Mamlūk Sultanate was plunged into a general crisis from which it would never fully recover.[1] The reasons for this mounting crisis are readily apparent. As the major faction among the governing élite, the Circassian mamlūks seized control of the empire in 783/1382, but only prolonged the internecine struggle for the sultanate, which may be dated from the death of an-Nāṣir in 741/1340. The factionalism led to civil wars in Egypt and Syria, while the undisciplined Circassians abused or abandoned a number of the characteristic features of the mamlūk institution.

Economically, the cultivated regions of the Sultanate were subjected to destruction by warring armies and by increased bedouin unrest. Apart from this disruption of agricultural production, famines caused by exceptional fluctuations of the

[1] *Muslim Cities*, pp. 25-38.

Nile in the century after the Black Death and increased taxation forced the peasantry to flee the land. The contraction of the vital agrarian economy, as evidenced by the cadastral surveys, brought about the decline in incomes for the mamlūk élite and, consequently, the decline in consumption of crafts and trade, accompanied by monetary chaos and inflation of prices. The decrease of agricultural revenues entailed, in a vicious circle, the neglect of irrigation and other rural investments by the government and the individual mamlūk amirs. The decline of the Mamlūk Empire may be attributed, in this manner, to the protracted crisis in the countryside. But the carious agricultural economy only points out most forcibly what was common to all facets of mamlūk society after the mid-fourteenth century: the impairment of the state by prolonged depopulation. Along with other unfavorable demographic factors, plague helped to destroy the most abundant resource of the Mamlūk Sultanate.

While there was a rehabilitation of political conditions from 1420 to 1470, it was severely handicapped by a continually declining population and was heavily burdened by the unremitting drain on Egypt's and Syria's dwindling economic resources for military enterprises. At this time, the regime was faced with the re-emergence of external dangers: Turkoman advances from Anatolia, the invasion of Timūr in the East, and Christian piracy at sea. The increased military demands, including that of manpower, on the contracting economy diverted surplus wealth from consumption and internal investment to enormous military expenditures, which were economically unproductive. The final defeat of Egypt by the Ottomans, in the early sixteenth century, found the country economically prostrate[2] and the population greatly depleted. We can date this striking economic deterioration from the Black Death.

In the immediate aftermath of the Black Death in Middle Eastern and European societies, the short-term economic effects were significant and very much in line with what modern

[2] *Ibid.*, p. 39 and n. 71.

economic theory would predict: a rapid rise in wages and per capita incomes of the laboring classes and downward pressure on rents and incomes of the propertied classes. Aggregate economic production declined in both societies from their previous levels. For urban workers, the century following the Black Death was a prosperous one, but the rural laborers in Egypt did not share in this prosperity, as did those in Western Europe. While the pandemic may have accelerated the decline of European manoralism and the shift to modern contractual relationships, no such change took place in the centralist landholding system of Egypt and Syria or in the nature of its agricultural production. It remains questionable whether the following century witnessed an actual decline in per capita well-being in European society; for the Middle East, the issue is far less doubtful. Except for the urban laborers, the economic evidence of the later Mamlūk Period indicates a marked decline in per capita income, together with an overall economic depression.[3]

At the same time that the Black Death and its recurrent epidemics had profound consequences for the economy and, therefore, the future of the Mamlūk Sultanate, they evoked the distinctive and dramatic communal reactions that we have described. As a means of both summing up and assessing the Muslim response to plague, it is instructive to relate this response to the simultaneous European Christian reaction to the pandemic.[4]

On the basis of contemporary Arabic and Latin sources for

[3] Cf. Hirshleifer, *Disaster and Recovery*, pp. 10-18, 27-28.

[4] There is a need for caution because of the lack of research on the demographic history of the Middle East. It is impossible to prove that the dramatic difference in the contemporary reactions of Muslim and Christian societies was due to a marked difference in population decline. It is improbable, in my opinion, that there was a greater decline in European population that would have caused greater social tension and alarm. A general assessment of the urban populations and the etiological conditions for plague in the Middle East would tend to suggest the opposite: a higher mortality rate in Muslim society and, almost certainly, a greater aggregate number of deaths.

the Black Death, we can be certain of the existence of the three major forms of plague (bubonic, pneumonic, and septicaemic) in these regions. In any historical comparison of the role of the pandemic in Muslim and Christian societies, therefore, we can assume as a constant the medical nature of the disease itself. In addition, almost all the medieval physicians believed that its immediate cause was a pestilential miasma; this belief was broadly accepted in both societies, as a result of their common reliance on the theory of epidemics found in Hippocrates and elaborated upon by Galen and Ibn Sīnā, the greatest medical authorities for the fourteenth-century doctors. Therefore, in the Oriental and Western plague treatises, there is similar advice for improving or changing the air in a plague-stricken community.

This medical advice is only one element of the defensive communal reactions of the two societies. A study of the more general communal responses to the same disaster delineates the respective values and practices of late medieval European and Middle Eastern societies.[5] After reviewing the European Christian understanding of the Black Death and the remarkable reactions to it, as well as the Muslim response, it will become evident that they were quite dissimilar, and the comparison of these differences tells us much about what is essential to the identity of each culture.[6] Faced with the

[5] The psychological impact of historical disasters, such as the Black Death, was the topic of William L. Langer's presidential address to the American Historical Association in 1957 ("The Next Assignment," *The American Historical Review*, vol. 63 [January, 1958], pp. 283-304, and "The Black Death," pp. 114-122).

[6] I am conscious that there is another natural way to cope with disease, or suffering and death in general, apart from the conscious human attempts at understanding: one can simply ignore them. Temporary or partial oblivion is, perhaps, not without merit; I am less convinced of the merit or even existence of complete oblivion. In one instance, obliviousness has been used as an explanation for a society's reaction to collective disaster: Robert Lifton has described the "psychic numbing" of those subjected to the atomic attack on Hiroshima (*Death in Life* [New York, 1969], pp. 500, 503). Concerning the Black Death in Europe and the Middle East, I have found very little evidence of

specter of death in a particularly horrible form, the values and attitudes around which lives were constructed met their severest test. We shall be drawn to re-examine the *religious* roots of each culture in order better to understand their differing responses. As Professor Lapidus has written about the long history of communal life in the Middle East: "In each epoch, the prevailing religions represented a different set of values and understandings, a different type of organization, and a different form of society; but in all ages, ancient, Christian, and Muslim, community life seems to have been inextricably bound up with religion. From religious teachings come the ideals and the norms of social action; from religious organization, the structuring of social life."[7]

In Europe the Black Death was interpreted on various levels by contemporary writers. However, the pandemic was considered by most European observers to result directly from a pestilential miasma, and it was believed that the disease was contagious, which accounts for the important protective measures taken by the Italian cities and the widespread advocacy of flight as the best means of escaping the disease. The physicians emphasized natural causations of the disease (such as an unfavorable conjunction of the planets or earthquakes) among the remote causes of the miasma. However, only one European treatise gives a concrete remedy against the astrological causes of plague; the customary recommendations were flight and prayer.[8] The most important thing to bear in mind

---

communal or individual indifference to the disaster. There seems to be a real danger here that must be resisted; the nature of the Muslim reaction to the Black Death should not be interpreted simply as psychic avoidance of or obliviousness to a real calamity.

[7] "Traditional Muslim Cities: Structure and Change," *From Madina to Metropolis*, ed. by L. Carl Brown (Princeton, 1973), p. 57.

[8] Campbell, p. 65. Campbell's monograph is devoted in part to an examination of the opinions on the Black Death by contemporary Europeans, particularly physicians. Although instructive about medical theory and practice, this examination is highly restrictive and cannot be said to reflect the general European interpretation of the disease. The physicians' views should be balanced by other sources, such as chron-

is not the precise mechanisms contrived by men to explain contagion (which were wrong) but the fact that in the Middle Ages—whether in Christian or in Muslim society—one simply could not separate the physiological from the mental and moral processes.

The real cause of the plague pandemic was believed to be a moral one: the European Christian viewed the Black Death as an overwhelming punishment from God for his sins and those of his fellow Christians.[9] Despite other interpretations of the disease, this view is the only one that satisfactorily explains the extraordinary forms of communal behavior in many parts of Europe during the Black Death. This supernatural explanation was propagated by the Church and is reflected in contemporary European art and literature.[10] The chronicles of the fourteenth century almost always attribute the affliction to divine retribution for the wickedness of European society.[11] Langland sum-

icles, vernacular literature, and art. Particularly the homiletic literature should be studied since the medieval homilists, in general, were the disseminators of the patristic understanding of plague; through preachers' manuals, sermon collections, and devotional writings, they conveyed to the popular culture the ecclesiastical idea of plague. See, for example, G. R. Owst, *Preaching in Medieval England* (Cambridge, 1926).

9 Explicitly or implicitly, all diseases were believed by medieval European observers to come ultimately from God; the common moral justification for disease was that God inflicted disease on the unrepentant sinner as punishment; see Stanley Rubin, *Medieval English Medicine* (New York, 1974), p. 16. For specific examples, see the interpretation of madness in medieval European society by P.B.R. Doob, *Nebuchadnezzar's Children: Conventions of Madness in Middle English Literature* (New Haven, 1974), pp. 1-53, and Judith S. Neaman, *Suggestion of the Devil: The Origins of Madness* (New York, 1975), pp. 50-51 *et passim*; for leprosy, S. N. Brody, *The Disease of the Soul: Leprosy in Medieval Literature* (Ithaca, 1974), pp. 11-12, 60-61, 104-106, 112-189; and for epilepsy, Owsei Temkin, *The Falling Sickness* (Baltimore, 1971), pp. 85-117.

10 Johannes Nohl, *The Black Death* (London, 1961), pp. 78-79; Crawfurd, *Plague and Pestilence.*

11 Ziegler, p. 35.

marizes the common view succinctly: "These pestilences were for pure sin."[12]

Based directly on Biblical and classical precedents,[13] a conviction of personal guilt and a need for individual and collective expiation were engendered in the faithful Christian. His attitude to the Black Death is well illustrated by the European communal response. This response took the forms of the flagellant movement, the persecution of alien groups (particularly the Jews), and a pessimistic preoccupation with imminent death.

The flagellant movement was based on a belief in the mortification of the flesh as suitable penance for men's sins. Beginning in mid-thirteenth-century Italy, a series of natural disasters convinced many that God's wrath was visiting men as a punishment for their sinfulness. This concept was acted out in expiatory pilgrimages and processions in an attempt to divert or allay God's chastisement. The processions recurred continually during the later Middle Ages.[14] From its inception, an implicit element of the flagellant movement was its participation in the millennial ideas that Professor Cohn has shown to be a significant theme of late medieval Christendom, stemming especially from the millennial scheme of Joachim of Fiore.[15] Self-flagellation was "a collective *imitatio Christi*, a redemptive sacrifice which protected the world from final overwhelming catastrophe, and by virtue of which they themselves [the flagellants] became a holy élite."[16]

During the Black Death, this holy élite became a messianic crusade without a putative messiah. A recent historian of the Black Death in Europe has described the movement in the following manner:

[12] *Piers Plowman*, Version B, v. 13.

[13] See Hirst, pp. 6-16.

[14] Ziegler, pp. 87-88; Norman Cohn, *The Pursuit of the Millennium*, rev. ed. (New York, 1970), pp. 127-147.

[15] Cohn, *The Pursuit of the Millennium*, pp. 108-113; see Marjorie Reeves, *The Influence of Prophecy in the Later Middle Ages: A Study in Joachimism* (Oxford, 1969).

[16] Cohn, *The Pursuit of the Millennium*, p. 142.

As the fervor mounted the messianic pretensions of the Flagellants became more pronounced. They began to claim that the movement must last for thirty-three years and end only with the redemption of Christendom and the arrival of the Millennium. Possessed by such chiliastic convictions they saw themselves more and more, not as mortals suffering to expiate their own sins and humanity's, but as a holy army of Saints.[17]

The flagellant movement was a complex social phenomenon. Its apocalyptic ambitions proved to be an incentive to personal mysticism, anti-clericalism, and revolutionary social ideas, such as the destruction of private wealth. The flagellants were also intimately associated with the second major feature of the European reaction to the pandemic: the persecution of the Jews.

The massacres of the Jews during the Black Death were unprecedented in their extent and ferocity until the twentieth century. The first attacks on the Jews resulted from the accusation that this unassimilable community had caused the pestilence by poisoning wells; this was neither new (Jews had been accused and massacred in southern France and Spain during the plague epidemics of 1320 and 1333), nor confined to the Jews alone. Lepers,[18] gravediggers and other social outcasts, Muslims in Spain, or any foreigners were liable to attack; the hunting-down of plague salvers continued well into the seventeenth century. But in September 1348 the forced confessions from ten Jews in Chillon were adduced to support the accusation and to implicate all European Jews.[19] A second wave of

[17] Ziegler, p. 92.

[18] Ernest Wickersheimer, "Les Accusations d'empoisonnement portées pendant la première moitié du XIVe siècle contre les lépreux et les juifs; leur relations avec les épidémies de peste," *Comptes-rendus du quatrième congrès international d'histoire de la médecine,* ed. by Tricot-Royer and Laignel-Lavastine (Anvers, 1927), pp. 76-83.

[19] The analysis by H. R. Trevor-Roper, *The European Witch-Craze of the Sixteenth and Seventeenth Centuries and Other Essays* (New York, 1969), pp. 90-192, is remarkably suitable to the interpretation of this "craze."

massacres from the middle of 1349 was instigated by the propaganda of the flagellants. In many cities of Germany and the Low Countries (Frankfort, Mainz, Cologne, Brussels) the destruction of the Jewish population was led by the flagellants, aided by the masses of the poor.[20] Pope Clement VI finally condemned the flagellants in 1349, after two bulls in the same year against the persecution of the Jews had been ineffectual.

Besides the immediate economic and social causes that have been pointed out for the Jewish persecution,[21] we must also consider the image of the Jew as Antichrist, commonplace in Europe during the later Middle Ages. As closely related to Christian millennial ideology as the reverse is to the obverse, this image was fostered by the Roman Catholic Church and gained considerable momentum from the time of the First Crusade. At its origin was a predisposition to seek a weak, unpopular, and easily identifiable scapegoat as the source of evil—the enemy of militant Christendom.

In general, European Christians reacted to the Black Death with profound guilt and fear, which religious attitudes about the mortification of the flesh often transformed into extreme penance.[22] There seems to have been a deep pessimism and sometimes a renunciation of life itself.[23] The frenetic character of religious life in the fourteenth century was magnified by the preoccupation with death. "The Dance of Death, the Art of Dying, the Council of Florence's definition of the doctrine

[20] Cohn, *The Pursuit of the Millennium*, p. 139.

[21] Ziegler, pp. 97-109.

[22] Langer, "The Black Death," p. 122: "Boccaccio, a few years after writing his *Decameron*, was overcome by repentance and a sense of guilt verging on panic. Martin Luther suffered acutely from guilt and fear of death, and Calvin, terror-stricken by the plague, fled from each epidemic. Indeed, entire communities were afflicted with what Freud called the primordial sense of guilt, and they engaged in penitential processions, pilgrimages and passionate mass preaching."

[23] Ziegler, pp. 274-276; Meiss, *Painting in Florence and Siena after the Black Death*, pp. 74-78; J. Huizinga, *The Waning of the Middle Ages* (New York, 1954), pp. 27-52; Langer, "The Next Assignment," p. 298; George Rosen, *Madness in Society* (New York, 1969), p. 8.

of purgatory, the practice of indulgences—all suffered life to be seen increasingly from the perspective of death."[24]

Professor Huizinga has suggested that a "vision of death" pervades late fourteenth- and fifteenth-century European literature; the macabre weighed heavily on men's souls.[25] The awareness of imminent death and of the transitory nature of life is extraordinarily prominent in a variety of late medieval documents, as seen in sermons and poems, testaments and endowments.[26] It is not illogical, however, to find the opposite reaction—hedonism—as a form of defiance to this *danse macabre*.[27] No doubt it was a desperate kind of reassertion of life in the presence of death. Moreover, the natural desire of survivors to escape the threat of death by fleeing from a plague-stricken region was encouraged by European physicians and clerics. The pandemic brought to the fore the discontinuous view of human existence in Christianity—that is, the end of all things in the Apocalypse.

In the complex psychological response to the Black Death, the natural preoccupation with death was therefore not inconsistent with a vision of the Biblical Apocalypse.[28] Many believed that the end of the world had come, plague being the apocalyptic rider on the white horse. In an account of the island of Cyprus during the pandemic, an Arabic chronicler testified to the Christian belief by his remark that the Christian Cypriots "feared that it was the end of the world."[29] The Black Death did not create these forms of reaction or the ideology that lay behind them; it was a stimulus, despite its irregularity of attack, which excited the nerve system of late medieval Christian society.

[24] John M. Headley, "The Continental Reformation," *The Meaning of the Renaissance and Reformation*, ed. by Richard L. DeMolen (Boston, 1974), pp. 141-142.

[25] *The Waning of the Middle Ages*, pp. 138-151.

[26] *Ibid*., pp. 31ff; Campbell, pp. 171-174.

[27] I have found no evidence for a comparable abandonment of morality in Muslim society during the Black Death or later plague epidemics.

[28] Rosen, *Madness in Society*, pp. 9-10.

[29] *as-Sulūk*, part 2, vol. 3, p. 776.

The Middle Eastern interpretations of the Black Death display a diversity of opinions similar to that of the European accounts. Yet the dominant view of plague was religious and was set forth primarily in the three religio-legal principles that directly affected communal behavior as we have seen.

It would be unreasonable to assume that these three religio-legal tenets were totally characteristic of the Muslim response to the Black Death. While there was no question that the ultimate cause of plague was divine, the legal scholars argued both for and against these precepts in their plague treatises. As for the first principle, there is historical and literary evidence that plague was considered by some men as a warning or punishment by God. There is an obvious incompatibility between the beliefs in plague as a divine punishment and as a divine reward. Within this spectrum of beliefs, there was also the deterministic view, which finds support in the Qur'ān, that plague was a calamity decreed by an unknowable God. The latter interpretation is most consistent with the historical accounts and represents the consensus of the jurists and popular attitudes. As for the unique theological claim that plague was a mercy and martyrdom, it may have been both comforting and confounding for the distressed Muslim; it had the virtue of preserving the belief in a compassionate and merciful God.[30] At the very least, there was no unanimity of opinion

[30] The only comparable instance of a disease's being interpreted as a divine blessing or mercy, to my knowledge, is the medieval Christian belief in leprosy as a divine promise of salvation (Brody, *The Disease of the Soul*, pp. 68, 101-104). Both ideas were propagated by the religious establishments and posed similar inconsistencies. Medieval Europe, according to Brody, "accommodated two incompatible ideas of leprosy: the disease was the sickness both of the damned sinner and of one given special grace by God" (*Ibid.*, pp. 100-101). Unlike the Muslim treatment of plague victims, the Christian notion of sin and punishment prevailed over the pious assurances of salvation. The different treatments of the plague victim in Muslim society and the leper in Christian society may be explained in numerous ways, but the simple fact that plague was a short-term disease compared to the lifelong suffering of leprosy must account to some extent for Muslim society's receptivity to the idea of immediate salvation for the plague victim and its rejection by Christian society for the leper.

about the specific reason for plague; this lack of agreement had its virtue in removing the possibility of a single ideological basis for social activism.

Much the same may be said for the issue of flight from a plague-stricken community. Some jurists disagreed with the prohibition against fleeing, and there is historical evidence that clearly shows that there was flight from the countryside to the major cities. The Black Death and the recurrent plagues accelerated a pattern of rural depopulation that was perceptible to Arabic historians in the following century and a half.

On the other hand, there was at least temporary evacuation of the cities as well. Yet, despite the enormous problems created by the pandemic, there is no evidence that suggests that the machinery of government and religion broke down altogether in the most important cities, such as Damascus, Cairo, and Alexandria. The historical narratives that relate the attempts by the government to count the dead, either in the mosques or at the city gates, argue strongly in favor of the maintenance of urban organization. Indeed, such activities are rare examples in Muslim urban life of what could be called "municipal" organization. The popular religious ceremonies are equally indicative of municipal activity; they also argue against massive flight from the urban regions and against a popular belief in contagion. As late as the severe plague epidemic in Cairo in 1835, Edward Lane, a keen observer of traditional Muslim society, noted during the epidemic—for which he observed no unusual popular reaction—that "from a distrust in fate some Muslims even shut themselves up during the period of plague, but this practice is generally condemned. A Syrian friend of mine who did so nearly had his door broken open by his neighbors."[31] Concerning this third problem of contagion,

[31] *Arabian Society in the Middle Ages*, p. 10. For the same plague epidemic in the Middle East, we have the travel account of Kinglake—*Eothen*—which is virtually "A Journal of the Plague Year." Kinglake observed, particularly, the high mortality rate in Cairo and the traditional Muslim funeral practices. Compared with the massive flight of the Europeans due to their obsession with contagion, "the Orientals, however, have more quiet fortitude than Europeans under afflictions of

the Andalusian scholar Ibn al-Khaṭīb has attracted European attention for his observation and forceful statement of the contagious nature of the Black Death. However, this points to the exceptional nature of Ibn al-Khaṭīb's belief and the weight of opinion against him.

The importance of these three principles to Muslim society was in what they did *not* affirm: they did not declare that plague was God's punishment; they did not encourage flight; and they did not support a belief in the contagious nature of plague—all prevalent beliefs in Christian Europe. These principles appear to be borne out by the reports of the general communal responses to the Black Death in the major cities of the Middle East.

The comparison of Christian and Muslim societies during the Black Death calls attention to the appreciable disparity in their general communal responses. But has not the description of the Christian reaction stressed the exceptional rather than the typical responses? For were there not comparable magical beliefs and practices, religious services and prayers? Undoubtedly there were, although mass communal funeral services, processions, and journeys to the cemeteries were greatly limited by the common European belief in contagion, as seen in the *statuti sanitari* of the Italian cities,[32] and the advisability of flight.[33] Conversely, the Arabic sources do not attest to the "striking manifestations of abnormal collective psychology, of

---

this sort, and they never allow the plague to interfere with their religious usages (pp. 250-251). . . . There were no outward signs of despair nor violent terror (p. 268)."

[32] É. Carpentier, *Une ville devant la peste: Orvieto et la Peste Noire* (Paris, 1962), pp. 131-134.

[33] See, for example, *ibid.*, pp. 124-126, and W. M. Bowsky, "The Impact of the Black Death upon Sienese Government and Society," *Speculum*, vol. 39, no. 1 (January, 1964), pp. 1-34. These two excellent regional monographs represent the most profitable manner of further investigation of the Black Death in Europe. They are based on very rich archival material; unfortunately, comparable records are not extant for the major cities of the Middle East and North Africa for the same period, which places a severe limitation on similar research.

dissociation of the group mind,"[34] which occurred in Christian Europe. Fear of the Black Death in Europe activated what Professor Trevor-Roper has called, in a different context, a European "stereotype of fear";[35] the collective emotion played upon a mythology of messianism, anti-Semitism, and man's culpability for his sins.[36]

Why are the corresponding phenomena not found in the Muslim reaction to the Black Death?[37] The stereotypes did not exist. There is no evidence for the appearance of messianic movements in Muslim society at this time that might have associated the Black Death with an apocalypse. In Islamic history the religious leader who heralds the final judgment and the end of the world is known as the *mahdī*. The doctrine and the growth of mahdist movements usually gained adherence on the fringe of Muslim civilization and are characteristic of popular Muslim culture, for there is no dogma of an all-encompassing expectation of an apocalypse in *sunnī* or orthodox Islam corresponding to its role in medieval Christianity. Orthodox Islam, as opposed to shīʿism and other millennial Muslim sects, has never developed a doctrine of an apocalypse.[38] This feature of Islamic theology may be due to the lack of a Qur'ānic basis[39] comparable to the Christian Book of Revelation.[40] Our sources for the Black Death in the Middle

[34] Hirst, p. 17.

[35] *The European Witch-Craze*, p. 165.

[36] *Ibid.*, pp. 98, 185; demonology and witchcraft may be added to this mythology.

[37] Von Kremer has attempted to minimize the differences between the reactions of Christian and Muslim societies to the Black Death. While he concedes that there was no persecution of Jews (or Christians) in the Orient, he uncritically associates the religious fanaticism of the flagellants in Europe with the dervish orders in Muslim society ("Ueber die grossen Seuchen," p. 102).

[38] For the esoteric apocalyptical literature of *shīʿah*, see *EI*²: "djafr" (T. Fahd).

[39] See Gibb and Kramers, *Shorter Encyclopaedia of Islam*: "ʿĪsā."

[40] On this point, the Book of Revelation was the least popular book of the New Testament in Byzantine or Greek Christian theology, which may help to explain a corresponding lack of apocalyptic expectations or

East, North Africa, and Andalusia were written, admittedly, mainly by the articulate urban *'ulamā'* or religious scholars, but they would certainly have been sensitive to the development of messianic movements in the hinterland, since they were generally opposed to violent socio-religious innovation, not to say social revolution.[41] Furthermore, the fact that there was no certainty that plague was a divine punishment for sin removed the impetus for a cohesive puritanical and revivalist popular movement.[42]

The impact of the Black Death poses the question of the

---

popular movements reported in the Byzantine chronicles, either for the Plague of Justinian or the Black Death. Trevor-Roper suggests a similar contrast: the Greek Orthodox Church, unlike the Catholic Church, "built up no systematic demonology and launched no witch-craze" (*The European Witch-Craze*, p. 185). Moreover, there is a closer parallel between the fatalistic Muslim attitude toward the disease and the Byzantine Greek concept of blind and arbitrary *tyche* that directs the affairs of men (see Speros Vryonis, *The Decline of Medieval Hellenism in Asia Minor and the Process of Islamization from the Eleventh through the Fifteenth Century* [Berkeley and Los Angeles, 1971], pp. 409, 418).

[41] Poliak, "Les Révoltes populaires," p. 255.

[42] There is a large literature on the history of the millennium but very little investigation of comparative Semitic (Christian, Judaic, and Muslim) apocalyptical literature and its relation to messianic movements. Particularly, the nature of apocalyptic doctrines and their relation to millennial movements in Islamic history have not been the subject of any modern study. A clear presentation of the popular belief in the *mahdī* in the fourteenth century is given by Ibn Khaldūn, which includes its association with *ṣūfī* beliefs (*The Muqaddimah*, vol. 2, pp. 156-200). See also Gibb and Kramers, *Shorter Encyclopaedia of Islam*: "al-Mahdī," "al-Dadjdjāl"; *EI*[1]: "al-kiyamā" (D. B. Macdonald); M.G.S. Hodgson, "A Note on the Millennium in Islam," *Millennial Dreams in Action*, ed. by S. L. Thrupp (New York, 1970), pp. 218-219; M. Galal, "Essai d'observations sur les rites funeraires," pp. 249-252; Ignaz Goldziher, *Mohamed and Islam* (New Haven, 1917), pp. 240-247, with bibliographical references to *mahdist* doctrine, p. 284; and L. C. Brown, "The Sudanese Mahdiya," *Protest and Power in Black Africa*, ed. by Robert I. Rotberg and Ali A. Mazrui (Oxford, 1970), pp. 145-168. For two mahdist movements during the Mamlūk Period, see Poliak, "Les Révoltes populaires," pp. 255-256.

Muslim attitude toward minorities. The unassimilated communities were tolerated in medieval Muslim society and, in this instance, were not held responsible for the ravages of the pandemic.[43] However theoretical, the legal tenet against contagion of plague would have militated against the accusation of minorities. In no case is there a direct causal relationship to be found between the Black Death (or subsequent plague epidemics) and the active persecution of minorities, as in Europe.[44]

The Christian belief in plague as a divine punishment for men's sins was preached by clergymen deeply committed to the idea of original sin and man's guilt arising from his essential depravity, as well as a fundamental contempt—both Christian and Stoic—for this world. Indeed, original sin was interpreted as the cause of human degeneration; it would incline men to sin and thus provoke divine punishment in the guise of an appropriate disease.[45] The ultimate threat of disease, death, is the final punishment for the Christian for having been born in sin. On the other hand, there is no doctrine of

[43] There were sumptuary laws against the *ahl adh-dhimmah* ("people of the covenant" or protected non-Muslims) in the Middle East, which were enforced with varying degrees of severity. During the Mamlūk Period in Egypt and Syria, Jews and particularly Christians (Copts) were subjected to increased discrimination and violence for various reasons. For a recent review of the position of the *dhimmīs* in the Mamlūk Period, see Bosworth, "Christian and Jewish Religious Dignitaries in Mamlūk Egypt and Syria," pp. 64-66; see also Poliak, "Les Révoltes populaires," pp. 269-271. For the general study of *dhimmī* status, see *EI*²: "dhimma" (C. Cahen) and Goitein, *A Mediterranean Society*, vol. 2, chap. 7.

[44] See Ibn Taghrī Birdī, who was strongly in favor of discriminatory practices against non-Muslims, for instances of sumptuary legislation: *an-Nujūm*, Popper trans., vol. 17, pp. 67-69; vol. 18, p. 5; vol. 19, pp. 109, 125, 137; vol. 23, p. 56. M. Perlmann, "Notes on Anti-Christian Propaganda in the Mamlūk Empire," *BSOAS*, vol. 10 (1942), p. 854, discusses a case of incendiarism at the beginning of the year of the Black Death in Syria (A.H. 749) taken from an anti-Christian tract by al-Asnawī (d. 772/1370); there does not appear to be any relation between the two events.

[45] Doob, *Nebuchadnezzar's Children*, pp. 7-10.

original sin and man's insuperable guilt in Islamic theology.[46] The Muslim writers on plague, therefore, did not dwell on the sins and guilt of their co-religionists even if they did admit that plague was a divine warning against sin. Prayer was supplication and not expiation.

If we compare the Judeo-Christian tradition with the Muslim religion, we can appreciate one of its major defects, the tendency to subsume death under punishment, to leave out the possibility of death which is not punishment. The Black Death in Europe was an occasion for the vigorous realization of these ideas about sin and punishment, suffering and death. Specifically, the European writers laid greater emphasis upon the punitive aspect of plague in God's plan than upon the monitory and purgative virtues of the disease found in Muslim society.

The general reaction of Muslim society to the Black Death was governed by its interpretation as only another common disaster. This was the view of the majority of the *'ulamā'*, as exemplified by the treatise of Ibn Ḥajar.[47] The Muslim attitude toward the cataclysmic nature of plague seems to be more closely related to the view found in Thucydides' description of the "Athenian Plague" rather than to the then contemporary European experience of the Black Death. A comparison may be drawn between the language in the accounts of plague in Thucydides and the Arabic historical sources, especially al-Maqrīzī. In both, detailed descriptions show the awful power of the disease as an incalculable disaster that defies human reason and control. Plague is spoken of as a permanent aspect of the human condition; for the Greeks, plague is *pathos*, like war.[48] For the Muslims, this incalculable event is fated by God for mankind, as are other diseases, droughts, or floods. It is possible to see in the Muslim communal ceremonies, as well as

[46] See Georges C. Anawati, "La notion de 'Péché originel' existe-t-elle dans l'Islam?" *Studia Islamica*, vol. 31 (1970), pp. 29-40.

[47] See above, chap. iv, part B.

[48] See A. Parry, "The Language of Thucydides' Description of the Plague," *Institute of Classical Studies, Bulletin* (University of London), no. 16 (1969), pp. 106-118.

the more popular belief in jinn and the veneration of saints, a relatively successful defense against natural anxiety and guilt for having survived the death of others: a stereotype of submission to divine order. The sense of reverent resignation pervades the accounts of the popular Muslim reaction to plague epidemics through the nineteenth century.[49]

The Muslim responses were not entirely external; the wellspring of communal activity was the personal conviction of resignation to divine order. The responses were thus *both* individual and communal; the descriptions of individual piety that took the forms of ritual purity and participation in organized religious services are proof of the unity of religious belief. If the communal activity in the urban centers has been stressed, it is because of the common emphasis that has too often been placed on the Muslims' individual means of defense and the fragmentary nature of the Islamic city.[50]

It may rightly be asked whether we can really explain the apparently pacific, collective, and controlled Muslim reaction to the Black Death as largely the result of theoretical theological principles. There is good reason to believe that we can. The essential link between theory and practice was the communal leadership of the *'ulamā'*, who were not only the religious élite but also the social and administrative élite in the late medieval Muslim city.[51] It is instructive that, unlike contemporary European treatises,[52] the Muslim tracts are the work not primarily of physicians, but of this communal élite. The Muslim and Christian treatises testify to a further contrast in the intellectual authority of the two religious establishments over their

[49] For a further example, see Lane, *Arabian Society in the Middle Ages*, pp. 88-92.

[50] Albert Hourani, "Introduction: The Islamic City in the Light of New Research," *The Islamic City*, ed. by A. H. Hourani and S. M. Stern (Oxford, 1970), pp. 13, 24.

[51] See the excellent sociological description of the *'ulamā'* during the Mamlūk Period in *Muslim Cities*, pp. 107-115, 130-142; see also Hodgson, "Islām and Image," pp. 232-233, 236.

[52] See Campbell, pp. 6-92.

societies during a period of crisis. On the whole, we are struck by the fact that the interpretations and arguments of the Muslim jurists take fuller cognizance of the beliefs and practices of their community than do those of the European treatise writers.[53] For example, the latter are almost entirely silent about the persecution of the Jews[54] and the flagellant movement. The *'ulamā'* in Muslim society were able to formulate normative attitudes and to guide the popular reaction toward the Black Death.

In this regard, the sixteenth-century plague treatise of the Ottoman jurist Ṭāshköprüzāde is particularly instructive. In his discussion of the question of flight from a plague epidemic, he states, as usual, that changing the air is most desirable during a plague epidemic because of the common belief in plague miasma; the author recommends that one should go to a place where the disease is ordinarily not to be expected. Due consideration must be given to certain conditions, however, such as not violating the requirements of civil responsibilities (*al-ḥuqūq al-madanīyah*) or the social ties within the family. Further, obedience to the decision of the communal leader (*mukhtār*) with regard to moving away or remaining must be preserved. Flight may not be possible because (1) the epidemic is universal; (2) the plague victims would be neglected; or (3) the commonweal must be preserved from disruption and disorder. In this case the people are simply to remain and

[53] A careful scrutiny of the legal treatises of the *'ulamā'* demonstrates the active application of Muslim scholarship to the problems arising from a plague-stricken community. For this reason, I take strong exception to von Kremer's interpretation of the Muslim treatises as proof of the decadent intellectual rigidity of late medieval Islam ("Ueber die grossen Seuchen," pp. 94-98). Von Kremer disregards the contemporary European views of plague and the fact that similar questions were being posed. The clerics of the Reformation, most notably Martin Luther, argue whether a Christian should flee from plague or whether his duty was to remain and trust in God.

[54] S. Guerchberg, "La Controverse sur les prétendus semeurs de la Peste Noire d'après les traités de peste de l'époque," *Revue des Études Juives*, n. s., vol. 8 (1948), pp. 3-40.

improve their circumstances by cleaning their houses and fumigating them with various scents and fresh fruits.[55]

Ṭāshköprüzāde's prescriptions for a Muslim community at the time of a plague epidemic bring into focus the contrasting orientations of the two religions. The Black Death affected the central theme of Christian teaching concerning evil and human suffering; Western man took the plague epidemic as an individual trial more than a collective social calamity. The Islamic tradition, however, has not concerned itself to the same degree with personal suffering; the central problem for the Muslim is the solemn responsibility for his decisions that affect other men's lives and fortunes within a purposeful creation.[56] The cosmic settings of the two faiths are wide apart in their emphasis: where the Muslim's primary duty was toward the correct behavior of the total community based on the sacred law, the Christian's was with personal salvation—resignation as opposed to redemption. For the Muslim, the Black Death was part of a God-ordered, natural universe; for the Christian, it was an irruption of the profane world of sin and excruciating punishment. It is indicative of something important in both the mind and the nature of Western culture that the dominant image in the history of European civilization has been that of a crucifixion. Orthodox Islam has no such central image.

In sum, it would be as great an error to discount the religious interpretations of plague as motives and limits to communal behavior as to discount the classical medical theories, which so clearly explain another level of defensive behavior. Taken together, the medieval Christian ideas of millennialism, militancy toward alien communities, punishment and guilt are raised to crucial significance in contrast to the Muslim understanding of the Black Death. The operative European Christian concepts were lacking in Muslim society, as

[55] Ṭāshköprüzāde, fol. 34a.

[56] M.G.S. Hodgson, "A Comparison of Islām and Christianity as Framework for Religious Life," *Diogenes*, no. 32 (1960), p. 70. See also Huston Smith's preface to S. H. Nasr, *Ideals and Realities of Islam* (Boston, 1972), p. 11.

were their unattractive consequences of religious fanaticism, persecution, and desperation. The predominant theological views of the two societies set the framework for normative attitudes and the prescriptions for communal behavior in which human nature found expression and form when confronted by the Black Death.

It is possible to describe and explain a generalized Muslim response to plague because the Arabic chroniclers of the Black Death have given us vivid descriptions of social behavior. On the other hand, they furnish us with no estimates of total population and only imprecise and exaggerated mortality figures. The mortality figures, even when they are reasonably reliable, are used merely to reinforce the general impression of severe crisis and, as a secondary descriptive device, putting the cause of the calamity after the effects and interpreting the cause by means of its results.

The reasons for the non-statistical attitude of the medieval chronicler—which sets him so far apart from the modern social scientist—are the lack of data and, more important perhaps, a lack of interest in the figures. In the first instance, precise mortality figures were meaningless for the chroniclers, as they are for us, when they cannot be correlated to total population. Second, there seems to have been a cultural aversion to numbering the faithful, which may be derived from a strictly religious attitude (also found in Judaism) and best illustrated by the familiar Biblical story of God's punishment—by plague?—of David for counting the Israelites. The aversion may also be due to superstitious fear, as observed by Volney[57] and others in the Middle East and North Africa. In any case, the late medieval Muslim descriptions of plague epidemics, and particularly the Black Death, emerge as documents without measurements. To make an architectural comparison, they are like the ancient Egyptian method of building self-supporting vaults without centering.[58]

Yet the medieval historians of the Black Death used their

[57] *Voyages*, p. 134.

[58] Fathy, *Architecture for the Poor*, pp. 6-10.

natural descriptive talents to narrate the cataclysmic nature of the event, and there can be little doubt that they achieved their purpose. In general, medieval chroniclers in both the Orient and the Occident were supremely aware of such natural disasters and devoted particular attention to them. What could be more understandable than to recount the events that touched everyone's lives and livelihoods most directly and profoundly?

Even if we did possess accurate mortality records, the statistics would still have to be translated into recognizable descriptions, like those of our medieval chroniclers, to convey the effect of the plague epidemics on human society. An account of the social responses in terms of the society's cultural values and practices is a legitimate reflection of imposed change, while the exact degree of depopulation is irretrievable. Equally, the repercussions of plague epidemics can be seen in the disruption and decline of the Egyptian and Syrian economies in the late fourteenth and the fifteenth centuries.

While we can confidently assert that plague was not endemic to Egypt and Syria for a substantial period before the Black Death, the pandemic initiated a series of plague epidemics that contributed to a marked decline in Middle Eastern population from the middle of the fourteenth century. What must be emphasized is that this decline was continual in large part because of the recurrence of severe epidemics that included pneumonic plague. This decrease in population was the essential phenomenon of the social and economic life of Egypt and Syria in the later Middle Ages.

APPENDICES

APPENDIX ONE
Recurrences of Plague in the Period Subsequent to the Black Death: 750-922/1349-1517

A number of medieval and modern works give chronologies of natural disasters, including plague, in the Middle East and North Africa.[1] The following compilation of data is taken mostly from primary sources and is strictly confined to citations for possible plague (*ṭāʿūn*) epidemics from the time of the Black Death to the Ottoman conquest of the Middle East in 922/1517. The source citations are not exhaustive.

Date (A.H.)	*Location*	*Sources*
761-762	Egypt	*Dafʿ an-niqmah*, fols. 76a, 83a-86a; *an-Nujūm*, Cairo ed., vol. 10, p. 311: "al-wabāʾ al-wasaṭī."
	Morocco	Ibn al-Khaṭīb, *Nufāḍat al-jirāb*, quoted in at-Tiṭuānī, *Ibn al-Khaṭīb min khilāl kutubihi*, vol. 1, p. 128.

[1] See: (1) Hautecoeur and Wiet, *Les Mosquées du Caire*, vol. 1, pp. 81-82; (2) "The Plague and Its Effects," p. 67, n. 1; (3) Wiet, "Le Traité des famines de Maqrīzī," pp. 1-90; (4) as-Suyūṭī, *Husn al-muḥāḍarah*, vol. 2, pp. 274-310; (5) Ḥasan Ḥabishī, "al-Iḥtikār al-mamlūkī wa ʿalāqatuhu bil-ḥālah aṣ-ṣiḥḥīyah," *Bulletin of the Faculty of Arts*, ʿAyn Shams University, Cairo (1959), pp. 155-156; (6) Guyon, *Histoire Chronologique*, pp. 174-205, particularly p. 200 for dates of plague recurrences in Spain during the fifteenth century; (7) "Ueber die grossen Seuchen," pp. 107-143; (8) Sticker, *Abhandlungen*, vol. 1, pp. 24-100, 108-127, 161-174, 209-350, vol. 2, pp. 83-85 (unfortunately, Sticker relies exclusively on von Kremer for the medieval Near East; however, his chronology offers a convenient correlation with possible European plague occurrences); (9) Darrag, p. 59; (10) Ashtor, *Histoire*, p. 272; (11) Marchika, *La Peste en Afrique Septentrionale*, pp. 21-186; and (12) Bloch, *La Peste en Tunisie*, pp. 1-13.

Date (A.H.)	*Location*	*Sources*
764	Egypt & Syria	*as-Sulūk*, part 3, vol. 1, pp. 81-82; *al-Bidāyah*, vol. 14, p. 312; *an-Nujūm*, Cairo ed., vol. 11, p. 17; *Badhl*, fols. 123b, 130a; *Mā rawāhu l-wā'ūn*, p. 155; *Daf' an-niqmah*, fols. 76a, 86b; *Durrat al-aslāk*, ed. Meursinge and Weijers, *Orientalia*, vol. 2, p. 412; al-Manbijī, *Fī akhbār aṭ-ṭā'ūn*, Dār al-Kutub al-Miṣrīyah MS no. 16 *ṭibb Ḥalīm*, fols. 152-231; adh-Dhahabī and al-Ḥusaynī, *Min dhuyūl al-'ibar*, p. 362. A.D. 1363: Frescobaldi, Gucci and Sigoli, *Visit to the Holy Places*, p. 172; Makhairos, *Recital*, vol. 1, pp. 118-121.
765	Syria	*as-Sulūk*, part 3, vol. 1, p. 92.
	Tlemcen	Ibn Khaldūn, *Histoire des Berbères*, vol. 3, p. 447.
	Astrakhan	A.D. 1364: Wu Lien-Teh, "The Original Home of Plague," p. 299.
771	Syria	*Badhl*, fol. 123b; *Mā rawāhu l-wā'ūn*, p. 155; *Durrat al-aslāk*, ed. by Meursinge and Weijers, *Orientalia*, vol. 2, p. 426.
774	Syria	*Kunūz adh-dhahab*, vol. 2, p. 11; *Durrat al-aslāk*, ed. by Meursinge and Weijers, *Orientalia*, vol. 2, p. 432; *as-Sulūk*, part 3, vol. 1, p. 202.
775-776[2]	Egypt & Syria	775 A.H.: *as-Sulūk*, part 3, vol. 1, p. 226; *Durrat al-aslāk*, ed. by Meursinge and Weijers, *Orientalia*, vol. 2, p. 434. A.H. 776: *as-Sulūk*, part 3, vol. 1, pp. 233-234,

[2] There remains some doubt whether this was an epidemic of plague; further investigation should clarify the issue.

Date (A.H.)	*Location*	*Sources*
		236, 239; *an-Nujūm*, Cairo ed., vol. 11, p. 66; Ibn Ḥajar, *Inbā' al-ghumr*, vol. 1, p. 72; Wiet, "Le Traité des famines," pp. 42-43.
	Mardin	Cahen, "Contribution à l'histoire du Diyār Bakr," p. 82 and n. 4.
	Manbij	al-Manbijī, *Tasliyat ahl al-maṣā'ib fī maut al-awlād wal-aqārib*, p. 3.
	Greater Armenia	Sanjian, *Colophons*, p. 99.
778-779[3]	Egypt	*as-Sulūk*, part 3, vol. 1, pp. 295, 326.
781	Egypt	*as-Sulūk*, part 3, vol. 1, p. 374; *Badhl*, fol. 123b; *Mā rawāhu l-wā'ūn*, p. 155; *an-Nujūm*, Cairo ed., vol. 11, pp. 202, 275.
782-783	Egypt & Syria	Ibn Ḥajar, *Inbā' al-ghumr*, vol. 1, p. 219 (Shawwāl-Dhū l-Ḥijjah 782 to Muḥarram-Rabī' I, 783 A.H.); *as-Sulūk*, part 2, vol. 1, pp. 402, 409, vol. 2, pp. 440-441, 460; *Durrat al-aslāk*, ed. by Meursinge and Weijers, *Orientalia*, vol. 2, pp. 453-454. A.D. 1381: Frescobaldi, Gucci and Sigoli, *Visit to the Holy Places*, p. 100.[4]
786	Greater Armenia	Sanjian, *Colophons*, p. 101.
787	Aleppo	Ibn Qāḍī Shuhbah, *adh-Dhayl 'alā ta'rīkh al-islām*, Paris MS Ar. no. 1599, fols. 9a, 10b; *Kunūz adh-dhahab*, vol. 2, p. 11; *Durrat al-aslāk*, ed. by Meursinge and Weijers, *Orientalia*, vol. 2, p. 464.

[3] Again, there is uncertainty whether it was a plague epidemic.

[4] I have interpreted the passage of Gucci as follows: "And we heard in the said Cairo an extraordinary thing, better indeed left unsaid, that in the plague of which we spoke of LXXXXIII [A.D. 1383] in Italy, which raged in Cairo two years before [1381/782-783], they say there were many days in which in Cairo over thirty thousand persons died a day."

Date (A.H.)	*Location*	*Sources*
788	Alexandria	Ibn Ḥajar, *Inbā' al-ghumr*, vol. 1, pp. 315, 329; al-Jawharī, *Nuzhat an-nufūs*, vol. 1, p. 131; *as-Sulūk*, part 3, vol. 2, p. 544; *Durrat al-aslāk*, ed. by Meursinge and Weijers, *Orientalia*, vol. 2, p. 464.
790	Egypt	Ibn Ḥajar, *Inbā' al-ghumr*, vol. 1, pp. 350, 353-354; *an-Nujūm*, Popper trans., vol. 13, p. 19; Ibn al-Furāt, *Ta'rīkh*, vol. 9, pp. 26-31; al-Jawharī, *Nuzhat an-nufūs*, vol. 1, pp. 168, 170, 172; *as-Sulūk*, part 3, vol. 2, pp. 575, 577-578, 580.
791	Egypt	*as-Sulūk*, part 3, vol. 2, pp. 600, 608, 683-687; al-Jawharī, *Nuzhat an-nufūs*, vol. 1, pp. 201-202, 274, 276, 278; *Badhl*, fol. 123b; *Mā rawāhu l-wā'ūn*, p. 155; *an-Nujūm*, Popper trans., vol. 13, pp. 28, 33, 105-106.
795	Syria & Alexandria	Ibn Qāḍī Shuhbah, *adh-Dhayl*, fol. 90a; Ibn Ṣaṣrā, *ad-Durrah al-muḍī'ah*, vol. 1, pp. 182-183, vol. 2, p. 137.
796	Tunis	Brunschvig, *La Berbérie Orientale*, vol. 2, p. 374.
795-796/1393	Cyprus	Makhairos, *Recital*, pp. 610-613.
800	Golden Horde & Eastern Mediterranean	Sticker, *Abhandlungen*, vol. 1, p. 81. A.D. 1398; Setton, ed., *A History of the Crusades*, vol. 3, p. 262.[5]
	Egypt	al-Jawharī, *Nuzhat an-nufūs*, vol. 1, p. 472; *as-Sulūk*, part 3, vol. 2, pp. 891-892.

[5] In 1398 "a serious plague was sweeping through the Morea and Crete, the sixth great pestilence to strike the Morea and the islands since the Black Death of 1348."

Date (A.H.)	*Location*	*Sources*
806	Egypt	Ibn Ḥajar, *Inbāʾ al-ghumr*, vol. 2, p. 260; *an-Nujūm*, Popper trans., vol. 14, p. 80; *al-Khiṭaṭ*, vol. 1, pp. 236-237; *as-Sulūk*, part 3, vol. 3, pp. 1124-1126.
808	Egypt, esp. Upper Egypt	*as-Sulūk*, part 4, vol. 1, pp. 6, 19-20; *an-Nujūm*, Popper trans., vol. 14, p. 128.
809	Egypt	*an-Nujūm*, Popper trans., vol. 14, p. 133; Ibn Ḥajar, *Inbāʾ al-ghumr*, vol. 2, pp. 360, 361, 368; *as-Sulūk*, part 4, vol. 1, pp. 42-43.
812	Syria	Ibn Ḥajar, *Inbāʾ al-ghumr*, vol. 2, p. 430; *an-Nujūm*, Popper trans., vol. 14, p. 148; *as-Sulūk*, part 4, vol. 1, p. 98.
	Cyprus	A.D. 1410: Makhairos, *Recital*, pp. 622-623.
813	Syria	Ibn Ḥajar, *Inbāʾ al-ghumr*, vol. 2, pp. 459, 463, 466; *an-Nujūm*, Popper trans., vol. 14, p. 169; *Badhl*, fol. 123b; *Mā rawāhu l-wāʿūn*, p. 155; *as-Sulūk*, part 4, vol. 1, pp. 132, 150, 165.
814	Syria	Ibn Ḥajar, *Inbāʾ al-ghumr*, vol. 2, pp. 482, 503; *an-Nujūm*, Popper trans., vol. 14, pp. 178, 198; *as-Sulūk*, part 4, vol. 1, p. 179.
817-818	Fez	Ibn Ḥajar, *Inbāʾ al-ghumr*, vol. 3, pp. 40, 41, 45; *as-Sulūk*, part 4, vol. 1, pp. 291-292, 351.
818	Egypt	*an-Nujūm*, Popper trans., vol. 17, p. 30; Ibn Ḥajar, *Inbāʾ al-ghumr*, vol. 3, p. 53; *as-Sulūk*, part 4, vol. 1, pp. 301, 310, 312.
819	Egypt & Syria	Ibn Ḥajar, *Inbāʾ al-ghumr*, vol. 3, pp. 87 (mentions Fez and Isfahan), 106-107, 111, 113, 115, 117-119, 121-122, 124; *an-Nujūm*, Pop-

Date (A.H.)	*Location*	*Sources*
		per trans., vol. 17, p. 40; *as-Sulūk*, part 4, vol. 1, pp. 344, 347-349, 351, 358, 362; *Badhl*, fol. 123b; *Mā rawāhu l-wā'ūn*, p. 155; al-Jawharī, *Nuzhat an-nufūs*, vol. 2, pp. 363, 368-369, 374-376, 379-380.
820	Egypt	Ibn Ḥajar, *Inbā' al-ghumr*, vol. 3, p. 139; *as-Sulūk*, part 4, vol. 1, pp. 388, 394.
822	Egypt	*an-Nujūm*, Popper trans., vol. 17, pp. 64-67; *Badhl*, fol. 123b (gives the years A.H. 821-822); *Mā rawāhu l-wā'ūn*, p. 156; Ibn Ḥajar, *Inbā' al-ghumr*, vol. 3, pp. 198-200, 207, 209; *as-Sulūk*, part 4, vol. 1, pp. 481, 483, 486-490; al-Jawharī, *Nuzhat an-nufūs*, vol. 2, pp. 442, 455-456, 459.
825	Syria	*an-Nujūm*, Popper trans., vol. 18, pp. 5, 9; *Kunūz adh-dhahab*, vol. 2, pp. 11-12; Ibn Ḥajar, *Inbā' al-ghumr*, vol. 3, pp. 282, 287, 294.
826	Egypt & Syria	*an-Nujūm*, Popper trans., vol. 18, p. 9; Sauvaget, "Décrets Mamelouks de Syrie," pp. 11-15; Ibn Ḥajar, *Inbā' al-ghumr*, vol. 3, pp. 304, 310, 312, 321-322.
832-833	Egypt, Syria, Asia & Europe	*an-Nujūm*, Popper trans., vol. 17, p. 171, vol. 18, pp. 69-77, 181-189; Ibn Iyās, vol. 2, pp. 18-19; Khalīl aẓ-Ẓāhirī, *Kitāb zubda kashf al-mamālik*, p. 112; *Badhl*, fol. 123b; *Mā rawāhu l-wā'ūn*, p. 156; Ibn Ḥajar, *Inbā' al-ghumr*, vol. 3, pp. 289-290, 435, 437-439, 441-453; al-Mu'minī, *Kitāb al-futūḥ*, vol. 2, p. 296; *as-Sulūk*, part 4, vol. 2, pp. 819, 821-822, 824-830, 836-837, 846, 848.

Date (A.H.)	Location	Sources
838	Harāt	'Abdallāh ibn 'Abd ar-Raḥmān al-Ḥusaynī, *Risālat-yi mazārāt-i Harāt*, ed. by F. Saljūqī (Kābul, 1967), part 1, pp. 87ff (nos. 180, 182-188); *EI*[1]: "Shāh Rukh Mīrzā"; A. C. Barbier de Meynard, "Extraits de la Chronique Persane d'Herat," *JA*, series 5, vol. 20, pp. 274-277: Rajab 7-Dhū l-Qa'dah 15.
	Astarābād	E. G. Browne, *A History of Persian Literature* (Cambridge, 1920), vol. 3, p. 488.
839	Abyssinia	Ibn Ḥajar, *Inbā' al-ghumr*, Add. MS no. 7321, fol. 293a.
841	Egypt, Syria & Iraq	Ibn Ḥajar, *Inbā' al-ghumr*, Add. MS no. 7321, fols. 332a-332b; *Badhl*, fol. 124a; *Mā rawāhu l-wā'ūn*, p. 156; *an-Nujūm*, Popper trans., vol. 18, pp. 144-147, 149-156, 210-217; Ibn Iyās, vol. 2, p. 21; *as-Sulūk*, part 4, vol. 2, pp. 1025, 1027-1029, 1031-1035, 1038, 1040-1048, vol. 3, pp. 1057, 1060.
842	Egypt & Yemen	*as-Sulūk*, part 4, vol. 3, pp. 1126-1127, 1147; Ibn Ḥajar, *Inbā' al-ghumr*, Add. MS no. 7321, fol. 341a.
	Cyprus	A.D. 1438: Makhairos, *Recital*, pp. 682-683.
847-848[6]	Egypt	*Badhl*, fol. 124a; Ibn Ḥajar, *Inbā' al-ghumr*, Add. MS no. 7321, fol. 365a; *an-Nujūm*, Popper trans., vol. 19, pp. 92-93, 216; Ibn Taghrī Birdī, *Ḥawādith*, ed. by Popper, vol. 8, p. 11; as-Sakhāwī, *at-Tibr al-masbūk*, pp. 76, 87.

[6] In 846-847/1443, Sticker reports an epidemic of plague (*tā'ūn*) in central India (*Abhandlungen*, vol. 1, p. 83).

Date (A.H.)	*Location*	*Sources*
849-850	Egypt	"Ueber die grossen Seuchen," p. 139 (p. 142 refers to the MS now in the British Museum, Or. MS no. 3026—Rieu, *Supplement,* no. 559).
852-853	Egypt	*an-Nujūm*, Popper trans., vol. 19, pp. 111, 113-115, 213; *Mā rawāhu l-wā'ūn*, p. 156; Ibn Iyās, vol. 2, p. 32; as-Sakhāwī, *at-Tibr al-masbūk*, pp. 221, 253-255.
858-859	Egypt	Ibn Taghrī Birdī, *Ḥawādith*, pp. 206, 224, 228, 230; Ibn Iyās, vol. 2, pp. 48-49.
863-864	Egypt & Syria	*an-Nujūm*, Popper trans., vol. 22, pp. 84, 87, 88, 90, 92-100; Ibn Taghrī Birdī, *Ḥawādith*, pp. 331, 332, 334-338; *Mā rawāhu l-wā'ūn*, p. 156; Ibn Iyās, vol. 2, p. 64; *Unpublished Pages of the Chronicle of Ibn Iyās*, ed. by M. Mostafa (Cairo, 1951), pp. 63, 66, 69-71, 73, 78.
865	Cyprus	*Unpublished Pages of the Chronicle of Ibn Iyās*, p. 80; cf. *an-Nujūm*, Popper trans., vol. 22, p. 104.
868	Harāt	Barbier de Meynard, "Extraits de la Chronique Persane d'Herat," p. 316.
871	Tlemcen	Marchika, *La Peste en Afrique*, pp. 21-22.
873	Egypt & Syria	al-'Ulaymī, *al-Uns al-jalīl*, vol. 2, p. 286; *Mā rawāhu l-wā'ūn*, p. 156; Ibn Taghrī Birdī, *Ḥawādith*, pp. 687-688, 699; Ibn Iyās, *Badā'i' az-zuhūr*, Mostafa rev. ed., vol. 5c, pp. 18, 21, 26, 28-31; al-Jawharī, *Inbā' al-haṣr bi-abnā' al-aṣr*, pp. 12, 31-32, 46, 55-56, 58-61, 64, 79, 84, 90.

Date (A.H.)	Location	Sources
	Tunisia	Ibn Abī Dīnār, *al-Mu'nis* (Tunis ed.), p. 158 (Pellisier trans., p. 265); see Brunschvig, *Le Berbérie Orientale*, vol. 2, p. 374 for the severe plague in North Africa in A.D. 1468-1469; Bloch, *La Peste en Tunisie*, p. 3.
881-882[7]	Egypt	Ibn Iyās, *Badā'i' az-zuhūr*, Mostafa rev. ed., vol. 5c, pp. 122-125; *Mā rawāhu l-wā'ūn*, p. 156; Shihāb al-Manṣūrī, Dār al-Kutub al-Miṣrīyah MS no. 102 *majāmī' m*, fol. 201a.
	Syria	al-'Ulaymī, *al-Uns al-jalīl*, vol. 2, p. 318.
892-893	Tabrīz	Minorsky, *Persia in* A.D. *1478-1490*, pp. 56, 87; see also pp. 107-109 for the fear of plague in Tabrīz in A.H. 895.
897-898	Egypt & Syria	al-'Ulaymī, *al-Uns al-jalīl*, vol. 2, p. 360; *Mā rawāhu l-wā'ūn*, p. 156 (plague was in Rūm in A.H. 896 and entered Aleppo at the beginning of A.H. 897 and then Egypt); Shihāb al-Manṣūrī, Dār al-Kutub al-Miṣrīyah MS no. 102 *majāmī' m*, fols. 201a-215b; Ibn Iyās, *Badā'i' az-zuhūr*, Mostafa rev. ed., vol. 5c, pp. 286-292, 294. A.D. 1497-1498 in Syria: Sanuto, *I Diarii*, tome 1, col. 756, 845, 914; Priuli, *I Diarii*, tome 24, part 3, vol. 1, p. 71; for Egypt: Sanuto, *I Diarii*, vol. 1, cols. 994, 1032-1033, vol. 2, col. 1043.
899	Tunisia	Bloch, *La Peste en Tunisie*, p. 3; Ibn Abī Dīnār, *al-Mu'nis* (Tunis

[7] The plague epidemic is reported in Majorca in 879-880/1475, having come from the Levant (Guyon, *Histoire Chronologique*, p. 197).

Date (A.H.)	*Location*	*Sources*
		ed.), p. 159 (Pellisier trans., pp. 266-267).
903	Syria	Priuli, *I Diarii*, tome 24, part 3, vol. 1, p. 71; Sanuto, *I Diarii*, vol. 1, col. 856.
905-906	Tlemcen	Marchika, *La Peste en Afrique*, pp. 22-23 (A.D. 1500).
	Jirbah (Tunisia)	Bloch, *La Peste en Tunisie*, p. 3.
909	Egypt	*Mā rawāhu l-wā'ūn*, p. 156; noted by Leclerc, *Histoire de la médecine arabe*, vol. 2, p. 298; Ibn Iyās, *Badā'i' az-zuhūr*, Mostafa rev. ed., vol. 5d, pp. 64-65, 302.
910	Egypt	Ibn Iyās, *Badā'i' az-zuhūr*, Mostafa rev. ed., vol. 5d, pp. 75-77, 79.
912	Upper Egypt	Ibn Iyās, *Badā'i' az-zuhūr*, Mostafa rev. ed., vol. 5d, p. 109.
914-915	Oran	Marchika, *La Peste en Afrique*, p. 23 (A.D. 1509).
915-916	Bourgie	Marchika, *La Peste en Afrique*, pp. 23-24 (A.D. 1510).
918-919[8]	Egypt	Ibn Iyās, *Badā'i' az-zuhūr*, Mostafa rev. ed., vol. 5d, pp. 295-299, 301-304, 306-310, 312, 320, 357; Sanuto, *I Diarii*, vol. 16, col. 649.
	Syria	Sanuto, *I Diarii*, vol. 17, col. 155, vol. 18, col. 155.

[8] Ibn Iyās, *Badā'i' az-zuhūr*, Mostafa rev. ed., vol. 5d, apparently refers to a brief epidemic in Sharqīyah province in A.H. 920, but the epidemic did not spread to the rest of the country.

APPENDIX TWO
The Arabic Terminology for Plague

The common designation of *plague* in Arabic is *ṭāʿūn* (pl. *ṭawāʿīn*).[1] It is derived from the verb *ṭaʿana*, which has the general meaning of "to strike" or "to pierce."[2] Similarly, most Hebrew words for plague indicate a blow or thrust. Our English word *plague* and the German *plage* are derived from the Latin *plaga*; originally, *plaga* meant a wound or sudden stroke, being derived from *plangere*, "to strike." The French *fléau*, "a flail" or "a plague," embodies the same idea of striking, taken from the Latin *flagellum*. The more commonly used terms *peste* in French and *pest* in German come from the Latin *pestis* meaning a deadly disease, possibly derived from *perdere*, "to ruin."

Although *ṭāʿūn* may have the generic sense of "an epidemic," it is used consistently in the late medieval Arabic texts in the specific sense of "a plague." Almost every plague treatise from the Black Death to the nineteenth century distinguishes between the general terminology for epidemic diseases and plague. The general term for "epidemic" or "pestilence" is *wabāʾ* or *wabaʾ*. The following statement, which is found in these treatises, makes the distinction clear: "Every *ṭāʿūn* is a *wabāʾ*, but not every *wabāʾ* is a *ṭāʿūn*."[3] Ibn Ḥajar al-ʿAsqalānī states that the designation of *ṭāʿūn* gives the sense of the "pricking" (*wakhz*) of the jinn,[4] while *wabāʾ*, *wajaʿ*, and *dāʾ*

[1] Lane, *An Arabic-English Lexicon*, pp. 1855-1856.

[2] *Badhl*, fol. 11b gives a full discussion of the etymology of *ṭāʿūn*. Ibn Sīnā correlates the Greek and Arabic terminology of plague in the *Qānūn*, vol. 3, p. 122.

[3] *Badhl*, fols. 12a, 14a, 15a; *Dafʿ an-niqmah*, fol. 41b; al-Ḥijāzī, *Juzʾ fī ṭ-ṭāʿūn*, fol. 148a; *Taḥṣīl*, fol. 87a, etc.

[4] Or *rimāḥ al-jinn* (see Lane, *An Arabic-English Lexicon*, p. 1856).

do not; the *wabā'* is more general than *ṭā'ūn*, whereas *waja'* and *dā'* designate pain from the *ṭā'ūn* or another illness.[5]

Despite these distinctions, these words and a number of others are used as synonyms for *plague* in the Arabic sources. In many cases it is difficult to determine whether an illness is plague without additional corroborative evidence. Particularly the word *wabā'* may refer to other epidemic diseases, such as typhus, typhoid, smallpox, etc. It would be unprofitable to cite the vast number of times that the words *wabā'* and *ṭā'ūn* are employed; however, the following designations for *plague* were also used during the Mamlūk Period.[6] This list is followed by a discussion of the terminology for the plague pustule and bubo from the same sources.

I. "PLAGUE"

1. *ṭa'n*: Ibn Iyās, vol. 2, pp. 18, 64; Mostafa rev. ed., vol. 5c, pp. 124-125, vol. 5d, pp. 79, 296, 299, 302, 306-307, 309-310, 312, 375; *Unpublished Pages of the Chronicle of Ibn Iyās*, ed. by Mostafa, pp. 71-73; *Mā rawāhu l-wā'ūn*, p. 146.

2. *faṣl*: Khalīl aẓ-Ẓāhirī, *Kitāb zubda kashf al-mamālik*, p. 112; Ibn Taghrī Birdī, *Ḥawārith*, Popper ed., p. 337; Ibn Iyās, vol. 2, p. 21; Mostafa rev. ed., vol. 5d, pp. 95, 289, 360; *an-Nujūm*, Cairo ed., vol. 10, p. 211.

3. *fanā'*: Ibn Ḥajar, *Inbā' al-ghumr*, vol. 1, p. 315; al-Jawharī, *Nuzhat an-nufūs*, vol. 1, p. 472; *an-Nujūm*, Cairo ed., vol. 10, p. 233, vol. 11, pp. 26, 66, 203; *al-Khiṭaṭ*, vol. 2, p. 637; *as-Sulūk*, part 2, vol. 3, pp. 779, 780; *Badhl*, fol. 45b; Ibn Iyās, vol. 2, p. 64; Mostafa rev. ed., vol. 5c, pp. 30, 37, 287, vol. 5d, p. 79.

4. *mautān*:[7] *as-Sulūk*, part 2, vol. 3, pp. 774, 777, part 3, vol.

[5] *Badhl*, fol. 16b.

[6] The following list incorporates the work on plague terminology found in "The Plague and Its Effects," p. 67, n. 2.

[7] In the *Kitāb adh-dhakhīrah* of Thābit ibn Qurrah (d. 288/901), plague is divided into three kinds: (1) *mautān*, a fatal epidemic; (2) *amrād wāfidah*, a moderate epidemic; and (3) *amrāḍ baladīyah*, a

2, p. 577, part 4, vol. 1, pp. 347ff; *Mā rawāhu l-wāʿūn,* p. 147; *Badhl*, fols. 25a (where the author compares *quʿās* as murrain plague to *mautān* in men), 100a; aṭ-Ṭabarī, *Taʾrīkh*, Cairo ed., vol. 4, p. 63.

5. *maut*: *an-Nujūm*, Cairo ed., vol. 10, pp. 196, 197, 199, 200, 201, 203; *as-Sulūk*, part 2, vol. 3, pp. 774-775, 777, 778; al-Jawharī, *Nuzhat an-nufūs*, vol. 1, p. 170; Ibn Iyās, Mostafa rev. ed., vol. 5c, pp. 290-291.

6. *dāʾ*: *as-Sulūk*, part 2, vol. 3, pp. 777, 781, 791; *al-Bidāyah* vol. 14, p. 226; *Badhl*, fols. 12b, 77a; *an-Nujūm*, Cairo ed., vol. 10, p. 200.

7. *balāʾ*: *al-Bidāyah*, vol. 14, p. 225; *Dafʿ an-niqmah*, fols. 3a-4a; al-Ḥijāzī, *Juzʾ fī ṭ-ṭāʿūn*, fol. 148b; *Badhl*, fols. 99b, 103b.

8. *al-maraḍ al-wābil*: Ibn Haydūr, *Risālah fī l-amrāḍ*, fol. 100a. Also *al-amrāḍ ad-damawīyah*: *Dafʿ an-niqmah*, fol. 64b; *amrāḍ aṭ-ṭawāʿīn*: *al-Bidāyah*, vol. 14, p. 226; and *al-maraḍ al-wāfid*: *Taḥṣīl*, fol. 49a.

9. *al-kharāb*: *as-Sulūk*, part 4, vol. 1, pp. 486-490.

10. *al-āfah*: Ṭāshköprüzāde, fol. 42b.

There is a medical distinction between the plague buboes and the pustules or cutaneous marks[8] on the body of the plague victim. Very rarely are these two symptoms clearly distinguished by contemporary observers; Ibn Khātimah is the only writer who gives a detailed clinical description of the pustules of the skin.[9] Before death, "earthy" stains or blotches appeared on the body—including reddish to black marks—and were caused by subcutaneous hemorrhaging. The pustules (*qurūḥ*) are described as distinct from the buboes (*ṭawāʿīn*);[10] the latter term for the plague boils is infrequent in the later Middle Ages

---

plague epidemic that is endemic to one region. The same classification is found in *Kitāb al-malakī* by al-Majūsī, vol. 1, p. 168, vol. 2, p. 62. See Ullmann, p. 245, for al-Majūsī's classification.

[8] *Hirst*, p. 33.

[9] *Taḥṣīl*, fol. 82a.

[10] *Ibid.*, fol. 74a.

although it is common in the early Arabic sources. The former, *qurūḥ*, is encountered frequently in the Middle Eastern treatises.[11] Ibn Khātimah states that the pustules resembled blistering (*tafqī'*) accompanied by inflammation.[12] The author also refers to dark spots (*dharrah sūd*), which resemble grains (*ḥubūb*) and exude watery fluid when broken.[13]

However, Ibn Khātimah cites an earlier source (Ibn 'Ayyād), where *qurūḥ* is used in a generic sense: "The origin of the plague is the *qurūḥ* arising in the body."[14] This lack of distinction between the glandular buboes and the cutaneous pustules is found in most of the other Arabic texts. For example, Ibn Ḥajar cites a commentary on Abū Muslim, where the pustules and buboes (*bathr wa waram*) are interpreted as one general symptom of plague. As Ibn Ḥajar states: "They appear enflamed with blackening around them; they become green or red, the dark redness of a violet. . . . They appear in the groin and armpits but mostly on the hands and fingers and the rest of the body."[15] Nevertheless, the following terms are generally used during the Mamlūk Period for the two different symptoms.

II. "CUTANEOUS PUSTULE"

1. *ḥabbah*: the most common term for pustule, used particularly in the poetic descriptions of plague as in Ibn al-Wardī's *Risālat an-naba'* (see chapter v, part C, n. 15); *ḥabb* (collective): *Durrat al-aslāk*, p. 359; *ḥubaybah*: *as-Sulūk*, part 2, vol. 3, p. 791; *ḥubūb*: *Taḥṣīl*, fol. 82a.
2. *qurūḥ*: see discussion above and n. 11.
3. *bathrah*: *Badhl*, fols. 13a, 129a; *Durrat al-aslāk*, p. 358; al-Azhar MS no. 251, fol. 14b; *Risālat an-naba'*, p. 185; *as-Sulūk*, part 2, vol. 3, p. 775 uses the term specifically to de-

[11] *Qarḥ*: *Badhl*, fols. 11b, 15a, 119a; *qurūh*: *Badhl*, fol. 12a, and Ibn Abī Sharīf, *Kitāb fī aḥkām aṭ-ṭā'ūn*, fol. 157a. However, *qarhah* in *Badhl*, fols. 11b and 13a may refer to either bubo or pustule.

[12] *Taḥṣīl*, fol. 82a.

[13] *Ibid.*

[14] *Ibid.*, fol. 87a.

[15] *Badhl*, fol. 12b.

scribe the bubo behind the ear; *bathr* (collective): *Badhl*, fols. 12a-12b; al-Ḥijāzī, *Juz' fī ṭ-ṭā'ūn*, fol. 148b; *Daf' an-niqmah*, fol. 142b; *Durrat al-aslāk*, p. 358; Ibn Ḥajar describes it as a small boil (*dummal*) in *Badhl*, fol. 45a.

4. *ḥalā'*: *Daf' an-niqmah*, fol. 80b.
5. *ṭulū'*: *as-Sulūk*, part 2, vol. 3, p. 774.
6. *tafqī'*: *Taḥṣīl*, fol. 82a.
7. *nafāṭah*: Ibn al-Furāt, *Ta'rīkh*, vol. 9, p. 26.

III. "BUBO"

1. *kubbah*: *Badhl*, fol. 128a; *as-Sulūk*, part 2, vol. 3, p. 775 *et passim*; Ibn al-Furāt, *Ta'rīkh*, vol. 9, p. 26; aṣ-Ṣafadī, Dār al-Kutub al-Miṣrīyah MS no. 102 *majāmī' m*, fols. 199b, 200a.
2. *khurāj*: Ibn Abī Sharīf, *Kitāb fī aḥkām aṭ-ṭā'ūn*, fol. 160a; *Daf' an-niqmah*, fol. 75a; *Badhl*, fols. 16a, 116a, 119a, 127b; *al-awrām al-khurrājah*: ash-Shaqūrī, *Taḥqīq*, fol. 111a; *khurjān*: *Badhl*, fol. 76b margin, fol. 100b identifies the term as *khurāj ad-dummal*; *Muqni'at*, fols. 39b, 44b.
3. *waram*: Ibn Sīnā, *al-Qānūn*, vol. 3, p. 121; *Badhl*, fols. 12a-12b, 45a; *Daf' an-niqmah*, fol. 145a; *awrām*: ash-Shaqūrī, *Taḥqīq*, fol. 111a; al-Azhar MS no. 251, fol. 14b.
4. *dummal*: *Badhl*, fols. 45a, 77a, 78a, 100b.
5. *jaghalah*: Ibn Abī Ḥajalah gives this term as the designation of the bubo in Abyssinia (*Daf' an-niqmah*, fol. 145a).
6. *khazzah*: *Badhl*, fol. 77a.
7. *dharab*: *Badhl*, fols. 78a, 100b.
8. *ghuddah*: the term used for the bubo on camels, al-Azhar MS no. 251, fol. 17a: "Plague is a bubo like a *ghuddah* of the camel, appearing in the groin and axillae."; *Taḥṣīl*, fol. 87a; al-Majūsī, *Kitāb al-malakī*, vol. 1, p. 169.
9. *ṭawā'īn*: the term for plague boils found in the early Arabic translations of Hippocrates and Galen; for the Black Death, see *Taḥṣīl*, fols. 64b, 73a; *Muqni'at*, fol. 39b.
10. *khiyārah*: the bubo in the groin is frequently referred to as a "cucumber"; see *Durrat al-aslāk*, p. 358; *Badhl*, fol. 129a; aṣ-Ṣafadī, Dār al-Kutub al-Miṣrīyah MS no. 102 *majāmī' m*, fols. 99b, 200a.

APPENDIX THREE
The Arabic Manuscript Sources for the History of Plague from the Black Death to the Nineteenth Century

There has been no systematic study of the Arabic manuscript material dealing with the Black Death or its recurrences comparable to Karl Sudhoff's collection and publication of European *pestschriften* in his *Archiv für Geschichte der Medizin.* Four helpful bibliographical references are: (1) Labib, *Handelsgeschichte*, p. 418, n. 313; (2) Sarton, *Introduction*, vol. 3, part 2, pp. 1650-1652; (3) Ullmann, pp. 242-250; and (4) Rabie, *The Financial System of Egypt*, p. 69, n. 2. In no sense can these references be regarded as comprehensive discussions of the pertinent Arabic material. For this reason, I have attempted to give the fullest possible yet concise outline concerning these manuscript sources. These manuscripts include only those works devoted exclusively to plague; they deal with literary, medical, legal, and theological aspects of it. The material has been grouped chronologically, beginning with the manuscripts related to the Black Death in 1347-1349.

There are three major manuscript collections, containing selections of Arabic plague treatises assembled by copyists irrespective of chronology. They are: (1) Escorial MS no. 1785; (2) Dār al-Kutub al-Miṣrīyah MS no. 102 *majāmī' m*; and (3) Berlin MS no. 6380 (Ahlwardt). The last, which contained eleven treatises[1] dealing with plague, cannot be located by the Staatsbibliothek, Berlin, West Germany.[2]

[1] Although the manuscript is reportedly lost, it contained a very important collection of treatises; there are no other extant copies of some of these works. The summary of its contents is taken from W. Ahlwardt, *Verzeichnis der arabischen Handschriften der Königlichen*

Escorial MS no. 1785 (not no. 1780 as it is given in Casiri and Campbell)[3] contains three works devoted to the Black Death in southern Spain in 1348-1349. These works have been relatively well studied by European medievalists. The first treatise is *Taḥṣīl al-gharaḍ al-qāṣid fī tafṣīl al-maraḍ al-wāfid*,[4] written in February 1349 by Aḥmad ibn ʿAlī ibn Khātimah, a physician and poet of Almería.[5] In addition to a fragment published by M. J. Müller,[6] this work has been partly translated by Taha Dinānah: "Die Schrift von Abī Ǧaʿfar ibn Aḥmed ibn ʿAlī ibn Muḥammad ibn ʿAlī ibn Ḫātimah aus Almeriah über die Pest," in K. Sudhoff and H. E. Sigerist, *AGM*, vol. 19 (Leipzig, 1927), pp. 27-81.[7] Although the work

---

Bibliothek zu Berlin, vol. 17, p. 604: (1) Hippocrates, *al-Abīdhīmīan fī l-amrāḍ al-wāfidah*. This apparently refers to an Arabic translation of all or part of his *Epidemics*. (2) Ibn al-Khaṭīb, *al-Kalām ʿalā aṭ-ṭāʿūn al-muʿāṣir*. Probably this is a summary of his *Muqniʿat*. (3) ʿAbd al-Wāḥid al-Maghribī (d. ca 900/1594), *ʿIqd al-jumān fīmā yalzamu min walī al-bīmāristān*. (4) Tāj ad-Dīn as-Subkī, *Risālah fī ṭ-ṭāʿūn*. (5) Badr ad-Dīn az-Zarkashī (d. 794/1392), *Risālah fī t-ṭāʿūn*. (6) Yūsif ibn Hasan ibn ʿAbd al-Hādī (d. 909/1503), *Funūn al-manūn fī l-wabāʾ wat-ṭāʿūn* (not mentioned in *GAL*). (7) Muṣṭafā ibn Awhad ad-Dīn al-Yārhisārī, *Risālat al-wabāʾ wa jawāz al-firār minhu* (not mentioned in *GAL*). (8) Ibn Kamāl Pashā, *Rāḥat al-arwāh fī dafʿ ʿāhat al-ashbāḥ* (see below). (9) Aḥmad ibn Muṣṭafā Ṭāshköprüzāde, *Risālat ash-shifāʾ fī dawāʾ al-wabāʾ* (see below). (10) ʿAbd ar-Raʾūf al-Munāwī (d. 1031/1621), *Risālah minḥat at-ṭālibīn li-maʿrifah asrār aṭ-ṭawāʿīn* (not mentioned in *GAL*). And (11) ʿAbd ar-Raḥmān ibn Muṣṭafā al-Bisṭāmī, *Waṣf ad-dawāʾ fī kashf āfāt al-wabāʾ* (*GAL*, vol. 2, p. 232, no. 15).

[2] Communication of Dr. D. George, Staatsbibliothek, Preussischer Kulturbesitz, Orientalische Abteilung, September 23, 1970.

[3] See H. Derenbourg and E. Lévi-Provençal, *Les Manuscrits Arabs de l'Escurial* (Paris, 1884-1941), vol. 3, p. 283.

[4] Fols. 49a-105b; fols. 113a-115b of MS no. 1785 give a brief summary.

[5] *EI*[2]: "Ibn Khātimah" (S. Gilbert); *GAL*, vol. 2, p. 259, *Supplement*, vol. 2, p. 369; Sarton, *Introduction*, vol. 3, part 1, p. 896; Ullmann, pp. 246-247; Max Meyerhof, "Science and Medicine," *The Legacy of Islam*, p. 340.

[6] See below for Müller's study of Ibn al-Khaṭīb's plague treatise.

[7] See "The Twenty-Second Critical Bibliography," *Isis*, vol. 10, no. 33 (1928), pp. 131-132 (George Sarton).

is the fullest contemporary medical explanation of plague in Arabic (based on Hippocrates and Galen in part), the translation is misleading, giving the impression that it is entirely a medical work. The non-medical segment (fols. 83b-105b), the last third of the work, has simply been omitted from the translation. This final section, like the Middle Eastern tracts, includes an interpretation of *ḥadīths*, primarily the prohibition against entering or leaving a land that has been stricken by plague and the tenet that there is no infection. There is, also, a short history of plague epidemics (fols. 90b-92a), covering its occurrences in Spain before the Black Death, which the translation has omitted as well. The later plague treatises, prompted by the recurrences of plague, usually give similar accounts of the history of plagues in Islamic history up to their own time but with special attention to the Black Death. This faulty translation by Dinānah without the Arabic text severely misrepresents the intention of the author, who was a noted theologian as well as physician. Because of the importance of Ibn Khātimah's work and of Ibn al-Khaṭīb's (see below), references in this study are made to the manuscript pages rather than to the published translations.

The second Andalusian treatise is the work of Muḥammad ibn 'Abdallāh ibn al-Khaṭīb, an important scholar of Granada. The work is entitled *Muqniʿat as-sā'il 'an al-maraḍ al-hā'il* (Escorial MS no. 1785, fols. 39a-48b).[8] Ibn al-Khaṭīb, who was a friend of Ibn Khātimah, deals concisely with the Black Death in Granada from a medical point of view and then proceeds to make the famous claim for the idea of contagion.[9] The text has been edited by M. J. Müller in the *Sitzungsberichte der Königl. Bayerischen Akademie der Wissenschäften zu München* (Munich, 1863), part 2, pp. 1-34: "Ibnulkhaṭīb's Bericht über die Pest." The Arabic text is accompanied by a brief introduction and followed by an interpretation—not a translation—

[8] Fols. 111b-113a of MS no. 1785 give a summary of this work.

[9] See *EI*²: "Ibn al-Khaṭīb" (J. Bosch-Vilá); *GAL*, vol. 2, p. 262; Sarton, *Introduction*, vol. 3, part 2, pp. 1762-1764; Ullmann, pp. 179, 246; Meyerhof, "Science and Medicine," *The Legacy of Islam*, p. 340.

of the text. At the end of the interpretation is appended an excerpt from Ibn Khātimah's account of plague in Almería (Arabic text and translation, pp. 28-34), which does not appear in the original manuscript of Ibn al-Khaṭīb and only confuses the reader. Although the text of Ibn al-Khaṭīb is undated, it must have been written after Ibn Baṭṭūṭah's visit to Granada between A.H. 750 and 753,[10] since Ibn Baṭṭūṭah's account of plague in the East is given by Ibn al-Khaṭīb (fol. 43b). At-Tiṭuānī suggests that this plague treatise was written during Ibn al-Khaṭīb's exile in Morocco from 760 to 763/1359 to 1362.[11]

The third work is *Taḥqīq an-naba' 'an amr al-waba'* (Escorial MS no. 1785, fols. 106a-111a) by Muḥammad ibn 'Alī ash-Shaqūrī, a physician of Granada and a student of Ibn al-Khaṭīb.[12] A copy of this manuscript by the Spanish orientalist F. J. Simonet exists in the Biblioteca Nacional de Madrid. The tract is generally a "layman's guide" to the treatment of the plague victims and has not been published or studied as the other two Andalusian authors have. Ash-Shaqūrī states that medical treatment is sanctioned by Islam and desirable in an epidemic. Because plague is a corruption of the air, the author

[10] *Voyages*, ed. by Defrémery and Sanguinetti, vol. 4, pp. 370-373.

[11] *Ibn al-Khatīb min ḵhilāl ḵutubihi*, vol. 2, pp. 98-99. On Ibn al-Khaṭīb's journey from Fez to Marrākesh, a short time before Jumādā II, 761/April-May 1360, he observed plague at Maḥallat Sufyān (*ibid.*, vol. 1, p. 128). at Tiṭuānī does not give his sources for the pertinent excerpts from Ibn al-Khaṭīb's works. In this case, the first part of the *Nufāḍat al-jirāb* is apparently lost, and the only extant MS (Escorial MS no. 1755) is the second part, beginning with Ibn al-Khaṭīb's return from Marrākesh to Salé. This extract from the first part is unexplained. (See Elizabeth A. M. Warburton, "The *Nufāḍat al-jirāb* of Lisān ad-Dīn b. al-Khatīb," unpubl. diss., Cambridge University, 1965. I am very grateful to Dr. Warburton for making her thesis available to me.)

[12] ash-Shaqūrī ends another of his medical tracts on catarrhal dysentery by excusing himself for not having been able to bring to its composition all the care he would have liked because of the "present, severe illness." This has been interpreted as being an allusion to the Black Death; see H.P.J. Renaud, "Un Medicin du royaume de Grenade: Muhammad aš-Šaqūrī," *Hespéris*, vol. 33 (1946), p. 59. For ash-Shaqūrī, see Ibn Khaldūn, *Histoire des Berbères*, vol. 4, p. 390; Ullmann, pp. 179, 247.

advises how to improve the air (fols. 107b-108b) and how to improve men's bodies to resist the disease (fols. 108b-110b). This is an expansion of a section from an earlier work by ash-Shaqūrī.[13]

Finally, concerning the Andalusian sources, a fourth author has been cited:[14] Muḥammad ibn Muḥammad ibn Giapharaeus Abī 'Abdallāh (d. A.H. 764), according to the catalogue of Casiri, *Bibliotheca Arabico-Hispana Escurialensis*, vol. 2, pp. 74-75. The alleged treatise on plague was entitled *Iṣlāḥ an-nihhah* and should be MS no. 1673. However, this manuscript corresponds to parts 8 and 9 of the *'Iḥātah* of Ibn al-Khaṭīb. It could not be located in the Escorial Library nor is it mentioned in the *GAL*. Perhaps further investigation in Spain and North Africa will recover this lost work. Moreover, no extant Andalusian manuscripts deal with later recurrences of plague. Again, further research on plague epidemics in Spain and North Africa may possibly discover later Arabic plague treatises, as in the Middle East.

The Middle Eastern manuscripts are more numerous and more diverse, and they are not confined to the initial outbreak of the pandemic. There exists a large corpus of *risālahs* concerning the Black Death, which are noted by the mamlūk historian Ibn Bahādur al-Mu'minī.[15] The earliest known collection of these poetic narratives is by Ibn Abī Ḥajalah, who composed a plague treatise during an epidemic of plague in 764/1362 in Cairo. His *Daf' an-niqmah fī ṣ-ṣalāt 'alā nabī ar-raḥmān* (Escorial MS no. 1772; see below for a fuller description of this work) concludes with a chapter composed of these narratives. The same and additional material is found in a much later collection of plague material for which there are two copies, one in London and the other in Cairo. The British Museum manuscript, Or. no. 3053 (Rieu, *Supplement*, no. 160; von Kremer Collection no. 53) contains a collection of poetic accounts as well as the fifteenth-century plague treatise of as-

[13] Fol. 111a. See the discussion of this work in chap. IV.

[14] Sarton, *Introduction*, vol. 3, part 2, pp. 1661, 1721.

[15] *Kitāb futūh an-naṣr min ta'rīkh mulūk Miṣr*, vol. 2, p. 296.

Suyūṭī (see below). The British Museum manuscript was written during as-Suyūṭī's lifetime and is almost certainly the source of the later Dār al-Kutub al-Miṣrīyah copy. The Dār al-Kutub manuscript no. 102 *majāmī' m* contains a large collection of manuscript material relating to plague, besides the poetic narratives and the as-Suyūṭī tract, which deals with the plague recurrences through the fifteenth century (fols. 141a-205b). According to the colophons of the various parts of the Cairo manuscript, the works were copied by Muḥammad ibn 'Abd ar-Raḥmān al-Ḥanafī from Sunday, 22 Rabī' II, 1076/1 November 1665 (fol. 146a) to Wednesday, 15 Jumādā II, 1076/23 December 1665 (fol. 205b). The British Museum manuscript corresponds to fols. 171a to 215b of the Cairo manuscript.

The literature of the Dār al-Kutub al-Miṣrīyah manuscript comprises: (1) Ibn al-Wardī's *Risālat an-naba' 'an al-waba'*[16] and his short *Qasīdah fī ṭ-ṭā'ūn* (fols. 197a-197b). (2) An "account" (*muṭāla'ah*) by Bahā' ad-Dīn as-Subkī (d. 756/1355),[17] the chief *qāḍī* of Damascus during the Black Death, to as-Salāḥ aṣ-Ṣafadī (d. 764/1363 of plague in Damascus)[18] on the Black Death in Egypt in A.H. 749 (fols. 197b-198b). (3) As-Subkī quotes a few verses of the poetry of Ibrāhīm al-Mi'mār (fol. 198b),[19] who died during the Black Death in Cairo.[20] (4) An essay by aṣ-Ṣafadī to as-Subkī describing the spread of plague in Palestine and Syria in A.H. 749, particularly in Damascus. (The Cairo version of this essay [fols. 198b-200a] is the more complete; sections of the work are to be found in *as-Sulūk*, part 2, vol. 3, pp. 788-791, and *Daf' an-niqmah*, fols. 79a, 80a.) This may be identified with the *risālah* cited by Ibn Ḥajar, *Badhl*, fol. 45b. (5) Two verses (fols. 200a, see also *Daf'*

16 Published text in the *Dīwān* of Ibn al-Wardī, *Majmū'at al-jawā'ib*, ed. by Fāris ash-Shidyāq, Istanbul, 1300 A.H., pp. 184-188; see my translation of the *risālah*: "Ibn al-Wardī's *Risālat an-naba' 'an al-waba'*."

17 *EI*[1]: "al-Subkī" (J. Schacht); *GAL*, vol. 2, p. 86.

18 *EI*[1]: "Ṣafadī" (F. Krenkow); *GAL*, vol. 2, pp. 31-32, *Supplement*, vol. 2, pp. 27-29.

19 Cited also in *Daf' an-niqmah*, fol. 78b.

20 *GAL*, vol. 2, p. 10, *Supplement*, vol. 2, p. 3; quoted in *as-Sulūk*, part 2, vol. 3, p. 791, with additional verses.

an-niqmah, fol. 78b) by Shihāb ad-Dīn Faḍlallāh about the Black Death in Damascus, where he died in Dhū l-Ḥijjah 749 A.H.[21] (6) A few verses (fol. 200a)[22] by Ibn Nubātah (d. 768/1366), a distinguished Damascene poet who taught aṣ-Ṣafadī.[23] And (7) a poem on the Black Death in Egypt by Ṣadr ad-Dīn ibn al-Haymī (fols. 200b-201a).[24] There is also a citation of the poetic work of Jamāl ad-Dīn al-Khaṭīb al-Qubbī an-Nābalusī on plague in Damascus in *Daf' an-niqmah*, fol. 80b.

There was a Berlin manuscript (Sprenger no. 1962; Ahlwardt no. 6376, fols. 70-77), a fragment without beginning or end, that dealt with the religious prohibition against leaving or entering a plague-stricken area. The work was probably written in the period immediately after the Black Death, for the author lived about 760/1359. Dr. D. George of the Staatsbibliothek, Berlin, West Germany, has reported (23 September 1970) that this manuscript was unfortunately lost during the war.

The plague epidemic of 764/1362 in Cairo caused Aḥmad ibn Yaḥyā ibn Abī Ḥajalah to write three works; he himself died of plague in 776/1375.[25] The first, *Jiwār al-akhyār fī dār al-qarār*[26] resulted from the death of his son, Muḥammad, in Rajab (fol. 3a) during the plague of 764/1362, who was buried in the cemetery of Qarāfah next to the shrine of 'Uqbah ibn 'Amir al-Juhanī.[27] The work is devoted to the history of

[21] Ibn al-Wardī, *Tatimmat*, vol. 2, p. 354; *GAL*, vol. 2, p. 141, *Supplement*, vol. 2, pp. 175-176.

[22] Quoted in *Daf' an-niqmah*, fol. 78a; see Ibn Nubātah, *Dīwān* (Cairo, 1905), p. 50.

[23] *GAL*, vol. 2, pp. 10-12; *EI*[1]: "Ibn Nubāta" (J. Rikabi); Ibn Ḥajar, *Durar al-kāminah*, vol. 4, p. 216.

[24] Quoted in *Daf' an-niqmah*, fol. 78b, and *as-Sulūk*, part 2, vol. 3, p. 796. The author mentions the death of Shaykh Rukn ad-Dīn (fol. 201a), who died of plague in 749 A.H.

[25] *GAL*, vol. 2, pp. 12-13, *Supplement*, vol. 2, pp. 5-6; Sarton, *Introduction*, vol. 3, part 2, pp. 1722-1723.

[26] *Fihrist al-kutub al-'arabīyah* (Cairo, 1308 A.H.), vol. 5, p. 41.

[27] A companion of the Prophet; governor of Egypt, where he died in 58 A.H.

'Uqbah, the desirability of burial next to holy men, the etiquette of visiting tombs, and a religious discussion about dying and death. Concerning the first topic, the treatise contains a large number of *ḥadīths* related by 'Uqbah. The present manuscript was copied on 13 Rajab A.H. 1073 by Muḥammad ibn Muḥammad as-Suwaysī al-Aḥmadī (fol. 337a).

The second work by Ibn Abī Ḥajalah is *Daf' an-niqmah fī ṣ-ṣalāt 'alā nabī ar-raḥmān.*[28] As the title states, its primary purpose is a religious one: the best defense against a plague epidemic is prayer. This treatise includes a discussion of three customary subjects of the religio-legal treatises: death by plague is a martyrdom for the faithful Muslim; a Muslim should not enter or flee from a plague-stricken area; and what is the nature of plague (*ṭā'ūn*) itself. While the work is largely a collection of *ḥadīths* and their interpretation, the author also considers the remedies for plague (fols. 55a-59b), the history of plague epidemics in Islamic history (fols. 59b-76b), and the poetic narratives about the Black Death, mentioned above. In addition to the latter, there is a *qaṣīdah* of Ibn Abī Ḥajalah regarding plague (fols. 76b-78b), a *maqāmah* written by the author when the people proceeded to the tomb of an-Nāṣir in Cairo during the epidemic of A.H. 761, entitled *'Ayn as-sāhirah* (fols. 83b-86b), and verse written to aṣ-Ṣafadī about the plague of 761 A.H. (fols. 86b-87a).

The third work is *Kitāb aṭ-ṭibb al-masnūn fī daf' aṭ-ṭā'ūn*;[29] it is a very brief summary of the author's *Daf' an-niqmah*. The Cairo manuscript was copied on 22 Rabī' II, A.H. 1076 (fol. 146a).

Because of the Black Death and recurrent plagues, Tāj ad-Dīn as-Subkī composed his *Risālah fī ṭ-ṭā'ūn*,[30] which is a basic source for all subsequent religio-legal discussions of plague.[31] Also, a source for later compilations is the fourteenth-

[28] Escorial MS no. 1772, fols. 1a-87b.

[29] Dār al-Kutub al-Miṣrīyah MS no. 102 *majāmī' m*, fols. 141a-146a; the author omits a large number of *ḥadīths*, the historical account of plagues in Islam, and the poetry.

[30] Berlin MS no. 6380 (Ahlwardt); not mentioned in *GAL*.

[31] E.g., *Badhl*, fols. 35b-36a, 43b, 111b, 129b.

century treatise by Badr ad-Dīn az-Zarkashī (d. 794/1392), *Risālah fī ṭ-ṭā'ūn*,[32] which agrees with as-Subkī[33] on the right of a Muslim to flee from plague. Both treatises are contained in the lost Berlin MS no. 6380 (Ahlwardt); I know of no other copies of them.

Tasliyat ahl al-maṣā'ib fī maut al-awlād wal-aqārib[34] by Muḥammad ibn Muḥammad al-Manbijī[35] is a theological work explaining the misfortune brought upon his people by a plague epidemic in Rajab 775 to Muḥarram 776/December 1373 to June 1374.[36] As Ibn Abī Ḥajalah does in his first treatise, the author discusses the prescribed behavior of a Muslim at the time of death, burial, and visiting of the tombs. Al-Manbijī states in the introduction that he wrote another work that dealt with the history of the plague epidemic of 765/1363-1364.[37] In 1975 I located this work in the Dār al-Kutub al-Miṣrīyah, and it will be the subject of a separate publication.

A plague tractate of the late fourteenth century or early fifteenth century is the *Risālah fī al-amrāḍ al-wabā'iyah al-kā'inah 'an fasād al-aghdhiyah* by Abū al-Ḥasan 'Alī ibn 'Abdallāh ibn Muḥammad ibn Haydūr at-Tādalī (d. 816/1413).[38] It is preserved, to my knowledge, only in a single Maghribī manuscript in the Dār al-Kutub al-Miṣrīyah MS no. 183 *majāmī' m*, fols. 99b-106b.[39] After an explanation that the

[32] Berlin MS no. 6380 (Ahlwardt); not mentioned in *GAL.*

[33] *Badhl*, fols. 89a, 92a.

[34] Cairo, 1347 A.H.

[35] *GAL*, vol. 2, p. 76, *Supplement*, vol. 2, p. 82; Sarton, *Introduction*, vol. 3, part 2, pp. 1724-1725.

[36] *Tasliyat*, p. 3.

[37] *Ibid.*, pp. 3, 201: *Fī akhbār aṭ-ṭā'ūn*, Dār al-Kutub al-Miṣrīyah MS no. 16 *ṭibb Ḥalīm*, fols. 152-231 (see S. K. Hamarneh, *History of Arabic Medicine and Pharmacy* [Cairo, 1967], part 1, pp. 60-61, part 2, pp. 22-23).

[38] Not mentioned in *GAL*; az-Ziriklī, *al-A'lām* (Cairo, 1954-1959), vol. 5, p. 122.

[39] *Fihrist al-kutub al-'arabīyah*, vol. 7, part 2, p. 668. I have given above the title as it appears in the *Fihrist*; however, the title clearly appears at the end of the manuscript (fol. 106a): *an-Nubadh al-kullīyah fī iṣlāḥ al-amrāḍ al-khaliṭīyah.*

epidemic is caused by the corruption of foods, the author devotes the major portion of the small treatise to remedies. These remedies are divided according to: (1) the secrets of letters and supplication (fols. 101b-104b) and (2) medical treatment (fols. 104b-106b). The work was written during the time of one of the plague recurrences (fol. 99b), but it is impossible to determine precisely which one. The discussion of the secrets of letters begins, however, with a report of his teacher's dream during the plague epidemic of A.H. 764 (fol. 102a) and may be dated to roughly that time.

The best-known treatise on plague during the later Middle Ages and the most complete is *Badhl al-māʿūn fī faḍl aṭ-ṭāʿūn* by Ibn Ḥajar al-ʿAsqalānī (773-852/1372-1449).[40] Ibn Ḥajar brings together most of the relevant historical and theological material on plague in Islam up to his own time, and his work is the primary source for all later treatise writers, particularly as-Suyūṭī. The treatise exists in a number of manuscript copies in the Middle East and Europe. There are two copies in the Dār al-Kutub al-Miṣrīyah. Manuscript no. 2353 *taṣawwuf* is the full text and the basis of my own study. Ibn Ḥajar states that he began a work on plague in A.H. 819 (fol. 109b) but later revised it completely. The last plague that he describes is the epidemic in Egypt in Ṣafar 848/May 1444 (fol. 124a); because Ibn Ḥajar died in 852/1449, the work must have been completed in the five years between these two dates. The present copy (MS no. 2353 *taṣawwuf*) was made on 3 Muḥarram 909/28 June 1503. The second Cairene copy (no. 2198 *taṣawwuf*) is an abbreviated version of the first, probably from a common parent manuscript. In addition to the manuscripts listed in *GAL*, there is another copy in the Damascus Library, MS no. 3158. The Berlin manuscript (Ahlwardt no. 6370), entitled *Tuḥfat ar-rāghibīn fī bayān amr aṭ-ṭawāʿīn*, contains only extracts from the treatise. (Because of the political situation in Egypt in 1969-1970, I was unable to use the Alexandrian manuscript.) A detailed analysis of this work is given in

[40] *EI*²: "Ibn Hajar al-Asḳalāni" (F. Rosenthal); *GAL*, vol. 2, p. 67, *Supplement*, vol. 2, p. 74; Ullmann, p. 248.

chapter IV, part B, dealing with the religious interpretation of plague.

The Cairo manuscript no. 102 *majāmī' m* contains a poetic description by Nawājī (d. 859/1455) of a plague epidemic in Egypt in the first half of the fifteenth century (fol. 201a).[41] In the same manuscript collection, Shihāb al-Manṣūrī relates in rhymed prose (*saj'*) the events of the plague epidemics in 881/1476-1477 and 897-898/1491-1492 in Egypt (fols. 201a-205b). For these two epidemics we also have the work of Ibn Abī Sharīf al-Kāmilī (d. 906/1500): *Fatāwā fī ṭ-ṭā'ūn*.[42] The author interprets the various theological problems presented by plague on the basis of the relevant *ḥadīths*; in general, he follows the interpretation of Ibn Abī Ḥajalah in *Daf' an-niqmah*. Ibn Abī Sharīf's *Kiṭab fī aḥḳām aṭ-ṭā'ūn*[43] is the same work divided into two parts: the first part (fols. 156b-164a) corresponds directly to the second half of the *Fatāwā* regarding questions about the plague of A.H. 897 (fols. 178b-185a). The Cairo manuscript states that this part was copied by al-Faqīr Aḥmad ibn as-Safīrī ash-Shāfi'ī on 10 Sha'bān 939/6 March 1533, and the present copy was made at the time of the mid-day prayer on Saturday, 6 Jumādā I, 1076/14 November 1665. The second part (fols. 164b-170b) corresponds to the first section of the *Fatāwā* (fols. 173a-178b), regarding the prohibition against fleeing from plague, which was questioned during the epidemic of A.H. 881. The second part of the Cairo manuscript was copied on Thursday, 11 Jumādā I, 1076/19 November 1665.[44]

Jalāl ad-Dīn as-Suyūṭī summarizes the historical content of Ibn Ḥajar's *Badhl* and Ibn Abī Ḥajalah's *Daf' an-niqmah* and brings the chronology of plagues up to his own time—the plague epidemic of 897/1491-1492, when the work was composed. The tract is entitled *Mā rawāhu l-wā'ūn fī akhbār aṭ-*

[41] *GAL*, vol. 2, p. 56, *Supplement*, vol. 2, pp. 8, 56.

[42] Cambridge University Library Add. MS no. 3257, fols. 173a-185b.

[43] Dār al-Kutub al-Miṣrīyah MS no. 102 *majāmī' m*, fols. 156b-171a.

[44] There follows directly in the Cairo MS a *fatwā* of Ibn Abī Sharīf (fols. 170b-171a) about rents, which is apparently unrelated to plague.

ṭāʿūn.[45] Alfred von Kremer has edited the text of the Dār al-Kutub al-Miṣrīyah manuscript[46] along with an introduction and compilation of epidemics: "Ueber die grossen Seuchen." There also exists another work by as-Suyūṭī on plague: *Fāʾidah fī l-wiqāyah min aṭ-ṭāʿūn* in Alexandria.[47] This may be the treatise referred to by Leclerc on the plague that ravaged Cairo in 909 A.H.[48]

The plague of 897/1492 in Egypt prompted the writing of *Juzʾ fī ṭ-ṭāʿūn* by Shaykh Shams ad-Dīn al-Ḥijāzī ash-Shāfiʿī.[49] The work is primarily a religio-legal one concerned with a discussion of *ḥadīths* related to plague. According to the colophon, the manuscript had been copied on 24 Jumādā I, 963/6 April 1556, and copied again in the present collection on 1 Jumādā I, 1076/9 November 1665 by Muḥammad al-Ḥaqīr.[50]

In 899/1493-1494, ʿAbd al-Qāhir ibn Muḥammad ibn ʿAbd ar-Raḥmān at-Tunisī wrote *Kitāb aṭ-ṭibb fī tadbīr al-musāfirīn wa-maraḍ aṭ-ṭāʿūn.*[51]

A short fifteenth-century discussion of plague is found in Mullā Luṭfallāh aṭ-Ṭuqātī's *Risālah fī taḍʿīf al-madhbaḥ.*[52] It begins with an explanation of a classical geometric problem, the doubling of a cube by Plato, which, if solved, would raise plague from the Greeks. The author then explains the cause of plague epidemics. The manuscript deals also with the efficacy of the divine names in prayers and talismans against the propagation of the disease, a discussion drawn largely from al-Būnī.

45 *GAL*, vol. 2, p. 146, *Supplement*, vol. 2, p. 182; Ullmann, p. 248.

46 MS no. 102 *majāmīʿ m*, fols. 172a-195a. In the manuscript the work is preceded by a short summary (fols. 171a-171b). This summary, in turn, is preceded by a short essay on the administration of *waqfs* by as-Suyūṭī (fol. 171b), which is apparently unrelated to plague.

47 *GAL*, vol. 2, p. 146, no. 32a.

48 *Histoire de la médecine Arabe*, vol. 2, p. 298.

49 Dār al-Kutub al-Miṣrīyah MS no. 102 *majāmīʿ m*, fols. 147a-155a; not mentioned in *GAL*.

50 Fol. 155a.

51 *GAL*, *Supplement*, vol. 2, p. 367; Ullmann, p. 248.

52 A. Adnan, *Les Sciences chez les Turcs Ottomans* (Paris, 1939), pp. 44-45; *GAL*, vol. 2, pp. 235-236, no. 10.

The manuscript copies are found in two libraries: Leiden[53] and Istanbul.[54]

During the reign of Bāyazīd II (d. 918/1512), an anonymous plague treatise was written, a short, undated manuscript entitled *Risālah fī wabā' aṭ-ṭā'ūn*. A beautiful eighteenth-century copy of the work in *nastaliq* script is located in al-Azhar Mosque Library, Cairo.[55] Plague is explained linguistically, medically, and legally; the author cites Ibn Ḥajar and follows his orthodox opinions about the subject.

Idrīs ibn Ḥusām ad-Dīn al-Badlīsī (d. 926/1520), a famous Ottoman historian, dedicated a plague treatise to sultan Selīm ibn Bāyazīd. The author had heard in Syria in 917/1511, on his way to Mecca, that plague had broken out in Egypt; he returned immediately to Istanbul. His work, *Risālat al-ibā' 'an mawāqi' al-wabā'*, is mainly a justification for fleeing a plague epidemic.[56]

Another plague tract also dedicated to sultan Selīm I was written by Ilyās ibn Ibrāhīm al-Yahūdī al-Isbānī: *Kitāb majannat aṭ-ṭā'ūn wa l-wabā'*.[57] Ilyās states that he decided to write this tract after studying the works of Hippocrates, Galen, Isḥāq al-Isrā'īlī, and Arab medical works, and to draw together all the pertinent material on plague. The immediate reason for the work was the author's fear that plague would follow the earthquakes of his time since, according to Aristotle, earthquakes unleash the pestilential air that is the vehicle of plague.

[53] P. de Jong and J. de Goeje, *Catalogus Codicum Orientalium* (Leiden, 1851-1877), vol. 3, p. 179: MS no. 1229, fols. 13a-19a.

[54] Sulaymanīyah Library, Es'ad Effendi MS no. 3596, fols. 1a-9b; copied on Shawwāl 5, 968 A.H. (fol. 9a).

[55] al-Azhar Library *Fihrist* (Cairo, 1950), chapter 6, p. 116: MS no. 251 *majāmī'* (7384), fols. 14b-18a. The date of composition can be placed during the reign of Bāyazīd II since the tract was written at his request (fol. 14b).

[56] Berlin MS Sprenger no. 727 (Ahlwardt no. 6371); also entitled *Risālat at-tā'ūn*, see *GAL, Supplement*, vol. 2, p. 325. See also *EI*²: "Bidlīsī" (V. L. Ménage) and Süheyl Ünver, "Sur l'histoire de la peste en Turquie," p. 479.

[57] Chester Beatty MS no. 3676, 6 (fols. 185-216).

Ullmann gives a brief outline of the contents of the work, pp. 348-349.

A *Risālah fī ṭ-ṭāʻūn wal-wabāʼ* or *Rāḥat al-arwāḥ fī dafʻ ʻāhat al-ashbāḥ* was written by Shams ad-Dīn ʻAlī ibn S. ibn Kamāl Pāshā, Shaykh of Islām in Istanbul (d. 941/1535).[58] The author advises the reader to avoid the areas contaminated by plague, in accordance with the decision of the famous Ottoman jurist, Abū s-Su'ud, and to flee from places infected by the disease.[59] The work contains a large number of prayers, amulets, and *materia medica.*

There exists in the manuscript collection of the National Library of Medicine, Bethesda, Maryland, a plague treatise entitled *ʻUmdat ar-rāwīn fī bayān aḥkām aṭ-ṭawāʻīn* by Yaḥyah ibn Muḥammad ibn M. al-Ḥaṭṭāb; the manuscript is dated 19 Rabīʻ A.H. 944.[60]

A plague in Egypt in 950/1543 was the occasion for the writing of a treatise by Zayn al-ʻAbidīn ibn Ibrāhīm ibn Nujaym al-Miṣrī (d. 950/1543): *Risālah fī ṭ-ṭaʻn waṭ-ṭāʻūn.*[61] The work is based on the tract of as-Suyūṭī (mentioned above) and an-Nawawī's commentary on the *Ṣaḥīḥ* of Abū Muslim.

A plague treatise entitled *Majmūʻat ash-shifāʼ li-adwiyat al-wabāʼ maʻ rasāʼil lil-Bisṭāmī*[62] is listed as anonymous in the Berlin collection but should be identified with the *Risālat ash-shifāʼ fī dawāʼ al-wabāʼ* by Abū l-Khayr A. ibn Muṣliḥ ad-Dīn Muṣṭafā Ṭāshköprüzāde ʻIṣmāddīn (901-968/1495-1560).[63] The

[58] *EI*[1]: "Kemāl-Pasha-Zāde" (F. Babinger); *GAL*, vol. 2, p. 452, no. 102; in addition, the manuscript is found in Berlin MS no. 6380 (Ahlwardt). The Dār al-Kutub al-Miṣrīyah MS no. 32 *majāmīʻ m* (fols. 37-41) is the earliest text in Cairo.

[59] Süheyl Ünver, "Sur l'histoire de la peste en Turquie," p. 480; Ullmann, p. 248.

[60] Schullian and Sommer, *A Catalogue of Incunabula and Manuscripts in the Army Medical Library*, pp. 323-324, MS no. A80.

[61] *GAL*, vol. 2, p. 311, *Supplement*, vol. 2, p. 426. I have used the Berlin MS Landberg no. 598 (Ahlwardt no. 6372), fols. 17b-19b; Ullmann, p. 249.

[62] Berlin MS Landberg no. 999 (Ahlwardt no. 6378).

[63] *GAL*, vol. 2, p. 426; published ed.: *ash-Shifāʼ li-adwāʼ al-wabāʼ* (Cairo, A.H. 1292); see Ullmann, p. 249, and *EI*[1]: "Ṭashköprüzāde" (F. Babinger).

work is largely theological but also incorporates a large section on magic and superstitions about plague, a history of plagues, and a portion from the tract on remedies by ʿAbd ar-Raḥmān al-Bisṭāmī al-Ḥanafī al-Ḥurūfī (d. 858/1454): *al-Adʿiyah al-muntakhabah fī l-adwiyah al-mujarrabah.*[64]

The treatise *Ẓuhūr ath-thurayā wa khafāʾ mā kāna wabiyā* by Sulaymān al-ʿUthmānī al-Ḥanafī al-Falakī[65] was written on 5 Rabīʿ II, 988/20 May 1580 about the epidemic in the previous year. Another sixteenth-century tract on plague by ʿAlī ibn Muḥammad ibn ʿAlī ash-Shahīd (d. 1004/1596)[66] is a discussion of religious law *(istiftāʾ)*. The substance of the argument is that plague is a consequence of bad air and not a divine punishment.

A treatise composed in 1028/1619, containing twenty medical and theological questions and answers about plague, was written by Marʿī ibn Yusūf al-Ḥanbalī al-Muqaddasī (d. 1033/1624); it is entitled *Kitāb taḥqīq aẓ-ẓunūn bi akhbār aṭ-ṭāʿūn.*[67]

The plague tractate *Khulāṣat mā taḥṣul ʿalaihi as-sāʿūn fī adwiyat dafʿ al-wabāʾ waṭ-ṭāʿūn*, by Muḥammad Fatḥallāh ibn Maḥmūd al-Baylūnī al-Ḥalabī (d. 1042/1632),[68] is devoted to the remedies against plague, including medicine, prayers, special foods, etc. The work was written at the end of Rabīʿ II, 1028/March 1619. Another copy in Cairo was made, according to the colophon, on Saturday, 13 Rabīʿ I, 1185/26 June 1771.[69]

Slightly later is a manuscript in the Damascus Library: *Suʾāl*

[64] *GAL*, vol. 2, p. 232, no. 18. Al-Bisṭāmī is also the author of *Wasf ad-dawā fī kashf āfāt al-wabāʾ* (*GAL*, vol. 2, p. 232, no. 15, *Supplement*, vol. 2, pp. 323-324) in which he gives a number of remedies for plague as well as a history of plague epidemics in Islam; see Leclerc, *Histoire de la médecine Arabe*, vol. 2, p. 297.

[65] *GAL*, vol. 2, p. 357, *Supplement*, vol. 2, p. 484; I have used the Cairo copy (*Fihrist*, vol. 7, p. 266).

[66] *GAL*, vol. 2, p. 312; no. 5c; I have used the Cairo copy (*Fihrist*, vol. 7, p. 68).

[67] Berlin MS no. 6373 (Ahlwardt), fols. 31-76; *GAL*, vol. 2, p. 369, *Supplement*, vol. 2, p. 496.

[68] *GAL*, vol. 2, p. 274, *Supplement*, vol. 3, p. 1278; I have used the Berlin MS no. 6374, fols. 161b-188a and the Cairo copies (*Fihrist*, vol. 7, pp. 4, 266).

[69] *Fihrist al-kutub al-ʿarabīyah*, vol. 7, p. 102.

fī ṭ-ṭā'ūn ma' jawāb by aṣ-Ṣadīqī, who died in A.D. 1626, according to the library handlist.[70]

The seventeenth-century *Kitāb maskin ash-shujūn fī ḥukm al-firār min aṭ-ṭā'ūn* by Ni'matallāh al-Jazā'irī (d. 1112/1700)[71] considers the justification for fleeing plague, in addition to some remedies described at the end of the treatise.

A report on the plague epidemic of 1124-1125/1712-1713, *Risālah taṭhīr ahl al-Islām biṭ-ṭa'n waṭ-ṭā'ūn al-'ām* is by 'Abd al-Mu'ṭī as-Saḥalāwī.[72] The tract gives medical treatment, superstitions, and a brief history of plague based on Ibn Ḥajar. Moreover, Dr. Galip Ata has drawn attention to a plague treatise of the early eighteenth century by Ḥayātī Zādah Muṣṭafā Fayḍī.[73]

It will suffice, perhaps, simply to note two manuscripts from the nineteenth century. *Ad-Durr al-maknūn fīmā yata'allaq bil-wabā' waṭ-ṭā'ūn* was written by Nāfi' ibn al-Jawharī ibn S. al-Khafājī[74] in 1281/1864 on the plague epidemic then raging in the Ḥijāz. Second, *as-Samm al-'adhāb lir-rajul al-kadhdhāb* by 'Alī al-Ḥashshāb is devoted to a plague that was anticipated in Egypt on 25 Sha'bān A.H. 1282.[75]

Finally, there is an anonymous and undated *Risālah fī ṭ-ṭā'ūn* in the Berlin Library, which could not be microfilmed.[76] It is reportedly a strictly theological interpretation of plague.

[70] Damascus Library MS no. 83.

[71] *GAL, Supplement,* vol. 2, p. 586 does not mention this work. See Berlin MS no. 6377 (Ahlwardt), fols. 147-150; Ullmann, p. 250.

[72] Ṭanṭā Library, section *kha*, no. 275, fols. 1-9; also section *'ayn*, no. 4893. Because of the political conditions in Egypt in 1969-1970, I was unable to visit the Ṭantā Library. However, through the kindness of Dr. 'Abd at-Tawwāb of the Egyptian Museum, I was able to obtain a copy of MS no. 275. See 'Alī Sāmī an-Nashār, *Fihrist makhṭūṭāt al-masjid al-Aḥmadī bi-Ṭanṭā* (Alexandria, 1964), p. 143, where the work is given the title: *Risālah fī t-ṭā'ūn.*

[73] Ata, "Évolution de la médecine en Turquie," p. 118.

[74] *GAL, Supplement,* vol. 2, p. 811; Olga Pinto, *Manoscritti arabi delle biblioteche governative di Firenze non ancora catalogati* (Florence, 1935-), Bibliofilia, vol. 37, pp. 234-246.

[75] Berlin MS Landberg no. 526 (Ahlwardt no. 6375), fols. 151-155.

[76] Berlin MS Landberg no. 671 (Ahlwardt no. 6379).

BIBLIOGRAPHY

The following bibliography for the history of the Black Death and recurrences of plague in the Middle East has been made as comprehensive as possible with regard to primary and secondary sources. The most complete, general guide to works dealing with Mamlūk Egypt and Syria may be found in the bibliography of Ira M. Lapidus' *Muslim Cities in the Later Middle Ages*, pp. 217-242.

Concerning the Black Death in Europe, I have selected for inclusion in this bibliography only those works that I have found to be pertinent to the Middle East because of their methodological approach or comparative value. The most useful bibliographies for the extensive scholarship on the European phase of the pandemic are Philip Ziegler, *The Black Death*, pp. 302-312, and Élisabeth Carpentier, "Autour de la Peste Noire: famines et épidémies dans l'histoire du XIVe siècle," *Annales*, vol. 17 (1962), pp. 1062-1092. More recent additions to the literature are cited in William M. Bowsky's collection of documents and articles: *The Black Death: A Turning Point in History?*, pp. 126-128.

CLASSIFICATION OF CONTENTS

A. Manuscripts
B. Bibliographical Sources
C. Primary Printed Sources
D. Secondary Printed Sources and Theses

A. MANUSCRIPTS

Aside from the plague treatises described in Appendix 3, I have used a number of historical sources still in manuscript form in 1969-1970. These general chronicles included:

(1) The unpublished portions of al-Maqrīzī's *as-Sulūk*. Professor Sa'īd 'Āshour (Cairo University) kindly allowed me to use the al-Maqrīzī texts, which he was editing, for my own work; these manuscripts included microfilm copies of the Paris MSS nos. 1726-1728 and the Aya Sofya, Istanbul, MSS nos. 3372, 3374, 3375. I have also consulted the British Museum MSS Or. no. 2902 (years A.H. 815-844) and Or. no. 9542 (years A.H. 718-761), and the Bodleian MSS Or. no. 458 (years A.H. 810-830) and Marsh no. 121 (years A.H. 831-844). Since that time, Professor 'Āshour has published this remaining portion of the *Sulūk* (Cairo, 1970-1973); therefore, my source citations are to the published text.

(2) The unpublished section of Ibn Ḥajar al-'Asqalānī, *Inbā' al-ghumr*. Again, the work was being edited by an Egyptian scholar, Professor Ḥasan Ḥabishī ('Ayn Shams University) in 1969-1970. The first volume was published in Cairo in 1969 and covered the years from A.H. 773 to 799. I am grateful to Professor Ḥabishī for allowing me to read his typescript of the entire work. In addition, I have consulted a complete British Museum manuscript, Add. MS no. 7321 (years A.H. 773-849); the Bodleian MS Huntington no. 123 and the British Museum MS Or. no. 5311 are vols. 1 and 2 of another copy of the work, covering the years A.H. 773 to 811 and A.H. 812 to 850 respectively. The British Museum Add. MS no. 7321 is earlier and more reliable than the second. At the present time, two further volumes of the history have appeared (Cairo, 1970-1972), and my source citations are made, where possible, to this edition of the text.

(3) Ibn Bahādur al-Mu'minī, *Kitāb futūḥ an-naṣr min ta'rīkh mulūk Miṣr*, Dār al-Kutub al-Miṣrīyah MS no. 2399 *ta'rīkh* (photographic copy).

(4) Ibn Ḥabīb al-Ḥalabī, *Durrat al-aslāk fī dawlat (mulk) al-atrāk*, Cairo University Library no. 22961 (photographic copy of Berlin MSS nos. 9723, 9724), and Ibn Ḥabīb's *Tadhkirat an-nabīh fī ayyām al-Manṣūr wa banīh*, British Museum Or. Add. MS 7335, which Professor Udovitch kindly studied for me.

(5) al-'Aynī, *'Iqd al-jumān fī ta'rīkh ahl az-zamān*, Dār al-Kutub al-Miṣrīyah MS no. 1574 *ta'rīkh*.

(6) Ibn Qāḍī Shuhbah, *adh-Dhayl 'alā ta'rīkh al-islām*, Paris MS no. 1599, which is being edited by Mr. Adnān Darwish. Mr. Darwish furnished me with copies of the pertinent folios.

(7) al-Waṣṣābī, *Kitāb al-i'tibār fī t-tawārīkh wal-'athār*, Dār al-Kutub al-Miṣrīyah microfilm no. 85.

(8) al-Khazrajī, *Kifāyah wal-i'lam fīman waliya al-Yaman*, Dār al-Kutub al-Miṣrīyah microfilm no. 2206.

B. BIBLIOGRAPHICAL SOURCES

Adnan, A., *La Science chez les Turcs Ottomans*, Paris, 1939.

Ahlwardt, W., *Verzeichnis der arabischen Handschriften der Königlichen Bibliothek zu Berlin*, nos. 6-9, 16-22, 10 vols., Berlin, 1882-1899.

Ashtor (Strauss), Eliyahu, "Some Unpublished Sources for the Baḥrī Period," *Scripta Hierosolymitana*, vol. 9, ed. by Uriel Heyd, Jerusalem, 1961, pp. 11-30.

Brockelmann, Carl, *Geschichte der Arabischen Litteratur*, 2 vols., 2nd ed., Leiden, 1945-1949; *Supplements*, 3 vols., Leiden, 1937-1942.

Casiri, Miguel, *Bibliotheca Arabico-Hispana Escurialensis*, 2 vols., Madrid, 1760-1770.

Dār al-Kutub al-Miṣrīyah, *Fihrist al-kutub al-'arabīyah*, 7 vols. in 4, Cairo, A.H. 1305-1310.

———, *Fihrist al-kutub al-'arabīyah al-mawjūdah bid-dār lighāyat sanat 1921-1955*, 9 vols., Cairo, 1924-1959.

Derenbourg, H., and E. Lévi-Provençal, *Les Manuscrits Arabes de l'Escurial*, 3 vols. in 4, Paris, 1884-1941.

Ebied, Rifaat Y., *Bibliography of Medieval Arabic and Jewish Medicine and Allied Sciences*, Publication of the Wellcome Institute of the History of Medicine, Occasional Series II, London, 1971.

Hamarneh, Sami K., *History of Arabic Medicine and Pharmacy*, Cairo, 1967.

al-Jāmi' al-Azhar, Cairo, *Fihrist al-kutub al-mawjūdah bilmaktabah al-Azharīyah*, 6 vols., Cairo, 1946-1952.

Jong, Pieter de, and J. de Goeje, *Catalogus Codicum Orientalium*, 6 vols., Leiden, 1851-1877.

Leclerc, Lucien, *Histoire de la medécine Arabe*, 2 vols., Paris, 1876.

Lewis, Bernard, and P. M. Holt, eds., *Historians of the Middle East*, London, 1962.

———, "Sources for the Economic History of the Middle East," *Studies in the Economic History of the Middle East*, ed. by M. A. Cook, London, 1970, pp. 78-92.

Little, D. P., *An Introduction to Mamlūk Historiography*, Wiesbaden, 1970.

an-Nadīm, Ibn Abī Ya'qūb, *al-Fihrist*, ed. by Gustav Flügel, Beirut, 1966 reprint.

———, *The Fihrist of al-Nadīm*, trans., by Bayard Dodge, 2 vols., New York, 1970.

an-Nashār, 'Alī Sāmī, *Fihrist Makhṭūṭāt al-masjid al-Aḥmadī bi-Ṭanṭā*, Alexandria, 1964.

Pinto, Olga, *Manoscritti arabi delle biblioteche governative di Firenze non ancora catalogati*, Florence, 1935.

Rieu, Charles, *Supplement to the Catalogue of the Arabic Manuscripts in the British Museum*, London, 1894.

Rosenthal, Franz, *A History of Muslim Historiography*, Leiden, 1952.

Sauvaget, Jean, *Introduction to the History of the Muslim East: A Bibliographical Guide*, ed. by Claude Cahen, trans. by von Grunebaum and Little, Berkeley and Los Angeles, 1965.

Schullian, D. M., and F. E. Sommer, *A Catalogue of Incunabula and Manuscripts in the Army Medical Library*, New York, 1950.

Sezgin, Fuat, *Geschichte der Arabischen Schrifttums*, 3 vols., Leiden, 1967-1971.

Wensinck, A. J., *Concordance et indices de la tradition musulmane*, Leiden, 1936.

Wüstenfeld, Ferdinand, *Geschichte der Arabischen Aerzte und Naturforscher*, Göttingen, 1840.

az-Ziriklī, Khayr ad-Dīn, *al-A'lām*, 10 vols., 2nd ed., Cairo, 1954-1959.

Ziyādah, M. M., *al-Mu'arrikūn fī Miṣr fī l-qarn al-khāmis 'ashar*, part 2, Cairo, 1954.

C. PRIMARY PRINTED SOURCES

Anonymous, *Beiträge zur Geschichte der Mamlūken-sultane in den Jahren 690-741 der Hegra*, ed. by K. V. Zetterstéen, Leiden, 1919.

'Abd al-Laṭīf al-Baghdādī, *The Eastern Key* (*Kitāb al-ifādah wal-i'tibār*), trans. by K. H. Zand, J. A. and I. E. Videan, London, 1964.

———, *Relation de l'Égypte par Abd-Allatif, medicin arab de Baghdad* (*Kitāb al-ifādah wal-i'tibār*), trans. by A. I. Silvestre de Sacy, Paris, 1810.

Abū Bakr al-Quṭbī al-Ahrī, *Ta'rīkh ash-Shaykh Uwais*, partial trans. by J. B. Van Loon, The Hague, 1954.

Abū l-Fidā', *al-Mukhtaṣar fī akhbār al-bashar*, 4 vols., Cairo, 1907.

'Alī ibn Ḥasan, al-Khazrajī, *al-'Uqūd al-lu'lu'īyah fī ta'rīkh al-dawlah ar-Rasulīyah*, 2 vols., Cairo, 1911-1914.

Atiya, Aziz S., "An Unpublished XIV Century Fatwā on the Status of Foreigners in Mamlūk Egypt and Syria," *Studien zur Geschichte und Kultur des Nahen und Fernen Ostens Paule Kahle*, Leiden, 1935, pp. 55-68.

Barbier de Meynard, A. C., ed. and trans., "Extraits de la Chronique Persane d'Herat," *JA*, series 5, vol. 16, pp. 461-520; vol. 17, pp. 438-457, 473-522; vol. 20, pp. 268-319.

Bartsocas, C. S., trans., "Two Fourteenth Century Greek Descriptions of the 'Black Death'," *Journal of the History of Medicine and Allied Sciences*, vol. 21, no. 4 (October, 1966), pp. 394-400.

Broquière, Bertrandon de la, *Early Travels in Palestine*, ed. by Thomas Wright, London, 1848.

Browne, W. G., *Travels in Africa, Egypt and Syria from the Years 1792 to 1798*, London, 1799.

al-Bukhārī, Muḥammad ibn Ismā'īl, *Kitāb al-Jāmi' aṣ-Ṣaḥīḥ*, 4 vols., Leiden, 1864.

———, *Le Recueil des traditions mahométanes*, ed. by M. Ludolf Krehl and T. W. Juynboll, 4 vols., Leiden, 1862-1908.

al-Būnī, Aḥmad ibn 'Alī, *Shams al-ma'ārif al-kubrā*, 4 vols. in 1, Cairo, 1874.

Caetani, Leone, Principe di Teano, *Annali dell'Islām*, 10 vols. in 11, Milan, 1905-1926.

Chavannes, Édouard, *Documents sur les Tou-Kiue (Turcs) Occidentaux*, Paris, 1942.

Cobham, C. D., ed. and trans., *Excerpta Cypria*, Cambridge, 1908, 1969 reprint.

adh-Dhahabī and al-Ḥusaynī, *Min dhuyūl al-'ibar*, ed. by M. Rashād 'Abd al-Muṭṭalib, Kuwait, n.d.

Evagrius, *The Ecclesiastical History*, ed. by J. Bider and L. Parmentier, London, 1898.

Evliyā, *Narrative of Travels in Europe, Asia and Africa in the Seventeenth Century by Evliya Efendi*, trans. by Joseph, Freiherr von Hammer-Purgstall, London, 1834, 1968 reprint.

al-Fāsī, Taqī ad-Dīn, *Shifā' al-gharām bi akhbār al-balad al-ḥarām*, Mecca, 1956.

Frescobaldi, Gucci, and Sigoli, *Visit to the Holy Places of Egypt, Sinai, Palestine and Syria*, trans. by T. Bellorini and E. Hoade, Jerusalem, 1948.

Galen, *Medicorum Graecorum Opera Quae Exstant*, ed. by C. G. Kühn, 20 vols., Leipzig, 1821-1833.

———, *On the Parts of Medicine, On Cohesive Causes, On Regimen in Acute Diseases in Accordance with the Theories of Hippocrates*, ed. and trans. by Malcolm Lyons, Berlin, 1969.

Hippocrates, Epidemics I and III, ed. and trans. by W.H.S. Jones, New York, 1923.

al-Ḥusaynī, 'Abdallāh ibn 'Abd ar-Raḥmān, *Risālat-yi mazārāt-i Harāt*, ed. by F. Saljūqī, Kābul, 1967.

Ibn Abī Dīnār, Muḥammad ibn Abī l-Qāsim ar-Ru'aynī al-

Qayrawānī, *al-Mu'nis fī akhbār Ifriqīyah wa Tūnis*, ed. by Muḥammad Shammān, Tunis, 1967.
——, *Histoire de l'Afrique de Mohámmed-ben-Abi-el-Raini-el-Kairouāni*, trans. by E. Pellissier and Rémusat; vol. 7 of *Exploration scientifique de l'Algérie pendant les années 1840, 1841, 1842*, Paris, 1845.
Ibn Abī Uṣaybi'ah, *'Uyūn al-anbā' fī ṭabaqāt al-aṭibbā'*, ed. by A. Muller, 2 vols., Cairo, 1882.
Ibn 'Asākir, 'Alī ibn al-Ḥasan, *Ta'rīkh madīnat Dimashq*, vols. 1, 2, and 10, Damascus, 1951-1963.
Ibn al-Athīr, *al-Kāmil fī t-ta'rīkh*, 14 vols., Beirut, 1965-1967 (reprint of Tornberg ed., Leiden, 1851-1883).
Ibn Baṭṭūṭah, *Voyages d'Ibn Batoutah*, ed. and trans. by C. Defrémery and B. R. Sanguinetti, 4 vols., Paris, 1853-1858.
——, *Travels, AD 1325-1354*, trans. by Sir Hamilton Gibb, 3 vols., Cambridge, 1958-1971.
——, *The Travels of Ibn Batūta*, trans. by Samuel Lee, London, 1829.
Ibn al-Bayṭār, *Traité des simples (Jāmi' fīṭ-ṭibb)*, trans. by L. Leclerc, 3 vols., Paris, 1877-1883.
Ibn Duqmāq, Ibrāhīm, *al-Intiṣār li-wāsiṭat 'iqd al-amṣār*, ed. by Vollers, Beirut, 1966 reprint.
Ibn al-Furāt, *Ta'rīkh ad-duwal wal-mulūk*, vols. 7-9, Beirut, 1936-1942.
Ibn Ḥabīb, al-Ḥalabī, *Durrat al-aslāk fī dawlat al-atrāk*, ed. by A. Meursinge and H. E. Weijers, *Orientalia*, vol. 2 (Amsterdam, 1846), ed. by Juynboll, Roorda, and Weijers.
Ibn Ḥajar al-'Asqalānī, *ad-Durar al-kāminah fī a'yān al-mi'ah ath-thāminah*, 4 vols., Hyderabad, A.H. 1348-1350.
——, *Inbā' al-ghumr bi-anbā' al-'umr*, 3 vols., Cairo, 1969-1972.
Ibn Iyās, *Badā'i' az-zuhūr fī waqā'i' ad-duhūr*, 3 parts in 2 vols., Būlāq, A.H. 1311-1312.
——, *Badā'i' az-zuhūr fī waqā'i' ad-duhūr*, ed. by P. Kahle M. Mostafa [Muṣṭafā] and M. Sobernheim, *Bibliotheca Islamica*, 3 vols., rev. ed. (vols. 5c, 5d, 5e), Cairo, 1960-1963.

Ibn Iyās, *Ṣafaḥāt lam tünshar min badā'i' az-zuhūr fī waqā'i' ad-duhūr (Unpublished Pages of the Chronicle of Ibn Iyās, AH 857-872/AD 1453-1468)*, ed. by Muḥammad Mostafa [Muṣṭafā], Cairo, 1951.

———, *Histoire des mamlouks Circassiens*, ed. by Gaston Wiet, vol. 2, Paris, 1945.

———, *Journal d'un Bourgeois du Caire, Chronique d'Ibn Iyās*, ed. by Gaston Wiet, 2 vols., Paris, 1955, 1960.

Ibn al-Ji'ān, Yaḥyā ibn al-Maqarr, *at-Tuḥfah as-sanīyah fī asma' al-bilād al-Miṣrīyah*, ed. by B. Moritz, Cairo, 1898.

Ibn Kathīr, *al-Bidāyah wan-nihāyah fī t-ta'rikh*, 14 vols., Cairo, n.d.

Ibn Khaldūn, *Kitāb al-'Ibār*, 7 vols., Būlaq A.H. 1284.

———, *Histoire des Berbères et des dynasties musulmanes de l'Afrique Septentrionale*, trans. by Baron de Slane and Paul Casanova, 4 vols., Paris, 2nd ed., 1925-1956.

———, *The Muqaddimah*, trans. by Franz Rosenthal, 3 vols., Princeton, 1967.

———, *at-Ta'rīf*, Cairo, 1951.

Ibn Khaldūn, Yaḥyā ibn Muḥammad, *L'Histoire des Beni 'Abd el-Wād, rois de Tlemcen*, ed. and trans. by A. Bel, vol. 1, Algiers, 1903.

Ibn al-Khaṭīb, Lisān ad-Dīn, "Ibnulkhatīb's Bericht über die Pest," ed. by M. J. Müller, *Sitzungsberichte der Königl. Bayerischen Akademie der Wissenschäften zu München*, Munich, 1863, part 2, pp. 1-34.

———, *Ibn al-Khaṭīb min khilāl kutubihi*, ed. by Muḥammad ibn Abī Bakr at-Tiṭuānī, Tiṭuān, Morocco, 2 vols., 1954, 1959.

———, *Nufādat al-jirāb*, ed. and trans. by Elizabeth A. M. Warburton, unpubl. diss., Cambridge University, 1965.

Ibn Khātimah, "Die Schrift von Abī Ja'far Aḥmed ibn 'Alī ibn Moḥammed ibn 'Alī ibn Ḫātimah aus Almeriah über die Pest," ed. by Taha Dinānah, *AGM*, vol. 19 (1927), pp. 27-81.

Ibn Nubātah, *Dīwān*, Cairo, 1905.

Ibn Qutaybah, *Kitāb ta'wīl mukhtalif al-ḥadīth*, ed. by al-Kurdī, al-Alūsī and Shābandārzāde, Cairo, A.H. 1326.

Ibn Qutaybah, *Le Traité des divergences du ḥadīth d'Ibn Qutayba*, trans. by G. Lecomte, Damascus, 1962.

———, *al-Maʿārif*, ed. by Saroite Okacha, Cairo, 1960.

Ibn Ṣaṣrā, Muḥammad ibn Muḥammad, *ad-Durrah al-muḍī'ah fī ad-dawlah az-zāhiriyyah*, ed. and trans. by William M. Brinner, *A Chronicle of Damascus, 1389-1397*, 2 vols., Berkeley and Los Angeles, 1963.

Ibn Sīnā, *al-Qānūn fī ṭ-ṭibb*, 4 vols., Cairo, 1877.

Ibn Taghrī Birdī, *al-Manhal aṣ-ṣāfī*, vol. 1, Cairo, 1957.

———, *an-Nujūm az-zāhirah fī mulūk Miṣr wal-Qāhirah*, 12 vols., Cairo, 1929-1956.

———, *an-Nujūm az-zāhirah fī mulūk Miṣr wal-Qāhirah, History of Egypt 1382-1469 AD*, ed. and trans. by William Popper, *University of California Publications in Semitic Philology*, vols. 5-7, 13-14, 17-19, 22-23, 24 (indices), Berkeley and Los Angeles, 1915-1963.

———, *Ḥawādith ad-duhūr fī madā al-ayyām wash-shuhūr*, ed. by William Popper, *University of California Publications in Semitic Philology*, vol. 8, Berkeley and Los Angeles, 1930-1931.

Ibn Ṭūlūn, *Les Gouverneurs de Damas sous les Mamlouks et les Premiers Ottomans (658-1156/1260-1744)*, trans. by Henri Laoust, Damascus, 1952.

Ibn al-Wardī, *Risālat an-naba' 'an al-waba'*, ed. by Fāris ash-Shidyāk, *Majmūʿat al-jawā'ib*, Istanbul, A.H. 1300, pp. 184-188.

———, "Ibn al-Wardī's *Risālah al-naba' 'an al-waba'*, A Translation of a Major Source for the History of the Black Death in the Middle East," trans. by Michael W. Dols, *Near Eastern Numismatics, Iconography, Epigraphy and History: Studies in Honor of George C. Miles*, ed. by Dickran K. Kouymjian, Beirut, 1974, pp. 443-456.

———, *Ta'rīkh*, 2 vols., Baghdad, 1969.

———, *Tatimmat al-mukhtaṣar fī akhbār al-bashar*, 2 vols., Cairo, A.H. 1285.

Ignatius of Smolensk, "The Pilgrimage," *Itinéraires Russes en Orient*, trans. by B. de Khitrowo, vol. 1, Paris, 1889, pp. 149-157.

al-Jāḥiẓ, ʿAmr ibn Baḥr, *Kitāb al-Ḥayawān*, ed. by ʿAbd as-Salām Muḥammad Hārūn, Cairo, 1966-1969.

———, *The Life and Works of Jāhiẓ*, partial trans. by Charles Pellat, Berkeley and Los Angeles, 1969.

al-Jawharī, ʿAlī ibn Dāʿūd, *Inbāʾ al-haṣr bi-abnāʾ al-aṣr*, vol. 1, Cairo, 1970.

———, *Nuzhat an-nufūs wal-abdān*, 2 vols., Cairo, 1970-1971.

Julien, Stanislas, "Documents historiques sur les Tou-Kioue (Turcs), extraits du Pien-t-tien, et traduits du Chinois," *JA*, series 6, vol. 4 (1864), pp. 200-242, 391-430, 453-477.

Khalīl aẓ-Ẓāhirī, *Kitāb zubda kashf al-mamālik*, ed. by P. Ravaisse, Paris, 1894.

———, *La Zubda Kachf al-mamālik de Khalīl az-Zāhirī*, ed. by Jean Gaulmier, Beirut, 1950.

al-Khazrajī, *Kitāb al-ʿuqūd al-luʾluʾīyah*, 2 vols., Cairo, 1914.

Kinglake, A. W., *Eothen*, Lincoln, Nebraska, 1970 reprint.

Leo Africanus, *The History and Description of Africa*, ed. by Robert Brown, 3 vols., Hakluyt Society, London, 1896.

Ludolfus de Suchem, *Description of the Holy Land, and the Way Thither*, trans. by Aubrey Stewart, Palestine Pilgrims' Text Society, vol. 12, part 3, London, 1895.

al-Majūsī, ʿAlī ibn al-ʿAbbās, *Kāmil aṣ-ṣināʿah aṭ-ṭibbīyah* [*Kitāb al-malakī*], 2 vols., Būlāq, A.H. 1294.

Makhairos, Leontios, *Recital Concerning the Sweet Land of Cyprus*, ed. and trans. by R. M. Dawkins, 2 vols., Oxford, 1932.

al-Manbijī, Muḥammad ibn Muḥammad, *Tasliyat ahl al-maṣāʾib fī maut al-awlād wal-aqārib*, Cairo, A.H. 1347.

al-Maqrīzī, *Ighāthat al-ummah bi kashf al-ghummah*, Cairo, 1937.

———, "Le Traité des famines de Maqrīzī," trans. by Gaston Wiet, *JESHO*, vol. 4 (1962), pp. 1-90.

———, *al-Mawāʿiẓ wal-iʿtibār bi-dhikr al-khiṭaṭ wal-athār*, 2 vols., Būlāq, 1854.

———, *as-Sulūk li-maʿrifat duwal al-mulūk*, 4 parts in 12 vols., Cairo, 1936-1958, 1970-1973.

———, *Histoire des Sultans Mamlouks de l'Égypte*, trans. by Étienne M. Quatremère, 4 vols. in 2, Paris, 1837-1845.

Māshā'allāh, *The Astrological History of Māshā'allāh*, trans. by E. S. Kennedy and David Pingree, Cambridge, Mass., 1971.

al-Mas'ūdī, 'Alī ibn Ḥusayn, *Les Prairies d'Or*, trans. by A. C. Barbier de Meynard and A.-J.-B. Pavet de Courteille, 9 vols., Paris, 1961-1977.

Medical Faculty of the University of Paris, *Compendium de Epidimia per Collegium Facultatis Medicorum Parisius* (1348), ed. by H. E. Rebouis, *Étude historique et critique sur la peste*, Paris, 1888.

Minorsky, Vladimir, *Persia in A.D. 1478-1490 (An Abridged Translation of Faḍlullah b. Rūzbihān Khunjī's Tārīkh-i 'Ālam-ārā-yi amīnī)*, Royal Asiatic Society, vol. 26, London, 1957.

Mufaḍḍal ibn Abī al-Faḍā'il, *an-Nahj as-sadīd wad-durr al-farīd*, ed. and trans. by E. Blochet, "Histoire des Sultans Mamlouks," *Patrologia Orientalis*, vol. 12 (1919), pp. 345-550; vol. 14 (1920), pp. 375-672; and vol. 20 (1929), pp. 1-270.

Muḥammad Haydar, Dughlāk, *Tarikh-i-Rashīdī: A History of the Moghuls of Central Asia*, trans. by E. D. Ross, London, 1895.

Mussi, Gabriele de', *Historia de Morbo s. Mortalitate quae fuit Anno Dni MCCCXLVII*, ed. by Henschel in H. Haeser, *Archiv für die Gesammte Medicin*, vol. 2 (Jena, 1842), pp. 26-59. Reprinted in H. Haeser, *Lehrbuch der Geschichte der Medicin und der epidemischen Krankheiten*, 3rd ed., vol. 3 (Jena, 1882), pp. 157-161. Text also in A. C. Tononi, "La peste dell'anno 1348," *Giornale Linguistico*, vol. 11, Genoa, 1884, pp. 144-152.

Niẓām al-Mulk, *Siyāsatnāmeh*, trans. by H. Darke, London, 1960.

———, *Siyāsatnāmah*, trans. by C. Schafer, Paris, 1891-1893.

Piloti, Emmanuel, "Traité d'Emmanuel Piloti d'Ile de Crète sur le passage dans la Terre Sainte," ed. by Baron de Reiffenberg, *Monuments pour servir à l'histoire des Provinces de Namur, de Hainaut et de Luxembourg*, vol. 4 (1846), pp. 312-419.

Piloti, Emmanuel, *L'Égypte au Commencement du Quinzième Siècle*, ed. by P.-H. Dopp, Cairo, 1950; Louvain and Leopoldville, 1958.

Poggibonsi, Niccolò da, *A Voyage Beyond the Seas*, trans. by T. Bellorini and E. Hoade, Jerusalem, 1946.

Priuli, Girolamo, *I Diarii*, ed. by L. A. Muratori, *Rerum Italicarum Scriptores*, tome 24, part 3, vol. 1, Lapi, 1912-1921.

Procopius, *History of the Wars*, trans. by H. B. Dewing, vol. 1, New York, 1914.

al-Qalqashandī, *Subḥ al-a'shā*, 14 vols., Cairo, 1914-1928.

Qur'ān, *Corani Textus Arabicus*, ed. by Gustav Flügel, Leipzig, 1841.

———, Gustav Flügel, *Concordantiae Corani Arabicae*, Leipzig, 1875.

———, *The Qur'ān*, trans. by Richard Bell, 2 vols., Edinburgh, 1937.

———, *The Holy Qur'ān*, trans. by M. Muḥammad 'Alī, Lahore, 1963.

ar-Rāzī, Bakr Muḥammad b. Zakarīyā', *Kitāb ḥāwī fī ṭ-ṭibb*, 21 vols. in 22, Hyderabad, 1955-1968.

Russell, Patrick, *A Treatise on the Plague: Containing an historical journal and medical account of the Plague, at Aleppo, in the years 1760, 1761, 1762*, London, 1791.

as-Sakhāwī, *aḍ-Ḍaw' al-lāmi'*, 12 vols., Cairo, A.H. 1353-1355.

———, *at-Tibr al-masbūḳ fī dhayl as-sulūḳ*, Būlāq, 1896.

Ṣāliḥ ibn Yaḥyā, *Ta'rīḳh Bayrūt*, ed. by P. L. Cheikho, 2nd ed., Beirut, 1927.

Sanjian, A. K., *Colophons of Armenian Manuscripts 1301-1480: A Source for Middle Eastern History*, Cambridge, Mass., 1969.

Sanuto, Marino, *I Diarii di Marino Sanuto*, 58 vols. in 59, Venice, 1879-1903.

Sauvaget, Jean, "Décrets Mamelouks de Syrie," *Bulletin d'Études Orientales*, Damascus, vol. 2 (1932), pp. 1-52, vol. 3 (1934), pp. 1-29, and vol. 12 (1947-1948), pp. 1-60.

Schimmel, Annemarie, *Die Chronik des Ibn Iyās, Indices, Bibliotheca Islamica*, vol. 5f, Istanbul, 1945.

Sibṭ ibn al-'Ajamī, *Kunūz adh-dhahab fī ta'rīkh Ḥalab (Les Trèsors d'Or)*, trans. by Jean Sauvaget, Institut Français de Damas, Beirut, 1950.

as-Suyūṭī, *Ḥusn al-muḥāḍarah fī ta'rīkh Miṣr wal-Qāhirah*, 2 vols., Cairo, 1968.

———, *Mā rawāhu l-wā'ūn fī akhbār aṭ-ṭā'ūn* [*Sard aṭ-ṭawā'īn al-wāqī'ah fī l-islām*], ed. by Alfred von Kremer, "Ueber die grossen Seuchen des Orients nach arabischen quellen," *Sitzungsberichte der Kaiserlichen Akademie der Wissenschaften (Philosophisch-Historische Classe)*, vol. 96, book 1, Vienna, 1880, pp. 144-156.

aṭ-Ṭabarī, *Ta'rīkh aṭ-Ṭabarī*, 10 vols., Cairo, 1960-1969.

aṭ-Ṭabarī, 'Alī ibn Rabban, *Firdausu l-Ḥikmat or Paradise of Wisdom*, ed. by M. Z. Siddiqī, Berlin, 1928.

Tāshköprüzāde, Aḥmad, *ash-Shifā' li-adwā' al-wabā'*, Cairo, A.H. 1292.

Tha'ālibī, *The Laṭā'if al-ma'ārif of Tha'ālibī,* trans. by C. E. Bosworth, Edinburgh, 1968.

Thābit ibn Qurrah, *Kitāb adh-dhakhīrah*, ed. by G. Sobhy, Cairo, 1928.

Tiesenhausen, Woldemar, ed., *Sbornik materialov otnosjaščichsja k istorii Zolotoj ordy* [*Documents Concerning the History of the Golden Horde*], 2 vols., St. Petersburg, 1884.

al-'Ulaymī, 'Abd ar-Raḥmān, *al-Uns al-jalīl bi-ta'rīkh al-Quds wal-Khalīl*, 2 vols., Baghdad, 1968.

Umārah, ibn 'Alī, al-Ḥakamī, *Yaman, Its Early Mediaeval History*, trans. by H. C. Kay, London, 1892.

al-'Umarī, Ibn Faḍlallāh, *Masālik al-abṣār fī mamālik al-amṣār*, vol. 1, Cairo, 1924.

———, *at-Ta'rīf bil-muṣṭalaḥ ash-sharīf*, Cairo, A.H. 1312.

Volney, *Voyage en Égypte et en Syrie*, ed. by Jean Gaulmier, Paris, 1959.

Wiet, Gaston, trans., "La Grande Peste Noire en Syrie et en Égypte," *Études d'orientalisme dédiées à la mémoire de Lévi-Provençal*, vol. 1, Paris, 1962, pp. 367-384.

al-Yāfi'ī, 'Abdallāh ibn As'ad, *Mir'āt al-jinān wa 'ibrat al-yaqẓān*, 4 vols., Beirut, 1970 reprint.

Yule, Sir Henry, ed. and trans., *Cathay and the Way Thither*, rev. ed. by Henri Cordier, 4 vols., Hakluyt Society, London, 1913-1916.

Zafer-name, trans. by A.L.M. Petis de la Croix, *Histoire de Timur-Bec*, Paris, 1722.

Zucchello, Pignol, *Lettere di Mercanti a Pignol Zucchello (1336-1350)*, Venice, 1957.

D. SECONDARY PRINTED SOURCES AND THESES

Abu-Lughod, Janet L., *Cairo: 1001 Years of "the City Victorious,"* Princeton, 1971.

Adams, Robert, *Land Behind Baghdad: A History of Settlement on the Diyala Plains*, Chicago, 1965.

Ackerknecht, E. H., "Anticontagionism between 1821 and 1867," *Bulletin of the History of Medicine*, vol. 22 (1948), pp. 562-593.

Anawati, G. C., "La notion de 'Péché originel' existe-t-elle dans l'Islam?" *Studia Islamica*, vol. 31 (1970), pp. 29-40.

Antuña, M. M., "Abenjátima de Almeria y su tratado de la peste," *Religión y Cultura* (El Escorial and Madrid), vol. 1, no. 4 (1928), pp. 68-90.

Arnold, T. W., and A. Guillaume, ed., *The Legacy of Islam*, Oxford, 1931.

'Āshour, Sa'īd 'Abd al-Fattāḥ, *al-'Aṣr al-mamālīkī fī Miṣr wash-Sham*, Cairo, 1964.

———, *Miṣr fī 'aṣr dawlat al-mamālīk al-baḥrīyah*, Cairo, 1959.

———, *al-Mujtama' al-Miṣrī fī aṣr salāṭīn al-mamālīk*, Cairo, 1962.

Ashtor (Strauss), Eliyahu, "Le Coût de la vie dans l'Égypte médiévale," *JESHO*, vol. 3 (1960), pp. 56-77.

———, "Le Coût de la vie dans le Syrie médiévale," *Arabica*, vol. 8 (1961), pp. 59-72.

———, "An Essay on the Diet of the Various Classes in the Medieval Levant," *Biology of Man in History*, ed. by R.

Forster and O. Ranum, Baltimore, 1975, pp. 125-162; reprinted and translated from *Annales* (1968), pp. 1017-1053.

———, "L'Évolution des prix dans le Proche-Orient à la basse-époque," *JESHO*, vol. 4 (1961), pp. 15-46.

———, *Histoire des prix et des salaires dans l'Orient médiéval*, Paris, 1969.

———, "Matériaux pour l'histoire des prix dans l'Égypte médiévale," *JESHO*, vol. 6 (1963), pp. 158-189.

———, *Les Métaux précieux et la balance des payments du Proche-Orient à la basse-époque*, Paris, 1971.

———, "Prix et salaires à l'époque Mamlouke," *REI*, 1949, pp. 49-94.

———, "Quelques indications sur les revenues dans l'Orient musulman au haut moyen âge," *JESHO*, vol. 2 (1959), pp. 262-280.

———, "The Social Isolation of the Ahl al-Dhimma," *Études orientales à la mémoire de P. Hirschler*, ed. by O. Komolos, Budapest, 1950, pp. 73-94.

Ata, Galip, "Évolution de la médicine en Turquie," *Comptes-Rendus*, The Ninth International Congress of the History of Medicine (Bucharest, September, 1932), ed. by Victor Gomoin and Victorica Gomoin, pp. 95-131; also to be found in the *Bulletin de la société française d'histoire de la médicine*, vol. 26 (1932).

Aubin, Jean, "Les Princes d'Ormuz du XIII au XV siècle," *JA*, vol. 241 (1953), pp. 77-137.

Ayalon (Neustadt), David, "The Circassians in the Mamlūk Kingdom," *JAOS*, vol. 69 (1954), pp. 135-147.

———, "A Comparison between the Mamluk Societies of Egypt in the Mamluk Kingdom and under the Ottomans," *Proceedings of the 23rd International Congress of Orientalists*, ed. by D. Sinor, Cambridge, 1954, pp. 333ff.

———, "Discharges from service, banishments and imprisonments in Mamluk society," *Israel Oriental Studies*, vol. 2, Tel Aviv, 1972, pp. 25-50.

———, *L'Esclavage du Mamelouk*, The Israel Oriental Society, *Oriental Notes and Studies*, no. 1, Jerusalem, 1951.

Ayalon (Neustadt). David, "The European-Asiastic Steppe—A Major Reservoir of Power for the Islamic World," *Proceedings of the 25th International Congress of Orientalists (Moscow, 1960)*, vol. 2, Moscow, 1963, pp. 47-52.

———, "The Muslim City and the Mamluk Military Aristocracy," *Proceedings of the Israel Academy of Sciences and Humanities*, Jerusalem, vol. 2 (1968), pp. 311-329.

———, "Notes on the Furūsiyya Exercises and Games in the Mamluk Sultanate," *Scripta Hierosolymitana*, ed. by Uriel Heyd, vol. 9, Jerusalem, 1961, pp. 31-62.

———, "The Plague and Its Effects upon the Mamlūk Army," *JRAS* (1946), pp. 67-73.

———, "Le Règiment Baḥriya dans l'armée Mamlouke," *REI* (1951), pp. 133-141.

———, "Studies on the Structure of the Mamluk Army," *BSOAS*, vol. 15 (1953), pp. 203-228, 448-476, vol. 16 (1954), pp. 57-90.

———, "Studies on the Transfer of the 'Abbāsid Caliphate from Baghdād to Cairo," *Arabica*, vol. 7 (1960), pp. 41-59.

———, "The System of Payment in Mamlūk Military Society," *JESHO*, vol. 1 (1957-1958), pp. 37-65, 257-296.

———, "The Wafidiya in the Mamluk Kingdom," *Islamic Culture*, vol. 25, part 1 (1951), pp. 89-104.

'Azzawī, 'Abbās, *Ta'rīkh al-'Irāq bayn iḥtilālayn*, 8 vols., Baghdad, 1935-1956.

Bahgat, Aly, and A. Gabriel, *Fouilles d'al-Foustat*, Paris, 1921.

———, and F. Mossoul, *La Céramique musulmane de l'Égypte*, Cairo, 1930.

Balbas, L. Torres, "Extensione y demografia de las Ciudades Hispano-musulmanas," *Studia Islamica*, vol. 3 (1955), pp. 35-59.

Balog, Paul, *The Coinage of the Mamlūk Sultans of Egypt and Syria*, American Numismatic Society, Numismatic Studies, vol. 12, New York, 1964.

———, "Études numismatiques de l'Égypte musulmane," *BIE*, vol. 34 (1951-1952), pp. 17-55.

Balog, Paul, "History of the Dirhem," *Revue Numismatique*, Paris, series 3, vol. 6 (1961), pp. 109-146.

Baltazard, M., and B. Seydian, "Enquête sur les conditions de la pest au Moyen-Orient," *Bulletin of the World Health Organization*, vol. 23, nos. 2-3 (1960), Geneva, pp. 157-169.

——, "Recherches sur la peste en Iran," *Bulletin of the World Health Organization*, vol. 23, nos. 2-3 (1960), Geneva, pp. 141-156.

Barkan, Ömer L., "Essai sur les données statistiques des registres de recensement dans l'empire Ottoman aux XVe et XVIe siècles," *JESHO*, vol. 1 (1957), pp. 9-36.

Basset, René, *Mille et un contes, récits de légendes Arabes*, 2 vols., Paris, 1924.

Bean, J.M.W., "Plague, Population and Economic Decline in England in the Later Middle Ages," *The Economic History Review*, 2nd series, vol. 15 (1962-1963), pp. 423-437.

Belyaev, E. A., *Arabs, Islam and the Arab Caliphate in the Early Middle Ages*, trans. by A. Gourevitch, New York, 1969.

Biraben, J.-N., "La Peste dans l'Europe Occidentale et le Bassin Méditérranéen: principales épidémies, conceptions médicales, moyens de lutte," *Concours Medical*, vol. 35, Paris, 1963, pp. 781-790.

——, and J. LeGoff, "La Peste dans le haut moyen âge," *Annales*, vol. 24, part 6 (1969), pp. 1484-1510.

Björkman, Walter, *Beiträge zur Geschichte des Staatskanzler im Islamischen Ägypten*, Hamburg, 1928.

Bloch, Édouard, *La Peste en Tunisie (aperçu historique et épidémiologique)*, (diss., Faculty of Medicine, Paris), Tunis, 1929.

Bosworth, C. E., "Christian and Jewish Religious Dignitaries in Mamlūk Egypt and Syria: Qalqashandī's Information on Their Hierarchy, Titulature and Appointment," *IJMES*, vol. 3, nos. 1-2 (1972), pp. 59-74, 199-216.

——, *The Ghaznavids*, Edinburgh, 1963.

Bowsky, W. M., ed., *The Black Death: A Turning Point in History?* New York, 1971.

Bowsky, W. M., "The Impact of the Black Death upon Sienese Government and Society," *Speculum*, vol. 39, no. 1 (1964), pp. 1-34.

Braudel, Fernand, *La Méditerranée et le monde méditerranéen à l'époque de Philippe II*, Paris, 1949.

Bretschneider, E. V., *Mediaeval Researches from Eastern Asiatic Sources*, 2 vols., London, 1910.

Brian, Doris, "A Reconstruction of the Miniature Cycle in the Demotte Shah Namah," *Ars Islamica*, vol. 6 (1939), pp. 96-112.

Bridbury, A. R., "The Black Death," *The Economic History Review*, 2nd series, vol. 26, no. 4 (1973), pp. 577-592.

Brody, S. N., *The Disease of the Soul: Leprosy in Medieval Literature*, Ithaca, 1974.

Brown, L. Carl, "The Sudanese Mahdiya," *Protest and Power in Black Africa*, ed. by Robert I. Rotberg and Ali A. Mazrui, Oxford, 1970, pp. 145-168.

Brown, Peter, *The World of Late Antiquity: AD 150-750*, London, 1971.

Browne, E. G., *Arabian Medicine*, Cambridge, 1921.

———, *A History of Persian Literature*, 4 vols., Cambridge, 1902-1924.

Brunschvig, R., *La Bérberie Orientale sous les Hafsides*, 2 vols., Paris, 1940.

Cahen, Claude, "Contribution à l'histoire du Diyār Bakr au quatorzième siècle," *JA*, vol. 243 (1955), pp. 65-100.

———, "L'Évolution de l'Iqṭā' de IXe au XIIIe siècle," *Annales*, vol. 8 (1953), pp. 25-52.

———, "Mouvements populaires et autonomisme urbain dans l'Asie musulmane de moyen âge," *Arabica*, vol. 5 (1958), pp. 225-250; vol. 6 (1959), pp. 25-56, 223-265.

———, "Quelques mots sur le déclin commercial de monde musulman à la fin du moyen âge," *Studies in the Economic History of the Middle East*, ed. by M. A. Cook, London, 1970, pp. 31-36.

Campbell, A. M., *The Black Death and Men of Learning*, New York, 1931.

Campbell, Donald, *Arabian Medicine and Its Influence on the Middle Ages*, 2 vols., London, 1926.

Canard, M., "Les Relations entre les Mérinides et les Mamelouks au XIVe siècle," *Annales de l'Institut d'Études Orientales*, Algiers, vol. 5 (1939-1941), pp. 41-81.

Carpentier, É., "Autour de la Peste Noire: famines et épidémies dans l'histoire du XIVe siècle," *Annales*, vol. 17 (1962), pp. 1062-1092.

———, *Une Ville devant la peste: Orvieto et la Peste Noire*, Paris, 1962.

Carra de Vaux, Bernard, *Les Penseurs de l'Islam*, 5 vols. in 4, Paris, 1921-1926.

Chelhod, Joeseph, *Le Sacrifice chez les Arabes*, Paris, 1955.

Clerget, M., *Le Caire: Étude de géographie urbaine et d'histoire économique*, 2 vols., Cairo, 1934.

Cohn, Norman, *The Pursuit of the Millennium*, rev. ed., New York, 1970.

Coulton, G. G., *The Black Death*, London, 1929.

———, *Mediaeval Panorama*, Cambridge, 1938.

Crawfurd, Raymond H. P., *Plague and Pestilence in Literature and Art*, Oxford, 1914.

Creighton, C., *A History of Epidemics in Britain*, Cambridge, 1894.

Creswell, K.A.C., *A Brief Chronology of the Muḥammadan Monuments of Egypt to A.D. 1517*, Cairo, 1919.

Dąbrowski, Leszek, "Two Arab Nécroples Discovered at Kom el Dikka, Alexandria," *Études et Travaux*, no. 2, vol. 3 (1966), pp. 171-180.

Darrag, Aḥmad, *L'Égypte sous le règne de Barsbay 825-841/1422-1438*, Damascus, 1961.

———, *al-Mamālīk wal-Franj*, Cairo, 1961.

ad-Darwish, M., "Analysis of Some Estimates of the Population of Egypt before the Nineteenth Century," *L'Égypte Contemporaine*, vol. 20 (1929), pp. 273-286.

———, and H. as-S. Azmi, "A Note on the Population of Egypt," *Population*, vol. 2 (1934), pp. 34-56.

Deaux, George, *The Black Death 1347*, London, 1969.

D'Irsay, Stephen, "Defense Reactions during the Black Death, 1348-1349," *Annals of Medical History*, vol. 9 (1927), pp. 169-179.

——, "Notes to the Origin of the Expression 'atra mors'," *Isis*, vol. 8 (1926), pp. 328-332.

Dols, Michael W., "Plague in Early Islamic History," *JAOS*, vol. 94, no. 3 (1974), pp. 371-383.

——, "The Comparative Communal Responses to the Black Death in Muslim and Christian Societies," *Viator: Medieval and Renaissance Studies*, vol. 5 (1974), pp. 269-287.

Donaldson, B. A., *The Wild Rue*, London, 1938.

Doob, P.B.R., *Nebuchadnezzar's Children: Conventions of Madness in Middle English Literature*, New Haven, 1974.

Dozy, R.P.A., *Supplément aux Dictionnaires Arabes*, 2 vols., Paris, 1967 reprint.

Dufourcq, Charles-Emmanuel, *L'Espagne Catalane et le Maghrib aux XIIIe et XIVe siècles*, Paris, 1966.

Dzierżykray-Rogalski, T., "An Anatomical and Anthropological Analysis of Human Skeletal Remains from the Arab Nécroples at Kom el-Dikka, Alexandria (Egypt)," *Études et Travaux*, no. 2, vol. 3 (1966), pp. 200-216.

——, "Human Bones from Trench F and G of the Moslem Nécroples at Kom el-Dikka, Alexandria (Egypt)," *Études et Travaux*, no. 2, vol. 6 (1968), pp. 229-242.

——, and E. Promińska, "Studies of Human Bones from Sector M-IX of the Moslem Nécroples at Kom el-Dikka, Alexandria (Egypt)," *Études et Travaux*, no. 2, vol. 6 (1968), pp. 173-228.

Ebers, Georg, *L'Égypte, Alexandrie et la Caire*, 2 vols., Paris, 1880-1881.

Ehrenkreutz, Andrew S., *Saladin*, Albany, New York, 1972.

Elgood, Cyril, *A Medical History of Persia and the Eastern Caliphate, from the Earliest Times until AD 1932*, Cambridge, 1951.

Ettinghausen, Richard, *Arab Painting*, Geneva, 1962.

Faraj, Fu'ād, *al-Qāhirah*, 3 vols., Cairo, 1943-1946.

Fathy, Hassan, *Architecture for the Poor*, Chicago, 1973.

Fedorov, V. N., "Plague in Camels and Its Prevention in the USSR," *Bulletin of the World Health Organization*, vol. 23, nos. 2-3 (1960), pp. 275-282.

Fenyuk, B. K., "The Epizootic and Epidemic Situation in the Natural Foci of Plague in the USSR and the Prophylactic Measures Taken," *Bulletin of the World Health Organization*, vol. 23, nos. 2-3 (1960), pp. 401-404.

———, "Experience in the Eradication of Enzootic Plague in the North-West Part of the Caspian Region of the USSR," *Bulletin of the World Health Organization*, vol. 23, nos. 2-3 (1960), pp. 263-274.

Galal, M., "Essai d'observations sur les rites funéraires en Égypte actuelle," *REI*, vol. 11 (1937), pp. 131-299, plates I-XVIII.

Gasquet, F. A., *The Black Death of 1348 and 1349*, 2nd ed., London, 1908.

Gaudefroy-Demombynes, Maurice, *La Syrie au début du quinzième siècle*, Paris, 1923.

Génicot, Léopold, "On the Evidence of Growth of Population in the West from the Eleventh to the Thirteenth Century," *Change in Medieval Society*, ed. by S. L. Thrupp, New York, 1964, pp. 14-29.

Gibb, Sir Hamilton, "The Achievement of Saladin," *Bulletin of the John Rylands Library*, vol. 35, no. 1 (Manchester, 1952), pp. 44-60.

———, "The Armies of Saladin," *Cahiers d'Histoire Égyptéenne*, series 3, fasc. 4 (Cairo, 1951), pp. 304-320.

———, and J. H. Kramers, *Shorter Encyclopaedia of Islam*, Leiden, 1953.

———, *Studies on the Civilization of Islam*, ed. by S. J. Shaw and W. R. Polk, Boston, 1968.

Glubb, John B., *Soldiers of Fortune: the Story of the Mamlukes*, London, 1973.

Goitein, S. D., *A Mediterranean Society*, 2 vols., Berkeley and Los Angeles, 1967-1971.

Goldziher, Ignaz, *Mohamed and Islam*, New Haven, 1917.

Gottheil, Richard J. H., "Dhimmis and Moslems in Egypt," *Old Testament and Semitic Studies in Memory of William Rainey Harper*, ed. by R. F. Harper, F. Brown, and G. F. Moore, 2 vols., Chicago, 1908, pp. 351-414.

Grabar, Oleg, *The Formation of Islamic Art*, New Haven, 1973.

———, "The Illustrated Maqāmāt of the Thirteenth Century: The Bourgeoisie and the Arts," *The Islamic City*, ed. by A. Hourani and S. M. Stern, Oxford, 1970, pp. 207-222.

Greenwood, Major, *Epidemics and Crowd-Diseases*, London, 1935.

Grekov, B., and A. Iakoubovski, *La Horde d'Or*, trans. by F. Thuret, Paris, 1939.

Grousset, René, *The Empire of the Steppes: A History of Central Asia*, trans. by N. Walford, New Brunswick, N.J., 1970.

Grunebaum, G. E. von, *Islam*, London, 1961.

———, *Medieval Islam*, Chicago, 1966.

Guerchberg, S., "La Controverse sur les prétendus semeurs de la Peste Noire d'après les traités de peste de l'époque," *Revue des Études Juives*, n.s., vol. 8 (1948), pp. 3-40.

Guest, A. R., and E. T. Richmond, "Misr in the Fifteenth Century," *JRAS* (1903), pp. 791-816.

Guignes, Joseph de, *Histoire générale des Huns, des Turcs, des Mongols, etc.*, 4 vols. in 5, Paris, 1756-1758.

Guyon, J.-L.-G., *Histoire chronologique des épidémies du Nord de l'Afrique*, Algiers, 1855.

Ḥabishī, Ḥasan, "al-Iḥtikār al-mamlūkī wa 'alāqatuhu bil-ḥālah aṣ-ṣiḥḥīyah," *Bulletin of the Faculty of Arts*, 'Ayn Shams University, Cairo, 1959, pp. 133-157.

Haeser, Heinrich, *Lehrbuch der Geschichte der Medicin und der Epidemischen Krankheiten*, 3 vols., Jena, 1875-1882.

Hambis, Louis, "Le chapitre CVII du Yuan Che, les généologies impériales mongoles dans l'histoire chinoise officielle de la dynastie mongole," *T'oung Pao, Supplement*, vol. 38 (Leiden, 1945).

Hamdan, G., "The Pattern of Medieval Urbanism in the Arab World," *Geography*, no. 47 (1962), pp. 121-134.

Hammer-Purgstall, Joseph, Freiherr von, *Geschichte der Goldenen Horde in Kiptschak*, Pest, 1840.

Hautecoeur, Louis, and Gaston Wiet, *Les Mosquées du Caire*, 2 vols., Paris, 1932.

Headley, John M., "The Continental Reformation," *The Meaning of the Renaissance and Reformation*, ed. by Richard L. DeMolen, Boston, 1974.

Hecker, J.F.C., *The Epidemics of the Middle Ages*, trans. by B. G. Babington, London, 1846.

Henschen, Folke, *The History of Diseases*, London, 1966.

Herlihy, David, "The Generation in Medieval History," *Viator: Medieval and Renaissance Studies*, vol. 5 (1974), pp. 347-364.

———, "Population, Plague and Social Change in Rural Pistoria, 1201-1430," *The Economic History Review*, 2nd series, vol. 18 (1968), pp. 225-244.

Herz Bey, Max, *La Mosquée du Sultan Hassan au Caire*, Cairo, 1899.

Heyd, W., *Histoire du commerce du Levant au moyen-âge,* trans. by Furey Raynaud, 2 vols., Leipzig, 1936.

Hill, Sir George, *A History of Cyprus*, 3 vols., Cambridge, 1948.

Hinton, M.A.C., *Rats and Mice as Enemies of Mankind*, London, 1918.

Hirshleifer, Jack, *Disaster and Recovery: The Black Death in Western Europe*, RAND Corp., Santa Monica, Calif., 1966.

Hirst, L. Fabian, *The Conquest of Plague. A Study of the Evolution of Epidemiology*, Oxford, 1953.

Hodgson, Marshall G. S., "A Comparison of Islām and Christianity as Framework for Religious Life," *Diogenes*, no. 32 (1960), pp. 49-74.

———, "Islām and Image," *History of Religions*, vol. 3 (1964) pp. 220-260.

———, "A Note on the Millennium in Islam," *Millennial Dreams in Action*, ed. by S. L. Thrupp (New York, 1970), pp. 218-219.

Hodgson, Marshall G. S., "The Unity of Later Islamic History," *Journal of World History*, vol. 5 (1960), pp. 879-914.

Holt, P. M., A.K.S. Lambton, and Bernard Lewis, ed., *The Cambridge History of Islam*, 2 vols., Cambridge, 1970.

Hoogstraal, H., and R. Traub, "The Fleas (Siphonaptera) of Egypt. Host-Parasite Relationships of Rodents of the Families Spalacidae, Muridae, Gliridae, Dipodidae, and Hystricidae," *The Journal of the Egyptian Public Health Association*, vol. 40, no. 5 (1965), pp. 343-379.

Hourani, Albert, and S. M. Stern, eds., *The Islamic City*, Oxford, 1970.

Howorth, Sir Henry H., *History of the Mongols*, 4 vols., London, 1876-1927.

Hughes, T. P., *A Dictionary of Islam*, 2nd. ed., London, 1896.

Huizinga, J., *The Waning of the Middle Ages*, New York, 1954.

Huzayyin, S. A., *Arabia and the Far East: Their Commercial and Cultural Relations in Graeco-Roman and Irano-Arabian Times*, Cairo, 1942.

Ibn Abī Rabī', *Sulūk al-mālik fī tadbīr al-mamālik*, Cairo, 1329 A.H.

Issawi, Charles, "The Decline of Middle Eastern Trade, 1100-1850," *Islam and the Trade of Asia*, ed. by D. S. Richards, Oxford, 1970, pp. 245-266.

Jomard, E., "Mémoire sur la population comparée de l'Égypte ancienne et moderne," *Description de l'Égypte*, vol. 9 (Paris, 1829), pp. 109-211.

Jorga, N., *Brève histoire de la Petite Arménie*, Paris, 1930.

Jorge, Ricardo, "Les Anciennes épidémies de Peste en Europe, comparées aux épidémies modernes," *Comptes-Rendus*, the Ninth International Congress of the History of Medicine (Bucharest, September, 1932), ed. by Victor Gomoin and Victorica Gomoin, pp. 361-375.

Julien, C.-A., *History of North Africa*, New York, 1970.

Kahle, Paul, "Die Katastrophe des mittelalterlichen Alexandria," *Mélanges Maspéro*, vol. 3 (Cairo, 1940), pp. 137-154.

Kawash, Sabri K., "Ibn Ḥajar al-'Asqalānī (1372-1449 A.D.): A Study of the Background, Education and Career of a 'Ālim in Egypt," unpubl. diss., Princeton University, 1969.

Knappert, Jan, *Sawahili Islamic Poetry*, Leiden, 1971.

Kremer, Alfred von, *Culturgeschichte der Orients unter den Chalifen*, 2 vols., Vienna, 1877.

———, "Ueber die grossen Seuchen des Orients nach arabischen Quellen," *Sitzungsberichte der Kaiserlichen Akademie der Wissenschaften (Philosophish-Historische Classe)*, vol. 96, book 1, Vienna, 1880, pp. 69-156.

Kriss, Rudolf, and Hubert Kriss-Heinrich, *Volksglaube im Bereich des Islam*, 2 vols., Wiesbaden, 1960-1962.

Kubiak, W., "Les Fouilles Polonaises à Kōm el-Dick en 1963 et 1964," *Bulletin de la Société Archéologique d'Alexandria*, no. 42 (Cairo, 1967), pp. 47-80.

———, "Stèles funéraires Arabes de Kōm el-Dick," *Bulletin de la Société Archéologique d'Alexandrie*, no. 42 (Cairo, 1967), pp. 17-26.

Labib, Subhi Y., "Egyptian Commercial Policy in the Middle Ages," *Studies in the Economic History of the Middle East*, ed. by M. A. Cook, London, 1970, pp. 63-77.

———, *Handelsgeschichte Ägyptens im Spätmittelalter (1171-1517)*, Vierteljahrschrift für Sozial- und Wirtschaftsgeschichte, no. 46, Wiesbaden, 1965.

Lane, E. W., *The Manners and Customs of the Modern Egyptians*, London, 1895.

———, *Arabic-English Lexicon*, London, 1874 (New York, 1955-1956 reprint), 8 vols.

———, *Arabian Society in the Middle Ages*, ed. by S. Lane-Poole, London, 1883.

Lane-Poole, Stanley, *A History of Egypt in the Middle Ages*, London, 1968 reprint.

Langer, W. L., "The Black Death," *Scientific American* (February, 1964), pp. 114-122.

———, "The Next Assignment," *American Historical Review*, vol. 63 (January, 1958), pp. 283-304.

Lapidus, Ira M., "The Grain Economy of Mamlūk Egypt," *JESHO*, vol. 12, part 1 (1969), pp. 1-15.

———, "Muslim Cities and Islamic Societies," *Middle Eastern Cities*, ed. by I. M. Lapidus, Berkeley and Los Angeles, 1969, pp. 47-79.

Lapidus, Ira M., *Muslim Cities in the Later Middle Ages*, Cambridge, Mass., 1967.

———, "Traditional Muslim Cities: Structure and Change," *From Madina to Metropolis*, ed. by L. Carl Brown, Princeton, 1973, pp. 51-69.

Laufer, Berthold, "Geophagy," *Field Museum of Natural History*, Publication no. 280, Anthropological Series, vol. 18, no. 2 (Chicago, 1930), pp. 97-198.

Leroy, Jules, "Un Témoignage inédit sur l'état du monastère des Syriens au Wadi'n Natrūn au début au XVIe siècle," *BIFAO*, vol. 65 (1967), pp. 1-23, plate 1.

Le Tourneau, R., "North Africa to the Sixteenth Century," *The Cambridge History of Islam*, ed. by P. M. Holt, A.K.S. Lambton, and Bernard Lewis, Cambridge, 1970, vol. 2, pp. 211-237.

Levey, Martin, *Early Arabic Pharmacology*, Leiden, 1973.

Lewis, Bernard, "Egypt and Syria," *The Cambridge History of Islam*, ed. by P. M. Holt, A.K.S. Lambton, and Bernard Lewis, Cambridge, 1970, vol. 1, pp. 201-230.

———, *Race and Color in Islam*, New York, 1971.

Lewis, R. E., "The Fleas (Siphonaptera) of Egypt: An Illustrated and Annotated Key," *The Journal of Parasitology*, vol. 53, no. 4 (1937), pp. 863-885.

Lifton, Robert, *Death in Life*, New York, 1969.

Lopez, Robert, and Harry Miskimin, "The Economic Depression of the Renaissance," *The Economic History Review*, 2nd series, vol. 14 (1962), pp. 397-407.

———, Harry Miskimin and Abraham Udovitch, "England to Egypt, 1350-1500: Long-Term Trends and Long-Distance Trade," *Studies in the Economic History of the Middle East*, ed. by M. A. Cook, London, 1970, pp. 93-128.

Lorinser, C. J., *Die Pest der Orients*, Berlin, 1837.

Lucas, H. S., "The Great European Famine and Epidemic in 1315, 1316, and 1317," *Speculum*, vol. 5 (1930), pp. 343-377.

Lyons, Malcolm, *Galen on the Parts of Medicine*, Berlin, 1969.

Makar, A., *Contribution à l'étude de l'épidémiologie de la peste*, diss., Faculty of Medicine, University of Lausanne, 1938.

Marcel, J. J., *Égypte depuis la conquête des Arabes jusqu'à la domination française*, Paris, 1877.

Marchika, Jean, *La Peste en Afrique Septentrionale: histoire de la peste en Algérie de 1363 à 1830*, Algiers, 1927.

Marks Geoffrey, *The Medieval Plague*, New York, 1971.

Marques, A. H. de Oliveira, *Daily Life in Portugal in the Later Middle Ages*, Madison, 1971.

Martinez, Montavez P., *La oscilación del precio del trigo en el Cairo durante el primer régimen mameluco (1252-1382)*, Madrid, 1964 (summary).

Marzouk, M. A., "The Tirāz Institution in Medieval Egypt," *Studies in Islamic Art and Architecture in Honor of Professor K. A. C. Cresswell*, Cairo, 1965, pp. 157-162.

Massignon, Louis, "La Cité des Morts au Caire (Qarāfa-Darb al-Aḥmar)," *Opera Minora*, vol. 3 (Beirut, 1963), pp. 233-285, plates I-X.

——, "Les 'Sept Dormants' Apocalypses de l'Islam," *Opera Minora*, vol. 3 (Beirut, 1963), pp. 104-180.

Mayer, L. A., *Mamlūk Costume*, Geneva, 1952.

Mehrez, Shahira G., "The Ghawriyya in the Urban Context: An Analysis of Its Form and Function," unpubl. M.A. thesis, American University in Cairo, 1972.

Meinardus, O.F.A., *Monks and Monasteries of the Egyptian Desert*, Cairo, 1961.

Meiss, Millard, *Painting in Florence and Siena after the Black Death*, New York, 1964.

Meyer, K. F., "Plague," *Encyclopaedia Britannica*, New York, 1956.

Meyerhof, Max, "Ali at-Tabari's 'Paradise of Wisdom,' One of the Oldest Compendiums of Medicine," *Isis*, vol. 16 (1931), pp. 1-54.

——, "The 'Book of Treasure,' An early Arabic Treatise on Medicine," *Isis*, vol. 14 (1930), pp. 55-76.

Meyerhof, Max, "Climate and Health in Old Cairo, According to 'Alī ibn Ridwān," *Comptes-Rendus du congrès international de médicine tropicale et d'hygiène*, Cairo, 1929, vol. 2, pp. 211-239.

———, "La Peste en Égypte à la fin du XVIIIe siècle et le médecin Enrico di Wolmar," *La Revue médicale d'Égypte*, vol. 1 (Cairo, 1913), nos. 4 and 5.

Michel, Bernard, "L'Organisation financière de l'Égypte sous les Sultans Mamelouks d'après Qalqachandi," *BIE*, vol. 7 (1925), pp. 127-147.

Miller, William, *Trebizond, The Last Great Greek Empire of the Byzantine Era*, Chicago, 1969.

Miskimin, Harry, *The Economy of Early Renaissance Europe, 1300-1460*, Englewood Cliffs, N.J., 1969.

Mols, R., *Introduction à la démographie historique des villes d'Europe du XIVe au XVIIIe siècle*, 2 vols., Louvain, 1954-1956.

Morris, Christopher, "The Plague in Britain," *The Historical Journal*, vol. 14, no. 1 (1971), pp. 205-215.

Moule, A. C., *Christians in China Before the Year 1550*, New York, 1930.

Muir, William, *The Caliphate: Its Rise, Decline and Fall*, Edinburgh, 1924.

———, *The Mameluke or Slave Dynasty of Egypt, 1260-1517*, London, 1896.

Nasr, S. H., *Ideals and Realities of Islam*, Boston, 1972.

Neaman, Judith S., *Suggestion of the Devil: The Origins of Madness*, New York, 1975.

Neustatter, Otto, "Mice in Plague Pictures," *The Journal of the Walters Art Gallery*, vol. 4 (1941), pp. 105-114.

Niemeyer, Wolfgang, *Ägypten zur Zeit der Mamluken*, Berlin, 1936.

Nohl, Johannes, *The Black Death*, trans. by C. H. Clarke, London, 1961.

Opitz, Karl, *Die Medizin im Koran*, Stuttgart, 1906.

Owst, G. R., *Preaching in Medieval England: An Introduction to Sermon Manuscripts of the Period c. 1350-1450*, Cambridge, 1926.

Padwick, C. E., *Muslim Devotions*, London, 1961.
Pareja, F. M. et al., *Islamologie*, Beirut, 1964.
Parry, Adam, "The Language of Thucydides' Description of the Plague," *Bulletin*, Institute of Classical Studies, University of London, no. 16 (1969), pp. 106-118.
Pastukhov, B. N., "The Epizootic and Epidemic Situation in the Natural Foci of Plague in the USSR and the Prophylactic Measures Taken," *Bulletin of the World Health Organization*, vol. 23, nos. 2-3 (Geneva, 1960), pp. 401-404.
Pellat, Charles, *Langues et littérature Arabes*, Paris, 1970.
Perlmann, Moshe, "Notes on Anti-Christian Propaganda in the Mamlūk Empire," *BSOAS*, vol. 10 (1942), pp. 843-861.
Petrie, F. F., R. E. Todd, R. Skander, and F. Hilmy, "A Report on Plague Investigation in Egypt," *The Journal of Hygiene*, vol. 23, no. 2 (November, 1924), pp. 117-150.
Pevzner, S. B., "Ikta' v Egipte v Kontse XIII-XIV Vekakh" ["The Iqṭā' in Egypt at the End of the 13th and 14th Centuries"], *Pamiati Akademika Ignatiia Iulianovicha Krachkovskogo*, ed. by I. A. Orbeli, Leningrad, 1958, pp. 176-191.
"Plague," *Bulletin of the World Health Organization*, vol. 23, nos. 2-3 (Geneva, 1960), pp. 130-422.
Planhol, Xavier de, *Les Fondements géographiques de l'histoire de l'Islam*, Paris, 1968.
Poliak, A. N., "Le Caractère colonial de l'état Mamelouk dans ses rapports avec la Horde d'Or," *REI* (1935), pp. 231-248.
———, "The Demographic Evolution of the Middle East; Population Trends Since 1348," *Palestine and Middle East*, vol. 10, no. 5 (May, 1938), pp. 201-205.
———, "La Féodalité Islamique," *REI*, vol. 10 (1936), pp. 247-265.
———, *Feudalism in Egypt, Syria, Palestine and the Lebanon, 1250-1900*, London, 1939.
———, "Les Révoltes populaires en Égypte à l'époque des Mamelouks et leurs causes économiques," *REI*, vol. 8 (1934), pp. 251-273.
———, "Some Notes on the Feudal System of the Mamluks," *JRAS* (1937), pp. 97-107.

Pollitzer, Robert, *Plague*, World Health Organization, Monograph Series, no. 22, Geneva, 1954.

———, *Plague and Plague Control in the Soviet Union*, Bronx, 1966.

———, "A Review of Recent Literature on Plague," *Bulletin of the World Health Organization*, vol. 23, nos. 2-3 (1960), Geneva, pp. 313-400.

Popper, William, "The Cairo Nilometer, Studies in Ibn Taghrī Birdī's Chronicles of Egypt," *University of California Publications in Semitic Philology*, vol. 12 (1951).

———, "Egypt and Syria Under the Circassian Sultans, 1382-1468 A.D.; Systematic Notes to Ibn Taghrī Birdī's Chronicles of Egypt," *University of California Publications in Semitic Philology*, vols. 15, 16 (1955, 1957).

Postan, M., "Some Economic Evidence of Declining Population in the Later Middle Ages," *Economic History Review*, 2nd series, vol. 2 (1950), pp. 221-246.

Powers, E., "The Opening of the Land Routes to Cathay," *Travel and Travellers of the Middle Ages*, ed. by A. P. Newton, London, 1926, pp. 124-158.

Rabie, Hassanein M., *The Financial System of Egypt, A.H. 564-741/*A.D. *1169-1341*, Oxford, 1972.

———, "The Size and Value of the Iqṭā' in Egypt, 564-741 A.H.," *Studies in the Economic History of the Middle East*, ed. by M. A. Cook, London, 1970, pp. 129-138.

Rall, Y. M., "The Geography and Some Peculiarities of the Natural Foci of Rodent Plague" (in Russian), *Zhournal Mikrobiologii*, vol. 29, no. 2 (Moscow, 1958), pp. 74-78.

Ramzī, Muḥammad, *al-Qāmūs al-jughrāfī*, 6 vols., Cairo, 1953-1968.

Raymond, André, "Les Grandes épidémies de peste au Caire aux XVIIe et XVIIIe siècles," *Bulletin d'Études Orientales*, Institut Français de Damas, vol. 25 (Damascus, 1973), pp. 203-210.

———, "Signes urbains et étude de la population des grandes villes Arabes a l'époque Ottomane," *Bulletin d'Études Orientales*, vol. 27 (Damascus, 1974), pp. 183-193.

Reeves, Marjorie, *The Influence of Prophecy in the Later Middle Ages: A Study in Joachimism*, Oxford, 1969.

Reinaud, M., *Description des monumens musulmans du cabinet de M. le Duc de Blacas*, 2 vols., Paris, 1828.

Reitemeyer, Else, *Beschreibung Ägyptens im Mittelalter*, Leipzig, 1903.

Renaud, H.P.J., "Les Maladies pestilentielles dans l'Orthodoxie Islamique," *Bulletin d'Institut d'Hygiène de Maroc*, vol. 3 (Rabat, 1934), pp. 5-16.

———, "Un Médicin du royaume de Grenade: Muḥammad ash-Shaqūrī," *Hespéris*, vol. 33 (1946), pp. 31-64.

Renouard, Y., "Conséquence et intérêt démographique de la Peste Noire de 1348," *Population*, vol. 3 (1948), pp. 459-466.

Richards, D. S., ed., *Islam and the Trade of Asia*, Oxford, 1970.

Riché, P., "Problèmes de démographie historique de haut moyen âge, (Ve-VIIIe siècles)," *Annales de demographie historique* (1966), pp. 37-55.

Riddle, John M., "Pomum ambrae. Amber and Ambergris in Plague Remedies," *Sudhoffs Archiv*, vol. 48, part 2 (June, 1964), pp. 111-122.

Robbins, Helen, "A Comparison of the Effects of the Black Death on the Economic Organization of France and England," *Journal of Political Economy*, vol. 36 (1928), pp. 447-479.

Robson, James, "Magic Cures in Popular Islam," *Moslem World*, vol. 24 (1934), pp. 33-43.

Rodinson, Maxime, "Histoire économique et histoire des classes sociales dans le monde musulman," *Studies in the Economic History of the Middle East*, ed. by M. A. Cook, London, 1970, pp. 139-155.

Rogers, J.E.T., *A History of Agriculture and Prices in England*, 7 vols., Oxford, 1866-1902.

Rosen, George, *Madness in Society*, New York, 1969.

Rosenthal, F., "The Defense of Medicine in the Medieval Muslim World," *Bulletin of the History of Medicine*, vol. 43 (1969), pp. 519-532.

Rosenthal, F., *Four Essays on Art and Literature in Islam*, Leiden, 1971.
Roulx, J. Delaville le, *Les Hospitaliers à Rhodes jusqu'à la mort de Philibert de Naillac*, Paris, 1913.
Rubin, Stanley, *Medieval English Medicine*, New York, 1974.
Russell, Josiah C., *British Medieval Population*, Albuquerque, 1948.
———, "Demographic Comparison of Egyptian and English Cities in the Later Middle Ages," *Texas A. & I. University Studies*, vol. 2 (1964), pp. 64-72.
———, "Effects of Pestilence and Plague, 1315-1385," *Comparative Studies in Society and History*, vol. 8 (1966), pp. 464-467.
———, "Late Ancient and Medieval Population," *Transactions of the American Philosophical Society*, Philadelphia, n.s., vol. 48, part 3 (1958).
———, *Medieval Regions and Their Cities*, Bloomington, 1972.
———, *Population in Europe 500-1500*, vol. 1, chapter 1 of *The Fontana Economic History of Europe*, London, 1969.
———, "The Population of Medieval Egypt," *Journal of the American Research Center in Egypt*, vol. 5 (1966), pp. 69-82.
———, "Recent Advances in Mediaeval Demography," *Speculum*, vol. 40 (1965), pp. 84-101.
———, "That Earlier Plague," *Demography*, vol. 5, part 1 (1968), pp. 174-184.
Sadeque, S. F., *Baybars the First of Egypt*, Dacca, 1956.
Saltmarsh, John, "Plague and Economic Decline in England in the Later Middle Ages," *Cambridge Historical Journal*, vol. 7 (1941), pp. 23-41.
Sarton, George, *Galen of Pergamon*, Kansas, 1954.
———, *Introduction to the History of Science*, 5 vols., Baltimore, 1927-1948.
Sauvaget, J., *La Poste aux chevaux dans l'empire dans Mamelouks*, Paris, 1941.
Saunders, J. J., *Aspects of the Crusades*, Christchurch, New Zealand, 1962.

Sauvaire, H., "Matériaux pour servir à l'histoire de la numismatique et de la métrologie musulmanes," *JA*, series 7, vol. 14 (1879), pp. 455-533; vol. 15 (1880), pp. 228-277, 421-478; vol. 18 (1881), pp. 499-516; vol. 19 (1882), pp. 23-77, 281-327.

Schacht, Joseph, *An Introduction to Islamic Law*, Oxford, 1964.

Schmitt, Heinrich G., *Die Pest des Galenos*, diss., Medical Faculty, University of Würzburg, 1936.

Schroeder, Eric, "Aḥmed Musa and Shams ad-Dīn: A Review of Fourteenth Century Painting," *Ars Islamica*, vol. 6 (1969), pp. 113-142.

Seibel, Valentin, *Die Epidemienperiode des fünften Jahrhundert vor Christus und die gleichzeitigen ungewöhnlichen Naturereignisse*, Dillingen, 1869.

——, *Die Grosse Pest zur Zeit Justinians und die ihr voraus und zur Seite gehenden ungewöhnlichen Naturereignisse*, Dillingen, 1857.

Seidel, Ernst, "Die Lehre von der Kontagion bei den Arabern," *AGM*, vol. 6 (Leipzig, 1913), pp. 81-93.

Seligmann, S., "Das Sieben schäfer-Amulett," *Der Islam*, vol. 5 (1941), pp. 370-388.

Setton, Kenneth M., ed., *A History of the Crusades*, 3 vols. (Madison, 1969-1975).

Shapiro, S. Ye., and Z. S. Barkagan, "History of Haemorrhagic Fever in Central Asia" (in Russian), *Voprosy Virusologii*, vol. 5, no. 2 (Moscow, 1960), pp. 245-247.

Sheperd, W. R., *Historical Atlas*, 9th ed., New York, 1964.

Shrewsbury, J.F.D., *A History of Bubonic Plague in the British Isles*, Cambridge, 1970.

Siegel, Rudolph E., *Galen's System of Physiology and Medicine*, Basel, 1968.

Siegfried, André, *Germs and Ideas: Routes of Epidemics and Ideologies*, London, 1965.

Smith, John M., *The History of the Sarbadār Dynasty 1336-1381 A.D. and Its Sources*, Paris, 1970.

Soberheim, M., "Das Zuckermonopol unter Sultan Barsbāī," *Zeitschrift für Assyriologie und Verwandte Gebiete*, Berlin, vol. 27 (1912), pp. 75-84.

Spies, Otto, "Zur Geschichte der Pocken in der Arabischen Literatur," *AGM, Supplement*, no. 7 (Wiesbaden, 1966), pp. 187-200.

Spuler, Bertold, *Die Goldene Horde: Die Mongolen in Russland, 1223-1502*, Wiesbaden, 1965.

——, *Die Mongolen in Iran, 1220-1350*, Berlin, 1955.

——, *The Muslim World: An Historical Survey*, trans. by F.K.C. Bagley, 3 vols., Leiden, 1960-1969.

Stewart, J., *The Nestorian Missionary Enterprise*, Edinburgh, 1928.

Sticker, Georg, *Abhandlungen aus der Seuchengeschichte und Seuchenlehre*, vol. 1: *Die Pest*, part 1: *Die Geschichte der Pest* (Giessen, 1908); vol. 2: *Die Pest*, part 2: *Die Pest als Seuche und als Plague* (Giessen, 1910).

Sublet, Jacqueline, "La Peste prise aux rêts de la jurisprudence: Le Traité d'Ibn Ḥağar al-'Asqalānī sur la peste," *Studia Islamica*, vol. 33 (Paris, 1971), pp. 141-149.

Süheyl Ünver, A., "Sur l'histoire de la peste en Turquie," *Comptes-Rendus*, The Ninth International Congress of the History of Medicine (Bucharest, September, 1932), ed. by Victor Gomoin and Victorica Gomoin, pp. 479-483.

Surūr, Jamāl ad-Dīn, *Dawlat Banī Qalā'ūn fī Miṣr*, Cairo, 1947.

——, *Miṣr fī 'aṣr dawlat al-mamālīk al-baḥrīyah*, Cairo, 1959.

——, *aẓ-Ẓāhir Baybars*, Cairo, 1938.

aṭ-Ṭabbakh, Muḥammad R., *I'lām an-nubalā' bi-ta'rīkh Ḥalab ash-Shahbā'*, 7 vols., A.H. 1341-1345.

Tarkhān, Ibrāhīm, *Miṣr fī 'aṣr dawlat al-mamālīk al-Jarākisah*, Cairo, 1960.

Temkin, Owsei, *The Falling Sickness: A History of Epilepsy from the Greeks to the Beginning of Modern Neurology*, Baltimore, 1971.

Thies, Dorothee, *Die Lehren der arabischen Mediziner Tabari und Ibn Hubal über Herz, Lunge, Gallenblase, und Milz*, Bonn, 1968.

Tholozan, J.-D., *Histoire de la peste bubonique au Caucase, en Arménie et en Anatolie dans le première moitié du dix-neuvième siècle*, Paris, 1876.

Tholozan, J.-D., *Histoire de la peste bubonique en Mésopotamie ou détermination de son origine, de sa marche, du cycle de ses apparitions et de la cause de son extinction spontanée*, Paris, 1874.

——, *Histoire de la peste bubonique en Perse ou détermination de son origine, de sa marche, du cycle de ses apparitions et de la cause de son extinction spontanée*, Paris, 1874.

Thompson, James W., "The Aftermath of the Black Death and the Aftermath of the Great War," *The American Journal of Sociology*, vol. 26 (1921), pp. 565-572.

Thorndike, Lynn, "The Blight of Pestilence on Early Modern Civilization," *The American Historical Review* (April, 1927), pp. 455-474.

——, *History of Magic and Experimental Science*, 8 vols., New York, 1923-1958.

Thrupp, S. L., ed., *Millennial Dreams in Action*, New York, 1970.

——, "Plague Effects in Medieval Europe," *Comparative Studies in Society and History*, vol. 8 (1966), pp. 474-479.

Toussoun, Prince Omar, *Mémoire sur les finances de l'Égypte depuis les Pharaons jusqu'à nos jours,* Mémoires présentés à l'Institut d'Égypte, vol. 6, Cairo, 1924.

Trevor-Roper, H. R., *The European Witch-Craze of the Sixteenth and Seventeenth Centuries and Other Essays*, New York, 1969.

Trimingham, J. S., *The Sufi Orders in Islam*, Oxford, 1971.

Udovitch, A. L., "The 'Law Merchant' of the Medieval Islamic World," *Logic in Classical Islamic Culture*, ed. by G. E. von Grunebaum, Wiesbaden, 1970, pp. 113-130.

Ullmann, Manfred, *Die Medizin im Islam*, in *Handbuch der Orientalistik, Supplement*, ed. by B. Spuler, no. 6, vol. 1, Leiden, 1970.

——, *Die Natur- und Geheimwissenschaften im Islam*, Leiden, 1972.

Vasiliev, A. A., *The Goths in the Crimea*, Cambridge, 1936.

——, *History of the Byzantine Empire*, 2 vols., Madison, 1964.

Verlinden, Charles, "Le Grande peste de 1348 en Espagne," *Revue Belge de philologie et d'histoire*, vol. 17 (1938), pp. 103-146.

Vernadsky, G., *The Mongols and Russia*, New Haven, 1959.

Vryonis, Speros, *The Decline of Medieval Hellenism in Asia Minor and the Process of Islamization from the Eleventh through the Fifteenth Century*, Berkeley and Los Angeles, 1971.

Wakil, A. W., *The Third Pandemic of Plague in Egypt: Historical, Statistical and Epidemiological Remarks on the First Thirty-Two Years of Its Prevalence*, Faculty of Medicine, Egyptian University, no. 3, Cairo, 1932.

Walker, John, *Folk Medicine in Modern Egypt*, London, 1934.

Weil, Gustav, *Geschichte des Abbasidenchalifats in Egypten*, vol. 4, part 1, Stuttgart, 1860.

Wellhausen, J., *The Arab Kingdom and Its Fall*, Beirut, 1963 reprint.

Westermarck, Edward, "The Belief in Spirits in Morocco," *Acta Academiae Aboensis Humaniora*, vol. 1 (Åbo, 1920), pp. 1-167.

——, *Ritual and Belief in Morocco*, 2 vols., London, 1926.

Wickersheimer, Ernest, "Les Accusations d'empoisonnement portées pendant la première moitié du XIVe siècle contre les lépreux et les juifs; leur relations avec les épidémies de peste," *Comptes-Rendus du quatrième congrès international d'histoire de la médecine*, ed. by Tricot-Royer and Laignel-Lavastine, Antwerp, 1927, pp. 76-83.

Wiet, Gaston, *L'Égypte Arabe de la conquête Arabe à la Conquête Ottomane 642-1517 de l'ère Chrêtiene*, vol. 4 of *Histoire de la nation Égyptienne*, ed. by Gabriel Hanotaux, Paris, 1937.

——, *L'Égypte musulmane de la conquête Arabe à la conquête Ottoman*, vol. 2, part 2 of *Précis de l'histoire d'Égypte par divers historiens et archéologues*, Cairo, 1932.

——, "Kindi et Maqrīzī," *BIFAO*, vol. 12 (1916), pp. 61-73.

Winkler, H. A., *Siegel und Charaktere in der Muhammedanischen Zauberei*, Berlin, 1930.

Winslow, C.E.A., *The Conquest of Epidemic Diseases: A Chapter in the History of Ideas*, Princeton, 1943.

Wolmar, Enrico di, *Abhandlung über die Pest*, Berlin, 1827.

Wu Lien-Teh, "The Original Home of Plague," *Far Eastern Association of Tropical Medicine: Transactions of the Fifth Biennial Congress* (Singapore, 1923), ed. by A. L. Hoops and J. W. Scharff, London, 1924, pp. 286-304.

———, J.W.H. Chun, R. Pollitzer, and C. Y. Wu, *Plague: A Manual for Medical and Public Health Workers*, Shanghai, 1936.

———, "Plague in Wild Rodents, Including the Latest Investigations into the Rôle Played by the Tarabagan," *Far Eastern Association of Tropical Medicine: Transactions of the Fifth Biennial Congress* (Singapore, 1923), ed. by A. L. Hoops and J. W. Scharff, London, 1924, pp. 305-340.

———, *A Treatise on Pneumonic Plague*, Geneva, 1926.

Wüstenfeld, F., *Maqrizi's Geschichte der Copten*, Göttingen, 1845.

Zambauer, E. von, *Manuel de genealogie et de chronologie pour l'histoire de l'Islam*, Hanover, 1927.

Zananiri, G., *L'Égypte et l'equilibre du Levant au moyen âge, 637-1517*, Marseilles, 1936.

Zakirov, S., *Diplomaticheskie otnosheniya Zolotoy Ordy s Egiptom (XIII-XIVvv.)*, Moscow, 1966.

Zbinden, Ernst, *Die Djinn des Islam und der altorientalische Geisterglaube*, Berne, 1953.

Ziegler, Philip, *The Black Death*, London, 1969.

Zinsser, Hans, *Rats, Lice and History*, Boston, 1967.

INDEX*

* The unpublished Arabic plague treatises are listed according to author.

Library of Congress Cataloging in Publication Data

Dols, Michael W 1942
The Black Death in the Middle East.

Bibliography: p.
Includes index.
1. Black death—Islamic Empire. 2. Islamic Empire—Social conditions. 3. Islamic Empire—Economic conditions. I. Title.
RC179.I6D64 616.9'232'00956 76-3254
ISBN 0-691-03107-X